# Drug Abuse: A Clinical Guide to Diagnosis and Treatment

# Drug Abuse: A Clinical Guide to Diagnosis and Treatment

Editor: Odin Mullin

AMERICAN
MEDICAL PUBLISHERS
www.americanmedicalpublishers.com

AMERICAN
MEDICAL PUBLISHERS
www.americanmedicalpublishers.com

**Cataloging-in-Publication Data**

Drug abuse : a clinical guide to diagnosis and treatment / edited by Odin Mullin.
p. cm.
Includes bibliographical references and index.
ISBN 979-8-88740-068-6
1. Drug abuse. 2. Drug abuse--Diagnosis. 3. Drug abuse--treatment. 4. Substance abuse.
5. Psychiatry. I. Mullin, Odin.
RC564 .D78 2023
616.86--dc23



American Medical Publishers,
41 Flatbush Avenue,
1st Floor, New York,
NY 11217, USA

ISBN 979-8-88740-068-6 (Hardback)

# Contents

# Preface

Drug abuse refers to the use of certain chemicals for the purpose of creating pleasurable effects in the brain. The drugs that are used for seeking pleasure can be classified into three categories, namely, depressants, stimulants and hallucinogens. Some common examples of drugs are alcohol, tobacco, opium, marijuana and cocaine. Drug abuse causes damage to the body in the long run and there is a risk of contracting infections like hepatitis B and HIV in people using needles. The diagnosis and treatment of drug abuse involves the screening and assessment of drug use behavior. CRAFFT screening test is a screening tool used to diagnose drug abuse in adolescents. CAGE questionnaire is another screening tool used to assess drug use in adults. There are several types of therapies and medications that help to suppress cravings and mental anxiety and reduce the chances of relapse. These treatment therapies include exposure therapy, community reinforcement approach, contingency management, etc. This book outlines the diagnosis and management of drug abuse in detail. It will serve as a reference to a broad spectrum of readers.

The information contained in this book is the result of intensive hard work done by researchers in this field. All due efforts have been made to make this book serve as a complete guiding source for students and researchers. The topics in this book have been comprehensively explained to help readers understand the growing trends in the field.

I would like to thank the entire group of writers who made sincere efforts in this book and my family who supported me in my efforts of working on this book. I take this opportunity to thank all those who have been a guiding force throughout my life.

**Editor**

# 1

# Neuronal Stress and Injury Caused by HIV-1, cART and Drug Abuse: Converging Contributions to HAND

**Ana B. Sanchez [1] and Marcus Kaul [1,2,*]**

1 Immunity and Pathogenesis Program, Infectious and Inflammatory Disease Center, Sanford Burnham Prebys Medical Discovery Institute, La Jolla, CA 92037, USA; asanchez@SBPdiscovery.org
2 Department of Psychiatry, University of California San Diego, San Diego, CA 92093, USA
* Correspondence: mkaul@SBPdiscovery.org;

Academic Editor: Jaime H. Vera Rojas

**Abstract:** Multiple mechanisms appear to contribute to neuronal stress and injury underlying HIV-associated neurocognitive disorders (HAND), which occur despite the successful introduction of combination antiretroviral therapy (cART). Evidence is accumulating that components of cART can itself be neurotoxic upon long-term exposure. In addition, abuse of psychostimulants, such as methamphetamine (METH), seems to compromise antiretroviral therapy and aggravate HAND. However, the combined effect of virus and recreational and therapeutic drugs on the brain is still incompletely understood. However, several lines of evidence suggest a shared critical role of oxidative stress, compromised neuronal energy homeostasis and autophagy in promotion and prevention of neuronal dysfunction associated with HIV-1 infection, cART and psychostimulant use. In this review, we present a synopsis of recent work related to neuronal stress and injury induced by HIV infection, antiretrovirals (ARVs) and the highly addictive psychostimulant METH.

**Keywords:** HIV-1; HAND; anti-retroviral; methamphetamine; neurotoxicity

---

## 1. Introduction

Thirty-five years ago infection with human immunodeficiency virus (HIV-1) and acquired immunodeficiency syndrome (AIDS) evolved into an acute epidemic [1,2]. However, the development and use of combination antiretroviral therapy (cART) since the mid-1990s has changed the course of HIV infection/AIDS, which is now considered a chronic and treatable disease, if therapy is accessible [3]. Still, each year, more than 1 million people die from AIDS-related causes and 2.1 million people become newly infected by HIV-1. Globally, an estimated 36.7 million persons were living with HIV/AIDS in 2015, including more than 1.2 million people in the USA alone [4–6]. HIV-infection of the central nervous system (CNS) often leads to neurological problems and HIV-associated neurocognitive disorders (HAND) [7]. The underlying neuropathological mechanisms in humans are not completely understood and persist despite the use of antiretrovirals (ARVs) and effective virological control [7–11]. A major comorbidity of HIV infection is the abuse of drugs, such as heroin, cocaine and methamphetamine (METH), which is a public health problem in its own right [12]. Therefore, opiates, cocaine and METH are all being intensely studied in order to better understand their effects on HIV infection and HAND [13–19], but for the purpose of this review we will focus on the role of METH as one example of a widely abused drug. As such, HIV infection is frequently linked with the recreational use of the psychostimulant METH [20–22] and diminished adherence to cART regimens [23]. Additionally, increased viral loads have been linked to METH use in ART–receiving HIV positive individuals. [23,24]. The combination of METH and HIV-1 appears to trigger more neurocognitive impairment and neuropathology than either agent alone but the presumed mechanistic interaction of virus, anti-viral treatment and the psychostimulant drug is incompletely understood [25–28].

Clearly, the incidence of HIV-associated dementia (HAD), the most severe form of HAND, has declined with the implementation of cART [29,30], but the prevalence of cognitive impairment milder than dementia remains high in HIV patients on cART [9,11,31]. In addition, recent clinical studies observed that discontinuation of cART in virologically controlled HIV patients unexpectedly resulted in significant improvement of neurocognitive function [32–35]. Furthermore, experimental evidence is accumulating that at least some ARV compounds may themselves have neurotoxic effects [36–40]. These observations raised the possibility that certain ARVs may have neurotoxic effects that could contribute to the development of HAND.

Therefore, METH-using HIV patients are at risk of exposure to a combination of potential contributors to neurotoxicity: HIV and its components, a psychostimulant drug and ARVs. Here we will discuss current information about those contributing factors, the combination of which is being encountered in the clinical setting while an understanding of the mechanisms at the cellular level is only beginning to emerge.

## 2. HIV Infection, Neurotoxicity and HAND

Humans of all ages infected with HIV-1 develop neurological symptoms that include motor and cognitive dysfunction which are now termed HIV-associated neurocognitive disorders (HAND) [7,41–43]. HAND defines three categories of disorders with increasing severity according to standardized measures of dysfunction: (i) asymptomatic neurocognitive impairment (ANI); (ii) mild neurocognitive disorder (MND) and (iii) HAD. With the advent of cART, the incidence of HAND's most severe form, dementia, decreased, suggesting a beneficial effect on cognitive function [29,30,44]. However, the prevalence of milder cognitive impairment (ANI, MND) remains high in HIV patients on cART, and HAND/HAD continues to be a significant independent risk factor for death due to AIDS [9,11,31,45]. Although improved control of peripheral viral replication and the treatment of opportunistic infections continue to extend survival times, cART fails to provide protection from HAND, or to reverse the disease in most cases [46–51]. One study found that in a group of 669 HIV patients who passed away between 1996 and 2001 more than 90% had developed HAD as an AIDS-defining condition during the last 12 months of life [52]. Moreover, the proportion of new cases of HAND/HAD displaying a cluster of differentiation 4$^+$ (CD4$^+$) T cell count greater than 200 $\mu L^{-1}$ is growing [50]. This situation and distinct patterns of viral drug resistance in plasma and cerebrospinal fluid (CSF) compartments might at least in part be explained by limited penetration into the CNS of HIV protease inhibitors and several of the nucleoside analogues [46,53,54]. Therefore, it is possible that as people live longer with HIV-1 infection the prevalence of dementia may continue to rise [43,46,50,53–56].

Pathological features of HIV-1 infection in the brain are often referred to as HIV encephalitis (HIVE) and include activated resident microglia, microglial nodules, multinucleated giant cells, infiltration predominantly by monocytoid cells, including blood-derived macrophages, and decreased synaptic and dendritic density, combined with selective neuronal loss, widespread reactive astrocytosis, and myelin pallor [57,58]. However, the pathologic features best correlating with *ante mortem* measures of cognitive dysfunction include increased numbers of microglia [59], decreased synaptic and dendritic density, selective neuronal loss [58,60,61], elevated tumor necrosis factor (TNF)-$\alpha$ mRNA in microglia and astrocytes [62], and evidence of excitatory neurotoxins in CSF and serum [63]. Furthermore, two reports provide evidence that the amount of proviral HIV DNA in circulating monocytes and macrophages correlates better than viral load with the risk of developing HAD [64,65].

HIV infection can be associated with neuronal damage and loss in distinct brain regions, including frontal cortex [66,67], substantia nigra [68], cerebellum [69], and putamen [70] and features of neuronal apoptosis have been found in brains of HAD patients [71–73]. Moreover, the localization of apoptotic neurons was correlated with signs of structural damage and closely associated with evidence of microglial activation, especially within subcortical deep gray structures [71].

With the introduction of cART, HIV neuropathology began to shift. Although the incidence of opportunistic infections seemed to decline, two *post mortem* studies observed increased macrophage/microglia infiltration and activation in hippocampus and basal ganglia of cART-treated HIV patients as compared to samples from the pre-cART era as well as a higher prevalence of HIVE at the time of autopsy [25,74]. Specimens from HIV patients who had failed cART displayed even more encephalitis and severe leukoencephalopathy [74]. In line with these reports are more recent neuropathological descriptions of various forms with severe HIVE and white matter injury, extensive perivascular lymphocytic infiltration, "burnt-out" forms of HIVE and seemingly aging-related beta-amyloid accumulation implying an Alzheimer's-like neuropathology [75,76].

HIV-1 appears to reach the brain soon after infection in the periphery, and then localizes primarily to perivascular macrophages and microglia [77–80]. Infection by HIV-1 of macrophages and lymphocytes in the periphery and microglia in the brain occurrs after the viral envelope protein gp120 binds to CD4 in conjunction with at least one of several possible chemokine receptors. Depending on the viral strain, different HIV-1 variants use CC chemokine receptor 5 (CCR5, CD195) and CCR3, or CXC chemokine receptor 4 (CXCR4, CD184), or a combination of these chemokine receptors to enter target cells [81–83]. Neurons and astrocytes in the brain also express chemokine receptors, including CCR5 and CXCR4 [84,85]. However these cells, in contrast to microglia, appear to be largely refractory to productive HIV-1 infection under in vivo conditions. However, several in vitro studies strongly suggest that CXCR4 is prominently involved in HIV-associated neuronal damage whereas CCR5 may play a dual role by being able to either serve a toxic or protective function [86–92]. Intact HIV-1, as well as picomolar concentrations of isolated viral envelope gp120, can induce neuronal death via CXCR4 and CCR5 receptors in neurons from humans and rodents [86,87,89,90,93–98].

While progress is being made in characterizing the neuropathological processes, how exactly HIV-1 infection provokes neuronal injury and death as well as neurocognitive and motor deficits remains controversial [43,53,54,79,99]. While it is generally agreed upon that HIV-1 does not infect post-mitotic, mature neurons, the mechanism of neuronal damage is a matter of debate and continuing investigation. Ample evidence exists that various viral proteins; including Tat, Nef, Vpr and the Env proteins gp120 and gp41, can initiate neuronal injury and death [43,53,93,99–104]. Moreover, we and others found more recently that HIV-1 and at least its gp120 can also compromise neurogenesis [8,105,106]. All these observations, in particular those related to neurotoxicity, have contributed to at least two different possible explanations of how HIV-1 initiates brain injury, the "direct injury" and the "indirect" or "bystander effect" hypothesis. These two hypothetical mechanisms are by no means mutually exclusive, and the available data suggest a role for both. However, under conditions where glial and neuronal cells are present, the indirect neurotoxicity mediated by macrophages and microglia may predominate [43,53,78,79,92,99,107–109].

The hypothesis that HIV proteins can directly injure neurons without any contribution of non-neuronal cells (microglia/macrophages and/or astrocytes) is supported by experiments showing that viral envelope protein gp120, Tat, and Vpr are toxic in serum free primary neuronal cultures [87,88] or in neuroblastoma cell lines [86,99,102]. The absence of non-neuronal cells permits the investigation of potential direct effects of viral proteins on neurons, but a predominantly indirect effect cannot be detected.

In mixed neuronal/glial cultures that recapitulate the cellular composition of the brain, HIV-1, gp120 and Tat appear to induce neuronal apoptotic death primarily in an indirect fashion via the release of toxins from macrophages/microglia [89,93–95,97,98,107,109,110]. Moreover, both the inactivation or depletion of macrophages and microglia basically abrogate neurotoxicity of HIV-1/gp120 in mixed neuronal/glial cultures [89,98,107,111] and it appears likely that stimulation of CXCR4 or CCR5 in macrophages/microglia is a prerequisite for the neurotoxicity of HIV-1 and gp120 [89,96,109].

At least some of the neurotoxins released by HIV-1 infected or gp120-stimulated macrophages/microglia stimulate an ionotropic glutamate and neurotransmitter receptor, the *N*-methyl-D-aspartate-type receptor (NMDAR) [97,112,113]. NMDAR antagonists can prevent neuronal cell death in vitro due to HIV-infected or gp120-activated macrophages [97,112]. Activation of ionotropic glutamate receptors in neurons initiates under normal physiological conditions a transient depolarization and excitation that plays an important role in neurocognitive function [114,115]. In contrast, excessive and/or extended NMDAR stimulation causes excitotoxicity via a mechanism involving a sustained elevation of intracellular $Ca^{2+}$ concentration, a subsequent compromise of mitochondrial function and cellular energy metabolism which in turn results in the production of free radicals [43,115,116]. In case of a mild but sustained insult, as it seems to occur in HIV infection, neurons eventually undergo programmed cell death (apoptosis) which has also been observed in *post-mortem* brains of HIVE/HAD patient [71,72,89,96]. Neuronal apoptosis triggered by HIV-1 or gp120 toxicity or a direct excitotoxic insult involves neuronal $Ca^{2+}$ overload, activation of p38 MAPK and p53, activation of cell cycle protein, caspases, release of cytochrome c and other molecules, such as apoptosis-inducing factor (AIF) from mitochondria, free radical formation, lipid release and peroxidation, and chromatin condensation [84,89,90,98,109,117–121]. Alterations of cellular lipid metabolism, and an increase in ceramide, sphingomyelin and hydroxynonenal as well as the activation of the unfolded protein response (UPR) have also been linked to oxidative processes and cellular distress in the neurotoxic pathways associated with HIV infection [99,122,123].

### 3. Neurotoxicity of Antiretroviral Drugs

ARV drugs are classified based on the mechanism action and currently include (i) nucleoside/nucleotide reverse transcriptase inhibitors (NRTI); (ii) non-nucleoside reverse transcriptase inhibitors (NNRTI); (iii) protease inhibitors (PI), (iv) integrase strand transfer inhibitors (INSTI); (v) a fusion inhibitor (FI); and (vi) an entry inhibitor (EI), blocking chemokine receptor CCR5. In addition, two drugs, ritonavir (RTV) and cobicistat (COBI) are used as pharmacokinetic enhancers [124] (reviewed in [125,126]). The Department of Health and Human Services (HHS) Panel on Antiretroviral Guidelines for Adults and Adolescents (a working group of the office of AIDS research) [124] keep updating the combination regimens, based on more than 25 antiretroviral drugs approved by the Food and Drug Administration (FDA) in order to guide to the right and best treatment for $HIV^+$ individuals. Currently recommended cART regimen consist of two NRTIs (usually abacavir/lamivudine (ABC/3TC), tenofovir alafenamide/emtricitabine (TAF/FTC) or tenofovir disoproxil fumarate/emtricitabine (TDF/FTC)) in combination with a third active ARV drug from one of three drug classes: INSTI, NNRTI or PI with a pharmacokinetic enhancer (RTV or COBI). Other combination and/or regimen are selected based primarily on antiviral efficacy, potential adverse effects (toxicity), pill burden, drug-drug interaction, comorbid conditions and cost (see [124] on 12/1/2016). As a result of effective cART, HIV-1 infection has become a chronic condition and infected individuals have a longer, near normal life span leading to aging with HIV as a new clinical phenomenon [51,127–129].

The introduction of cART clearly led to a decline in the incidence of the most severe form of HAND, HAD [29,30]. However, the occurrence of cognitive impairment milder than HAD persists in HIV patients on cART [9,11,31] and recent studies observed that discontinuation of cART in virologically controlled HIV patients unexpectedly resulted in significant improvement of neurocognitive function [32–35]. Furthermore, clinical and experimental evidence is accumulating that at least some ARV compounds may themselves have neurotoxic effects [36–40,125,130].

Certain ARV or combinations thereof (cART) have been reported to be toxic in the periphery but also the brain, which could contribute to the development of HAND [32,36–40,131,132]. Several other studies have provided direct evidence that anti-retroviral drugs can exert neurotoxic effects in connection with oxidative stress, dysregulation of $Ca^{2+}$ homeostasis and alteration of mitochondrial respiration [39,40,133–139].

NRTIs: These compounds have primarily been linked to peripheral neuropathy, in particular didanosine (ddI), stavudine (d4T) and zalcitabine (ddC) [140]. The main unintentional target appears to be mitochondrial polymerase $\gamma$, an enzyme required to maintain mitochondrial DNA (mtDNA) in axons and Schwann cells [141,142]. Examples of NRTIs that seem less or non-toxic in terms of peripheral neuropathy or cellular neurotoxicity are emtricitabine (FTC), lamivudine (3TC), tenofovir (TAF or TDF) and abacavir (ABC) [39]. The earliest anti-retroviral drug zidovudine (AZT) has also been linked to mitochondrial toxicity, impaired neurogenesis and damage to neuronal dendrites and presynaptic terminals [131,143–145]. Overall, CNS neurotoxicity of NRTIs seems limited but also compound- and cell-specific [39,125].

NNRTIs: Compounds, such as rilpivirine (TMC278) and delavirdine (DLV) are considered to be non-toxic in the CNS [125]. Etravirine (ETR) recently appeared to be clinically safe but was found to be neurotoxic in vitro [39,146]. However, Efavirenz (EFV) and nevirapine (NVP), which are FDA approved and used in NNRTI regimen [124], have been found to exert neurotoxicity [39,137,147]. EFV has also been linked in the clinical setting to deterioration of neurocognitive function [127,130,148]. One study found that EFV caused in neuron-like SHSY-5Y cells and primary rat striatal neurons a loss of ATP, depolarization and fragmentation of mitochondria and increased mitophagy and autophagy in general suggesting disturbance of energy homeostasis as a mechanism of toxicity [149,150]. EFV was also found to cause endoplasmic reticulum (ER) stress in human brain endothelial cells and in microvessels of the CNS in HIV-transgenic mice [151]. However, the latter study found that EFV inhibited autophagy by binding to a complex comprising Beclin 1, autophagy-related 14 (ATG14) and Phosphatidyl inositol 3 kinase III (PI3KIII) which is required for formation of an autophagosome. In addition, an enzyme of the cytochrome P450 (CYP) family, CYP2B6, affects the metabolism and therefore likely the concentration of EFV in the brain, which may contribute to functional impairment in the CNS as the 8-hydroxy metabolite of EFV has been found to be neurotoxic [148,152].

PIs: This group of ARV is very effective and part of most first line treatment regimen [153]. Saquinavir (SQV) and nelfinavir (NFV) were also found to be very well tolerated in HIV patients whereas ritonavir (RTV) was associated with adverse and toxic effects [154]. PI, NRTI, INSTI and the CCR5 blocker maraviroc are metabolized by enzymes of the CYP450 family. In fact, CYP450 enzymes are known to be involved in the metabolism/activation/inactivation of the majority of pharmaceutical drugs [155]. Most of the human CYP450s are primarily membrane-associated proteins located in the inner membrane of the mitochondria or in the endoplasmic reticulum of cells. Especially the subclasses CYP2 and CYP3 are involved in the metabolism of drugs and steroids, which explains the risk of drug-drug interactions in cases of polypharmacy, such as cART. However, those interactions can on occasion be harnessed for therapeutic purposes. As such RTV has been used as a booster for mono- or triple therapy [156]. Other PIs, namely amprenavir (APV), indinavir (IDV) and atazanavir (ATV) have also been implicated in neurotoxicity [157–159]. Moreover, a recent study demonstrated in non-human primates, rodents and in vitro neuroglial cell cultures that the PIs SQY and ATV in combination with the NRTI tenofovir (TDF) and an INSTI and RTV and SQV separately caused endoplasmic reticulum (ER) stress, activated β-site amyloid precursor protein cleaving enzyme-1 (BACE-1) and neuronal damage [160].

INSTIs: Several reports have indicated possible CNS toxicity for raltegravir (RAL) and elvitegravir (EVG) as the compounds triggered clinical psychiatric symptoms [161–163].

FI: The only FDA approved compound, enfuvirtide (T-20) has not displayed any conclusive evidence for neurotoxicity. Some earlier studies suggested sensory neuropathy [164,165] while others found no signs of toxicity [164,166,167].

EI: The CCR5 blocker maraviroc (MVC) is the only FDA-approved compounds in its class. There is currently no evidence of neurotoxicity, and on the contrary, several studies found evidence for a neuroprotective effect of MVC [39,92,168–170].

As discussed above, certain ARV and cART carry the risk of neurotoxicity. One of the major concerns using cART is the role of drug-drug interaction via various CYP450 enzymes, which could aggravate neurotoxicity and contribute to the development of HAND. Therefore the need exists for a better understanding of the mechanism of not only individual effects of ARV but their combinations in order to identify the most effective and least toxic cART for HIV-infected individuals.

## 4. Neurotoxicity of METH

METH is an addictive psychostimulant drug, and its abuse can cause a number of acute and chronic symptoms, including agitation, anxiety, paranoia, psychosis and aggression [20,22,171], a variety of cardiovascular problems [172,173], reactive microgliosis [174], and hyperthermia and convulsions [175]. Abuse of METH is also associated with behavioral symptoms, including increased engagement in high-risk activities, such as unprotected sex [20–22,176,177]. Neurocognitive sequelae of chronic METH abuse include deficits in attention, working memory and executive functions [28,176,178–181]. In combination, METH and HIV-1 appear to cause more neurocognitive deficits than either agent alone, but the potential mechanistic interaction of both the virus and the drug is still poorly understood [14,26,27].

The neuropathology resulting from METH abuse in humans includes a decrease of dopamine (DA) transporter (DAT) in cortex, caudate-putamen and other brain regions [182], reduction of DA and D2DA receptor in caudate-putamen [183,184], decreased density of serotonin transporter (5-HTT) in cortex [185], and abnormal glucose metabolism [186]. A pronounced interference with the nigrostriatal dopaminergic neuronal system suggests a far reaching effect on dopamine-rich fronto-striatal-thalamo-cortical circuits [187]. Moreover, a loss of gray matter in cingulate, limbic and paralimbic cortices, a significantly smaller hippocampus, and a hypertrophy of white matter and pronounced microglial activation occur as a consequence of METH use and point to pathological effects beyond the dopaminergic system [188,189].

In agreement with the findings in humans, animal studies show that METH injures presynaptic DA and 5-HT terminals [190,191], causes a decrease of tyrosine hydroxylase (TH) and tryptophan hydroxylase (TPH) [192], depletes DA and 5-HT [193], reduces DAT, 5-HTT [194–196] and vesicular monoamine transporter (VMAT)-2 [197]. METH also triggers neuronal cell death in cortex [198,199], striatum [198], hippocampus [200] and olfactory bulb [201]. In the striatum, METH destroys specifically gamma-amino butyric acid (GABA)-ergic neurons that express enkephalin, but not those containing substance P, neuronal nitric oxide synthase (nNOS) or cholinergic markers [202,203].

The psychostimulant effect of METH is believed to result from an elevated extracellular DA concentration in the striatum due to increased release and reduced reuptake into vesicles [179,204–206]. Possibly via the increase of DA, METH appears to indirectly affect glutamatergic, GABAergic and serotonergic neurotransmission. One possible link involves striatal medium spiny neurons which receive synaptic input from nigrostriatal DA-ergic and corticostriatal glutamatergic neurons [179,207].

On the other hand, in macrophages and dendritic cells, METH compromises phagocytosis and antigen processing, important processes in building and maintaining a functional and protective immune response [28,178,179,208–210].

Other cellular effects of METH in the brain are reflected by signs of oxidative stress, neuroinflammation and apoptosis [211,212]. Abuse of METH seems to cause excessive neuronal release of monoamine neurotransmitters, particularly DA, in the synapse, which can be toxic to nerve terminals [213,214]. As a result of DA accumulation, levels of free radicals increase inside neurons, dysfunction of the ubiquitin-proteasome system ensues, oxidative protein nitration occurs, endoplasmic reticulum stress (ERS) and expression of p53 and inflammatory cytokines is induced, and microtubules may be deacetylated [215–218]. All these processes promote neurotoxicity via damage and/or dysfunction of proteins or cellular organelles, resulting in up-regulation of autophagy, a vital homeostatic mechanism required for maintenance of healthy and functional neurons [215–218].

## 5. Neuronal Injury by HIV + cART + METH

HIV infection is frequently linked with the recreational use of drugs, such as the psychostimulant METH [20–22,219]. Moreover, the use of METH increases the risk of infection with HIV-1 [20–22]. Recent clinic-based surveys found that depending on the demographics between 16% of heterosexual men and 15% of women and up to 20% to 50% of HIV-infected men who have sex with men (MSM) reported METH use over the past 12 months [21,219,220]. Thus, the brain of many HIV patients is exposed to HIV-1, combinations of ARVs and psychostimulants, such as METH, at the same time.

Elevated viral loads have been linked to METH use in ART–receiving HIV positive individuals [23,24] and METH-users with HIV also have shown greater neuronal injury compared with patients who do not abuse the drug [25,27]. The combination of METH and HIV-1 seems to cause more neurocognitive deficits and neuropathology than either agent alone [28,219,221]. We and others have been able to recapitulate some of those combined effects in animal models [219,222–225]. However, the potential mechanistic interaction of virus and psychostimulant drug is still incompletely understood and further complicated by the multitude of cART regimen [28,145,219,221].

Therefore, our group set out to investigate in vitro the potential contribution of all these factors to neuronal injury and loss [145]. In our study, we exposed mixed neuronal-glial cerebrocortical cells to ARVs of four different pharmacological categories (NRTI: AZT, NNRTI: NVP, PI: SQV and INSTI 118-D-24) with and without METH, and in some experiments HIV-1 gp120, an established neurotoxicity inducing viral protein. The incubations lasted for 24 h and 7 days in order to assess more acute, short-term and long-term effects, respectively. Subsequently, we assessed neuronal injury using different approaches. First, the exposed cell cultures were analyzed by fluorescence microscopy using specific markers for neuronal dendrites and pre-synaptic terminals; Second, we analyzed the disturbance of neuronal ATP levels; and third, we assessed involvement of autophagy using immunofluorescence and Western blotting. We found that ARVs led to alterations of neurites and presynaptic terminals predominantly during the 7-day incubation and depending on the specific compounds and their combinations with and without METH. Similarly, specific drug combinations with and without METH or viral gp120 as well as METH and gp120 each alone, all caused a significant loss of neuronal ATP, but none of the ARV applied as a single drug. Loss of ATP was accompanied by activation of adenosine monophosphate-activated protein kinase (AMPK) and autophagy, which, however, did not suffice to restore neuronal ATP to normal levels. In contrast, enhancing autophagy with rapamycin averted the long-term drop of ATP during exposure to cART in combination with METH or gp120.

Our study yielded a number of unexpected findings pointing to the complexities of the overall effects of exposure to HIV + cART + METH [145]. The psychostimulant drug, cART and HIVgp120 each alone and in combination led to a similar loss of neuronal ATP but lacked any additive effect. Moreover, METH or HIV/gp120 or an ARV each could exert neurotoxicity in terms of compromising neuronal dendrites and presynaptic terminals or diminishing neuronal ATP or, in the case of gp120, triggering the loss of neurons themselves when applied separately, but not necessarily when combined with ARV. Certain ARV combinations did not affect neuronal dendrites or presynaptic terminal in any detectable fashion in the presence or absence of METH, yet caused significant reduction of neuronal ATP levels. Thus, neurons were able to maintain their overall dendritic and presynaptic structures despite a disruption of neuronal energy homeostasis, an event that may explain, at least in part, progressive neurological diseases, such as HAND. Strikingly, METH, which itself is toxic to neurons [28], lacked any detectable damaging effect on neurites and synapses in combination with several ARVs and even ameliorated a significant reduction of neuronal ATP in combination with a cocktail of four ARVs. However, the admixture of four therapeutic compounds and psychostimulant compromised neuronal dendrites and synapses during long-term exposure, an effect that has also been reported by others as a result of ARV treatment [39]. Moreover, diminished neuronal ATP levels resulted when four ARVs and METH were combined with HIV-1 gp120.

All those observations were in line with earlier reports that ARVs can compromise mitochondria at various levels by altering (i) mitochondrial membrane components, such as transporters; (ii) mitochondrial kinases, such as Thymidine kinase 2 (TK2) and deoxyguanosine kinase (dGK) [138]; (iii) mitochondrial bioenergetics, in particular membrane potential; and (iv) mitochondrial DNA homeostasis by inhibiting polymerase $\gamma$ [134–136] or promote major deletions in neuronal mtDNA [133,139]. Interestingly, our findings also suggested that neuronal energy homeostasis could significantly change without causing overt structural neuronal damage or loss. The regulatory mechanism allowing for such neuronal adaptation remains to be elucidated.

Mitochondria are the cellular organelles supplying energy in the form of ATP. The lack of ATP as an energy source could be one of the factors that compromise neuronal function before cell death occurs. Neurons are known to produce energy almost exclusively through mitochondrial oxidative phosphorylation (OXPHOS). In contrast, astrocytes can stimulate glycolysis by activation of 6-phosphofructo-2 kinase (PFK2) through AMPK in order to maintain ATP levels. However, expression of PFK2 is low in neurons rendering this pathway insufficient [226,227]. Neuronal stress, such as the above discussed excitotoxicity or disturbance of the ER, may cause a disruption of mitochondrial homeostasis and consequently diminish OXPHOS. This situation is often associated with production of more reactive oxygen species (ROS) than the intracellular redox system can detoxify and precedes neurite retraction and eventual cell death [228]. Oxidatively damaged mitochondria undergo constant remodeling and turnover in neurons, a process that also demands energy [229], as functional mitochondria are transported along the microtubules to remote axonal regions [230], and conversely dysfunctional mitochondria are returned to the cell body for degradation [231]. The induction of endogenous anti-oxidant factors can apparently block the toxicity of ARV drugs, but it is not known if those protective measures are associated with normal neuronal ATP levels [40]. Maintenance of a functional population of mitochondria is critical for postmitotic neurons, and is regulated mainly by autophagy of the damaged organelles, a process called mitophagy [232,233]. This clearance usually contributes to maintenance or the re-establishment of baseline cellular ATP levels [234,235] and is mainly controlled by AMPK and mTOR signaling pathways [236]. Since ARV drugs, METH and HIV-1 or its fragments, including gp120, all generate in neurons oxidative stress and loss of ATP, activation of autophagy seems to provide a suitable protective mechanism [40,145,216]. The importance of the cellular clearance process is supported by several studies showing that impaired autophagy in neurons contributes to the development of neurodegeneration [237,238].

Since neurons induced autophagy in the presence of in HIV gp120 or cART or METH and combination thereof but failed to recover homeostatic levels of ATP, we employed rapamycin to block mTOR, which is an inhibitor of autophagy [145,239]. In the presence of cART, METH and gp120, rapamycin helped to restore neuronal ATP to control levels. Thus, neurons were in principle able to restore ATP levels by autophagy but failed to do so when challenged separately with gp120 or the ARV cocktail or in the absence of rapamycin for reasons that need to be further explored. Strikingly, rapamycin also preserved normal neuronal ATP levels over 7 days in the presence of the combination of cART and gp120 without METH or the combination of METH and gp120 without cART. This outcome might be explained if cART and gp120 engaged different disturbance mechanisms to push neuronal ATP homeostasis off balance. Those mechanisms could however neutralize each other when ARVs and gp120 were combined or could be modified by the presence of METH. The loss of ATP associated with METH exposure was significantly ameliorated by rapamycin but not completely prevented [145]. A possible explanation may be related to the observation that autophagy can cause neurite degeneration in the presence of METH [216]. Thus, autophagy may not always be protective and perhaps be associated with a risk of damaging neuronal structure. Figure 1 provides a schematic summary of the various aspects of the brain's exposure to HIV + METH + cART.

While we are beginning to untangle the combined effects of HIV + cART + METH by characterizing the associated cellular events, more work lies ahead. Studying the combination of HIV and_cART with other abused drugs, such as heroin and cocaine, seems equally important as these substances may involve other pathways and affect HIV neuropathogenesis in different ways than METH [15–18,240]. Moreover, we largely focused on neuronal injury, but METH as well as other abused drugs also affect the immune system and HIV infection itself by compromising for example the interferon response [241–244]. Opioids, cocaine and METH are highly addictive and all seem to be able to influence gene expression in neural and immune cells via mechanisms that involve short, con-coding, regulatory microRNAs and compromise control of HIV infection as well as normal neuronal function [19,245]. Moreover, accumulating evidence suggests a critical role for exosomes, globular, membranous extracellular nanovesicles in HIV infection, HAND and also drug abuse-related neurodegenerative diseases [246–249]. A detailed discussion of the additional abused substances, microRNAs and exosomes is beyond the scope of this review, but those areas of research are poised to significantly contribute to our understanding of the combined effects of HIV + cART + abused drugs on the brain and may help to develop future, improved therapies for addiction and HAND.

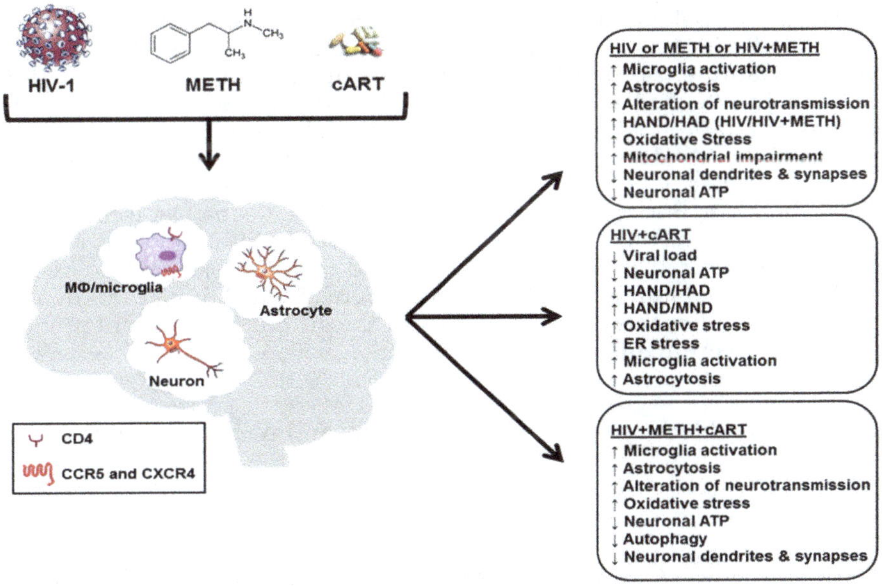


**Figure 1.** Treatment of HIV-1 infection with cART greatly reduces viral loads in periphery and the central nervous system (CNS), the incidence of HIV-associated dementia (HAD) and acquired immunodeficiency syndrome (AIDS)-related deaths. HIV-1 or its components, methamphetamine (METH) and some antiretrovirals used in combined antiretroviral therapy (cART) can induce oxidative and endoplasmic reticulum (ER) stress, compromise autophagy and neuronal energy homeostasis and trigger functional as well as structural neuronal injury. However, even without overt structural damage, diminished adenosine triphosphate (ATP) levels indicate that neurons may lose, at least in part, the energy reserve that is vital to maintaining their normal membrane potential and physiological functions, such as homeostatic regulation of neurotransmission. A compromised neuronal energy homeostasis may explain why cART permits the occurrence of HIV-associated mild neurocognitive disorders (MND). Interestingly, neuronal energy levels can apparently drop significantly during exposure to some drugs or combinations thereof without necessarily destructing neuronal dendrites and pre-synaptic terminals, suggesting that a restoration of full neuronal function may be possible.

## 6. Conclusions

The introduction of cART has transformed HIV-1 infection into a treatable, yet chronic disease that remains associated with a high probability for development of neurocognitive impairment, now termed HAND. Accumulating evidence points to the possibility that besides HIV-1 itself long-term exposure to cART can also contribute to the occurrence of HAND. The fact that HIV-1 infection is frequently associated with the abuse or recreational psychostimulant drugs further complicates the situation. Several lines of evidence indicate that similar to HIV-1 or its components and METH, some

ARV used in cART can also induce oxidative and ER stress, compromise neuronal energy homeostasis and trigger structural neuronal injury. However, even without overt structural damage, diminished ATP levels indicate that neurons may lose, at least in part, the energy reserve that is vital to maintaining their normal membrane potential and physiological function. Interestingly, neuronal energy levels can apparently drop significantly during exposure to some drugs or combinations thereof without necessarily destructing neuronal dendrites and pre-synaptic terminals, suggesting that a restoration of full neuronal function may be possible. Altogether, the available data suggest that the overall beneficial effect of cART against HIV infection can be accompanied by a discernable level of neurotoxicity that may be modified, but in the long-term primarily aggravated by the use of psychostimulant drugs, such as methamphetamine.

**Acknowledgments:** This work was supported by National Institutes of Health grants R25 MH081482 (Interdisciplinary Research Fellowship in NeuroAIDS to A.B.S.), R01 MH087332, MH104131, MH105330, R03 DA02948 and P50 DA026306 (Translational Methamphetamine AIDS Research Center (TMARC), Project 5) to M.K. The TMARC is affiliated with the University of California, San Diego (UCSD) and the Sanford Burnham Prebys Medical Discovery Institute (SBP). The TMARC is comprised of: Igor Grant; Ronald J. Ellis, Scott L. Letendre, and Cristian L. Achim; Steven Paul Woods; Aaron M. Carr, B.A.; Scott L. Letendre, Ronald J. Ellis, Rachel Schrier; Robert K. Heaton, J. Hampton Atkinson, M.D., Mariana Cherner, Thomas D. Marcotte, Erin E. Morgan; Gregory Brown. Terry Jernigan, Anders Dale, Thomas Liu, Miriam Scadeng, Christine Fennema-Notestine, Sarah L. Archibald, M.A.; Cristian L. Achim, Eliezer Masliah, Stuart Lipton, Virawudh Soontornniyomkij; Anthony C. Gamst, Clint Cushman, B.A.; Ian Abramson, Florin Vaida, Reena Deutsch, Anya Umlauf; J. Hampton Atkinson, Jennifer Marquie-Beck, M.P.H.; Project 1: Arpi Minassian, William Perry, Mark Geyer, Brook Henry, Jared Young; Project 2: Amanda B. Grethe, Martin Paulus, Ronald J. Ellis; Project 3: Erin Morgan, (Project Director), David M. Smith, M.D., M.A.S., Igor Grant; Project 4: Svetlana Semenova, Athina Markou, James Kesby; Project 5: Marcus Kaul. The views expressed in this article are those of the authors and do not reflect the official policy or position of the United States Government.

**Author Contributions:** A.B.S. and M.K. researched the literature and wrote the paper.

## References

1. Fauci, A.S. The aids epidemic—Considerations for the 21st century. *N. Engl. J. Med.* **1999**, *341*, 1046–1050. [CrossRef] [PubMed]
2. Piot, P.; Bartos, M.; Ghys, P.D.; Walker, N.; Schwartlander, B. The global impact of HIV/AIDS. *Nature* **2001**, *410*, 968–973. [CrossRef] [PubMed]
3. Fact Sheet November 2016. Available online: http://www.unaids.org/en/resources/fact-sheet (accessed on 9 January 2017).
4. The Joint United Nations Programme on HIV/AIDS (UNAIDS). Unaids Report on the Global Aids Epidemic 2013. Available online: http://www.unaids.org/sites/default/files/media_asset/UNAIDS_Global_Report_2013_en_1.pdf (accessed on 9 October 2013).
5. The Joint United Nations Programme on HIV/AIDS (UNAIDS). Global Aids Response Progress Reporting 2015. Available online: http://www.unaids.org/sites/default/files/media_asset/JC2702_GARPR2015guidelines_en.pdf (accessed on5 May 2015).
6. Centers for Disease Control and Prevention. Available online: https://www.cdc.gov/hiv/ (accessed on 11 January 2017).
7. Antinori, A.; Arendt, G.; Becker, J.T.; Brew, B.J.; Byrd, D.A.; Cherner, M.; Clifford, D.B.; Cinque, P.; Epstein, L.G.; Goodkin, K.; et al. Updated research nosology for HIV-associated neurocognitive disorders. *Neurology* **2007**, *69*, 1789–1799. [CrossRef] [PubMed]
8. Kaul, M. Hiv's double strike at the brain: Neuronal toxicity and compromised neurogenesis. *Front. Biosci.* **2008**, *13*, 2484–2494. [CrossRef] [PubMed]
9. McArthur, J.C.; Steiner, J.; Sacktor, N.; Nath, A. Human immunodeficiency virus-associated neurocognitive disorders: Mind the gap. *Ann. Neurol.* **2010**, *67*, 699–714. [PubMed]

10. Heaton, R.K.; Clifford, D.B.; Franklin, D.R., Jr.; Woods, S.P.; Ake, C.; Vaida, F.; Ellis, R.J.; Letendre, S.L.; Marcotte, T.D.; Atkinson, J.H.; et al. HIV-associated neurocognitive disorders persist in the era of potent antiretroviral therapy: Charter study. *Neurology* **2010**, *75*, 2087–2096. [CrossRef]
11. Saylor, D.; Dickens, A.M.; Sacktor, N.; Haughey, N.; Slusher, B.; Pletnikov, M.; Mankowski, J.L.; Brown, A.; Volsky, D.J.; McArthur, J.C. HIV-associated neurocognitive disorder—Pathogenesis and prospects for treatment. *Nat. Rev. Neurol.* **2016**, *12*, 234–248. [CrossRef] [PubMed]
12. Drugs of Abuse. Available online: https://www.drugabuse.gov/drugs-abuse (accessed on 10 January 2017).
13. Peterson, P.K.; Gekker, G.; Schut, R.; Hu, S.; Balfour, H.H., Jr.; Chao, C.C. Enhancement of HIV-1 replication by opiates and cocaine: The cytokine connection. *Adv. Exp. Med. Biol.* **1993**, *335*, 181–188. [PubMed]
14. Carey, C.L.; Woods, S.P.; Rippeth, J.D.; Gonzalez, R.; Heaton, R.K.; Grant, I. Additive deleterious effects of methamphetamine dependence and immunosuppression on neuropsychological functioning in HIV infection. *AIDS Behav.* **2006**, *10*, 185–190. [CrossRef] [PubMed]
15. Byrd, D.A.; Fellows, R.P.; Morgello, S.; Franklin, D.; Heaton, R.K.; Deutsch, R.; Atkinson, J.H.; Clifford, D.B.; Collier, A.C.; Marra, C.M.; et al. Neurocognitive impact of substance use in HIV infection. *J. Acquir. Immune Defic. Syndr.* **2011**, *58*, 154–162. [CrossRef] [PubMed]
16. Buch, S.; Yao, H.; Guo, M.; Mori, T.; Mathias-Costa, B.; Singh, V.; Seth, P.; Wang, J.; Su, T.P. Cocaine and HIV-1 interplay in CNS: Cellular and molecular mechanisms. *Curr. HIV Res.* **2012**, *10*, 425–428. [CrossRef]
17. Silverstein, P.S.; Shah, A.; Weemhoff, J.; Kumar, S.; Singh, D.P.; Kumar, A. HIV-1 gp120 and drugs of abuse: Interactions in the central nervous system. *Curr. HIV Res.* **2012**, *10*, 369–383. [CrossRef]
18. Chang, S.L.; Connaghan, K.P.; Wei, Y.; Li, M.D. Neurohiv and use of addictive substances. *Int. Rev. Neurobiol.* **2014**, *118*, 403–440. [PubMed]
19. Pilakka-Kanthikeel, S.; Nair, M.P. Interaction of drugs of abuse and microrna with HIV: A brief review. *Front. Microbiol.* **2015**, *6*, 967. [CrossRef] [PubMed]
20. Kapadia, F.; Vlahov, D.; Donahoe, R.M.; Friedland, G. The role of substance abuse in HIV disease progression: Reconciling differences from laboratory and epidemiologic investigations. *Clin. Infect. Dis.* **2005**, *41*, 1027–1034. [CrossRef] [PubMed]
21. Mitchell, S.J.; Morris, S.R.; Kent, C.K.; Stansell, J.; Klausner, J.D. Methamphetamine use and sexual activity among HIV-infected patients in care—San Francisco, 2004. *Aids Patient Care STDs* **2006**, *20*, 502–510. [CrossRef] [PubMed]
22. Urbina, A.; Jones, K. Crystal methamphetamine, its analogues, and HIV infection: Medical and psychiatric aspects of a new epidemic. *Clin. Infect. Dis.* **2004**, *38*, 890–894. [CrossRef] [PubMed]
23. Hinkin, C.H.; Barclay, T.R.; Castellon, S.A.; Levine, A.J.; Durvasula, R.S.; Marion, S.D.; Myers, H.F.; Longshore, D. Drug use and medication adherence among HIV-1 infected individuals. *AIDS Behav.* **2007**, *11*, 185–194. [CrossRef] [PubMed]
24. Ellis, R.J.; Childers, M.E.; Cherner, M.; Lazzaretto, D.; Letendre, S.; Grant, I. Increased human immunodeficiency virus loads in active methamphetamine users are explained by reduced effectiveness of antiretroviral therapy. *J. Infect. Dis.* **2003**, *188*, 1820–1826. [CrossRef] [PubMed]
25. Langford, T.D.; Letendre, S.L.; Larrea, G.J.; Masliah, E. Changing patterns in the neuropathogenesis of HIV during the haart era. *Brain Pathol.* **2003**, *13*, 195–210. [CrossRef] [PubMed]
26. Rippeth, J.D.; Heaton, R.K.; Carey, C.L.; Marcotte, T.D.; Moore, D.J.; Gonzalez, R.; Wolfson, T.; Grant, I. Methamphetamine dependence increases risk of neuropsychological impairment in HIV infected persons. *J. Int. Neuropsychol. Soc.* **2004**, *10*, 1–14. [CrossRef] [PubMed]
27. Chana, G.; Everall, I.P.; Crews, L.; Langford, D.; Adame, A.; Grant, I.; Cherner, M.; Lazzaretto, D.; Heaton, R.; Ellis, R.; et al. Cognitive deficits and degeneration of interneurons in HIV+ methamphetamine users. *Neurology* **2006**, *67*, 1486–1489. [CrossRef] [PubMed]
28. Cadet, J.L.; Krasnova, I.N. Interactions of HIV and methamphetamine: Cellular and molecular mechanisms of toxicity potentiation. *Neurotox. Res.* **2007**, *12*, 181–204. [CrossRef] [PubMed]
29. Eisfeld, C.; Reichelt, D.; Evers, S.; Husstedt, I. Csf penetration by antiretroviral drugs. *CNS Drugs* **2013**, *27*, 31–55. [CrossRef] [PubMed]
30. Heaton, R.K.; Franklin, D.R., Jr.; Deutsch, R.; Letendre, S.; Ellis, R.J.; Casaletto, K.; Marquine, M.J.; Woods, S.P.; Vaida, F.; Atkinson, J.H.; et al. Neurocognitive change in the era of HIV combination antiretroviral therapy: The longitudinal charter study. *Clin. Infect. Dis.* **2015**, *60*, 473–480. [CrossRef] [PubMed]

31. Heaton, R.K.; Franklin, D.R.; Ellis, R.J.; McCutchan, J.A.; Letendre, S.L.; Leblanc, S.; Corkran, S.H.; Duarte, N.A.; Clifford, D.B.; Woods, S.P.; et al. HIV-associated neurocognitive disorders before and during the era of combination antiretroviral therapy: Differences in rates, nature, and predictors. *J. Neurovirol.* **2011**, *17*, 3–16. [CrossRef] [PubMed]
32. Evans, S.R.; Ellis, R.J.; Chen, H.; Yeh, T.M.; Lee, A.J.; Schifitto, G.; Wu, K.; Bosch, R.J.; McArthur, J.C.; Simpson, D.M.; et al. Peripheral neuropathy in HIV: Prevalence and risk factors. *AIDS* **2011**, *25*, 919–928. [CrossRef] [PubMed]
33. Evans, S.R.; Lee, A.J.; Ellis, R.J.; Chen, H.; Wu, K.; Bosch, R.J.; Clifford, D.B. HIV peripheral neuropathy progression: Protection with glucose-lowering drugs? *J. Neurovirol.* **2012**, *18*, 428–433. [CrossRef] [PubMed]
34. Robertson, K.R.; Su, Z.; Margolis, D.M.; Krambrink, A.; Havlir, D.V.; Evans, S.; Skiest, D.J. Neurocognitive effects of treatment interruption in stable HIV-positive patients in an observational cohort. *Neurology* **2010**, *74*, 1260–1266. [CrossRef] [PubMed]
35. Underwood, J.; Robertson, K.R.; Winston, A. Could antiretroviral neurotoxicity play a role in the pathogenesis of cognitive impairment in treated HIV disease? *AIDS* **2014**, *29*, 253–261. [CrossRef] [PubMed]
36. Carr, A. Toxicity of antiretroviral therapy and implications for drug development. *Nat. Rev. Drug Discov.* **2003**, *2*, 624–634. [CrossRef] [PubMed]
37. Keswani, S.C.; Chander, B.; Hasan, C.; Griffin, J.W.; McArthur, J.C.; Hoke, A. Fk506 is neuroprotective in a model of antiretroviral toxic neuropathy. *Ann. Neurol.* **2003**, *53*, 57–64. [CrossRef] [PubMed]
38. Lewin, S.R.; Hoy, J.; Crowe, S.M.; McDonald, C.F. The role of bronchoscopy in the diagnosis and treatment of pulmonary disease in HIV-infected patients. *Aust. N. Z. J. Med.* **1995**, *25*, 133–139. [CrossRef] [PubMed]
39. Robertson, K.; Liner, J.; Meeker, R.B. Antiretroviral neurotoxicity. *J. Neurovirol.* **2012**, *18*, 388–399. [CrossRef] [PubMed]
40. Akay, C.; Cooper, M.; Odeleye, A.; Jensen, B.K.; White, M.G.; Vassoler, F.; Gannon, P.J.; Mankowski, J.; Dorsey, J.L.; Buch, A.M.; et al. Antiretroviral drugs induce oxidative stress and neuronal damage in the central nervous system. *J. Neurovirol.* **2014**, *20*, 39–53. [CrossRef] [PubMed]
41. Navia, B.A.; Jordan, B.D.; Price, R.W. The aids dementia complex: I. Clinical features. *Ann. Neurol.* **1986**, *19*, 517–524. [CrossRef] [PubMed]
42. Price, R.W.; Brew, B.; Sidtis, J.; Rosenblum, M.; Scheck, A.C.; Cleary, P. The brain in aids: Central nervous system HIV-1 infection and aids dementia complex. *Science* **1988**, *239*, 586–592. [CrossRef] [PubMed]
43. Kaul, M.; Garden, G.A.; Lipton, S.A. Pathways to neuronal injury and apoptosis in HIV-associated dementia. *Nature* **2001**, *410*, 988–994. [CrossRef] [PubMed]
44. Sacktor, N.; Lyles, R.H.; Skolasky, R.; Kleeberger, C.; Selnes, O.A.; Miller, E.N.; Becker, J.T.; Cohen, B.; McArthur, J.C. HIV-associated neurologic disease incidence changes: Multicenter aids cohort study, 1990–1998. *Neurology* **2001**, *56*, 257–260. [CrossRef] [PubMed]
45. Ellis, R.J.; Deutsch, R.; Heaton, R.K.; Marcotte, T.D.; McCutchan, J.A.; Nelson, J.A.; Abramson, I.; Thal, L.J.; Atkinson, J.H.; Wallace, M.R.; et al. Neurocognitive impairment is an independent risk factor for death in hiv infection. San Diego HIV neurobehavioral research center group. *Arch. Neurol.* **1997**, *54*, 416–424. [CrossRef] [PubMed]
46. Cunningham, P.H.; Smith, D.G.; Satchell, C.; Cooper, D.A.; Brew, B. Evidence for independent development of resistance to HIV-1 reverse transcriptase inhibitors in the cerebrospinal fluid. *AIDS* **2000**, *14*, 1949–1954. [CrossRef] [PubMed]
47. Cysique, L.A.; Maruff, P.; Brew, B.J. Variable benefit in neuropsychological function in HIV-infected haart-treated patients. *Neurology* **2006**, *66*, 1447–1450. [CrossRef] [PubMed]
48. Giancola, M.L.; Lorenzini, P.; Balestra, P.; Larussa, D.; Baldini, F.; Corpolongo, A.; Narciso, P.; Bellagamba, R.; Tozzi, V.; Antinori, A. Neuroactive antiretroviral drugs do not influence neurocognitive performance in less advanced hiv-infected patients responding to highly active antiretroviral therapy. *J. Acquir. Immune Defic. Syndr.* **2006**, *41*, 332–337. [CrossRef] [PubMed]
49. Nath, A.; Sacktor, N. Influence of highly active antiretroviral therapy on persistence of HIV in the central nervous system. *Curr. Opin. Neurol.* **2006**, *19*, 358–361. [CrossRef] [PubMed]
50. McArthur, J.C.; Haughey, N.; Gartner, S.; Conant, K.; Pardo, C.; Nath, A.; Sacktor, N. Human immunodeficiency virus-associated dementia: An evolving disease. *J. Neurovirol.* **2003**, *9*, 205–221. [CrossRef] [PubMed]
51. Brew, B.J.; Crowe, S.M.; Landay, A.; Cysique, L.A.; Guillemin, G. Neurodegeneration and ageing in the haart era. *J. Neuroimmune Pharmacol.* **2009**, *4*, 163–174. [CrossRef] [PubMed]

52. Welch, K.; Morse, A. The clinical profile of end-stage aids in the era of highly active antiretroviral therapy. *AIDS Patient Care STDs* **2002**, *16*, 75–81. [CrossRef] [PubMed]
53. Kaul, M.; Zheng, J.; Okamoto, S.; Gendelman, H.E.; Lipton, S.A. HIV-1 infection and aids: Consequences for the central nervous system. *Cell Death Differ.* **2005**, *12*, 878–892. [CrossRef] [PubMed]
54. Kramer-Hammerle, S.; Rothenaigner, I.; Wolff, H.; Bell, J.E.; Brack-Werner, R. Cells of the central nervous system as targets and reservoirs of the human immunodeficiency virus. *Virus Res.* **2005**, *111*, 194–213. [CrossRef] [PubMed]
55. Lipton, S.A. Treating aids dementia [letter; comment]. *Science* **1997**, *276*, 1629–1630. [CrossRef] [PubMed]
56. Jones, G.; Power, C. Regulation of neural cell survival by HIV-1 infection. *Neurobiol. Dis.* **2006**, *21*, 1–17. [CrossRef] [PubMed]
57. Petito, C.K.; Cho, E.S.; Lemann, W.; Navia, B.A.; Price, R.W. Neuropathology of acquired immunodeficiency syndrome (AIDS): An autopsy review. *J. Neuropathol. Exp. Neurol.* **1986**, *45*, 635–646. [CrossRef] [PubMed]
58. Masliah, E.; Heaton, R.K.; Marcotte, T.D.; Ellis, R.J.; Wiley, C.A.; Mallory, M.; Achim, C.L.; McCutchan, J.A.; Nelson, J.A.; Atkinson, J.H.; et al. Dendritic injury is a pathological substrate for human immunodeficiency virus-related cognitive disorders. Hnrc group. The HIV neurobehavioral research center. *Ann. Neurol.* **1997**, *42*, 963–972. [CrossRef] [PubMed]
59. Glass, J.D.; Fedor, H.; Wesselingh, S.L.; McArthur, J.C. Immunocytochemical quantitation of human immunodeficiency virus in the brain: Correlations with dementia. *Ann. Neurol.* **1995**, *38*, 755–762. [CrossRef] [PubMed]
60. Achim, C.L.; Wang, R.; Miners, D.K.; Wiley, C.A. Brain viral burden in HIV infection. *J. Neuropathol. Exp. Neurol.* **1994**, *53*, 284–294. [CrossRef] [PubMed]
61. Wiley, C.A.; Masliah, E.; Achim, C.L. Measurement of cns HIV burden and its association with neurologic damage. *Adv. Neuroimmunol.* **1994**, *4*, 319–325. [CrossRef]
62. Wesselingh, S.L.; Takahashi, K.; Glass, J.D.; McArthur, J.C.; Griffin, J.W.; Griffin, D.E. Cellular localization of tumor necrosis factor mrna in neurological tissue from HIV-infected patients by combined reverse transcriptase/polymerase chain reaction in situ hybridization and immunohistochemistry. *J. Neuroimmunol.* **1997**, *74*, 1–8. [CrossRef]
63. Heyes, M.P.; Brew, B.J.; Martin, A.; Price, R.W.; Salazar, A.M.; Sidtis, J.J.; Yergey, J.A.; Mouradian, M.M.; Sadler, A.E.; Keilp, J.; et al. Quinolinic acid in cerebrospinal fluid and serum in HIV-1 infection: Relationship to clinical and neurological status. *Ann. Neurol.* **1991**, *29*, 202–209. [CrossRef] [PubMed]
64. Shiramizu, B.; Gartner, S.; Williams, A.; Shikuma, C.; Ratto-Kim, S.; Watters, M.; Aguon, J.; Valcour, V. Circulating proviral HIV DNA and HIV-associated dementia. *AIDS* **2005**, *19*, 45–52. [CrossRef] [PubMed]
65. Shiramizu, B.; Ratto-Kim, S.; Sithinamsuwan, P.; Nidhinandana, S.; Thitivichianlert, S.; Watt, G.; Desouza, M.; Chuenchitra, T.; Sukwit, S.; Chitpatima, S.; et al. HIV DNA and dementia in treatment-naive HIV-1-infected individuals in bangkok, thailand. *Int. J. Med. Sci.* **2006**, *4*, 13–18. [CrossRef] [PubMed]
66. Ketzler, S.; Weis, S.; Haug, H.; Budka, H. Loss of neurons in the frontal cortex in aids brains. *Acta Neuropathol.* **1990**, *80*, 92–94. [CrossRef] [PubMed]
67. Everall, I.P.; Luthert, P.J.; Lantos, P.L. Neuronal loss in the frontal cortex in HIV infection. *Lancet* **1991**, *337*, 1119–1121. [CrossRef]
68. Reyes, M.G.; Faraldi, F.; Senseng, C.S.; Flowers, C.; Fariello, R. Nigral degeneration in acquired immune deficiency syndrome (AIDS). *Acta Neuropathol.* **1991**, *82*, 39–44. [CrossRef] [PubMed]
69. Graus, F.; Ribalta, T.; Abos, J.; Alom, J.; Cruz-Sanchez, F.; Mallolas, J.; Miro, J.M.; Cardesa, A.; Tolosa, E. Subacute cerebellar syndrome as the first manifestation of aids dementia complex. *Acta Neurol. Scand.* **1990**, *81*, 118–120. [CrossRef] [PubMed]
70. Everall, I.; Luthert, P.; Lantos, P. A review of neuronal damage in human immunodeficiency virus infection: Its assessment, possible mechanism and relationship to dementia. *J. Neuropathol. Exp. Neurol.* **1993**, *52*, 561–566. [CrossRef] [PubMed]
71. Adle-Biassette, H.; Chrétien, F.; Wingertsmann, L.; Héry, C.; Ereau, T.; Scaravilli, F.; Tardieu, M.; Gray, F. Neuronal apoptosis does not correlate with dementia in HIV infection but is related to microglial activation and axonal damage. *Neuropathol. Appl. Neurobiol.* **1999**, *25*, 123–133. [CrossRef] [PubMed]
72. Petito, C.K.; Roberts, B. Evidence of apoptotic cell death in HIV encephalitis. *Am. J. Pathol.* **1995**, *146*, 1121–1130. [PubMed]

73. Rostasy, K.; Monti, L.; Yiannoutsos, C.; Wu, J.; Bell, J.; Hedreen, J.; Navia, B.A. Nfkappab activation, TNF-alpha expression, and apoptosis in the aids-dementia-complex. *J. Neurovirol.* **2000**, *6*, 537–543. [CrossRef] [PubMed]
74. Anthony, I.C.; Ramage, S.N.; Carnie, F.W.; Simmonds, P.; Bell, J.E. Influence of haart on HIV-related cns disease and neuroinflammation. *J. Neuropathol. Exp. Neurol.* **2005**, *64*, 529–536. [CrossRef] [PubMed]
75. Everall, I.P.; Hansen, L.A.; Masliah, E. The shifting patterns of HIV encephalitis neuropathology. *Neurotox. Res.* **2005**, *8*, 51–61. [CrossRef] [PubMed]
76. Green, D.A.; Masliah, E.; Vinters, H.V.; Beizai, P.; Moore, D.J.; Achim, C.L. Brain deposition of beta-amyloid is a common pathologic feature in HIV positive patients. *AIDS* **2005**, *19*, 407–411. [CrossRef] [PubMed]
77. Ho, D.D.; Rota, T.R.; Schooley, R.T.; Kaplan, J.C.; Allan, J.D.; Groopman, J.E.; Resnick, L.; Felsenstein, D.; Andrews, C.A.; Hirsch, M.S. Isolation of HTLV-III from cerebrospinal fluid and neural tissues of patients with neurologic syndromes related to the acquired immunodeficiency syndrome. *N. Engl. J. Med.* **1985**, *313*, 1493–1497. [CrossRef] [PubMed]
78. Gartner, S. HIV infection and dementia. *Science* **2000**, *287*, 602–604. [CrossRef] [PubMed]
79. Gonzalez-Scarano, F.; Martin-Garcia, J. The neuropathogenesis of AIDS. *Nat. Rev. Immunol.* **2005**, *5*, 69–81. [CrossRef] [PubMed]
80. Koenig, S.; Gendelman, H.E.; Orenstein, J.M.; Dal Canto, M.C.; Pezeshkpour, G.H.; Yungbluth, M.; Janotta, F.; Aksamit, A.; Martin, M.A.; Fauci, A.S. Detection of aids virus in macrophages in brain tissue from aids patients with encephalopathy. *Science* **1986**, *233*, 1089–1093. [CrossRef] [PubMed]
81. Dragic, T.; Litwin, V.; Allaway, G.P.; Martin, S.R.; Huang, Y.; Nagashima, K.A.; Cayanan, C.; Maddon, P.J.; Koup, R.A.; Moore, J.P.; et al. HIV-1 entry into CD4+ cells is mediated by the chemokine receptor CC-CKR-5. *Nature* **1996**, *381*, 667–673. [CrossRef] [PubMed]
82. Oberlin, E.; Amara, A.; Bachelerie, F.; Bessia, C.; Virelizier, J.L.; Arenzana-Seisdedos, F.; Schwartz, O.; Heard, J.M.; Clark-Lewis, I.; Legler, D.F.; et al. The CXC chemokine SDF-1 is the ligand for LESTR/fusin and prevents infection by T-cell-line-adapted HIV-1. *Nature* **1996**, *382*, 833–835. [CrossRef] [PubMed]
83. He, J.; Chen, Y.; Farzan, M.; Choe, H.; Ohagen, A.; Gartner, S.; Busciglio, J.; Yang, X.; Hofmann, W.; Newman, W.; et al. CCR3 and CCR5 are co-receptors for HIV-1 infection of microglia. *Nature* **1997**, *385*, 645–649. [CrossRef] [PubMed]
84. Asensio, V.C.; Campbell, I.L. Chemokines in the CNS: Plurifunctional mediators in diverse states. *Trends Neurosci.* **1999**, *22*, 504–512. [CrossRef]
85. Miller, R.J.; Meucci, O. Aids and the brain: Is there a chemokine connection? *Trends Neurosci.* **1999**, *22*, 471–479. [CrossRef]
86. Hesselgesser, J.; Taub, D.; Baskar, P.; Greenberg, M.; Hoxie, J.; Kolson, D.L.; Horuk, R. Neuronal apoptosis induced by HIV-1 gp120 and the chemokine SDF-1 alpha is mediated by the chemokine receptor CXCR4. *Curr. Biol.* **1998**, *8*, 595–598. [CrossRef]
87. Meucci, O.; Fatatis, A.; Simen, A.A.; Bushell, T.J.; Gray, P.W.; Miller, R.J. Chemokines regulate hippocampal neuronal signaling and gp120 neurotoxicity. *Proc. Natl. Acad. Sci. USA* **1998**, *95*, 14500–14505. [CrossRef] [PubMed]
88. Meucci, O.; Fatatis, A.; Simen, A.A.; Miller, R.J. Expression of CX3CR1 chemokine receptors on neurons and their role in neuronal survival. *Proc. Natl. Acad. Sci. USA* **2000**, *97*, 8075–8080. [CrossRef] [PubMed]
89. Kaul, M.; Lipton, S.A. Chemokines and activated macrophages in HIV gp120-induced neuronal apoptosis. *Proc. Natl. Acad. Sci. USA* **1999**, *96*, 8212–8216. [CrossRef] [PubMed]
90. Kaul, M.; Ma, Q.; Medders, K.E.; Desai, M.K.; Lipton, S.A. HIV-1 coreceptors CCR5 and CXCR4 both mediate neuronal cell death but CCR5 paradoxically can also contribute to protection. *Cell Death Differ.* **2007**, *14*, 296–305. [CrossRef] [PubMed]
91. Zheng, J.; Thylin, M.R.; Ghorpade, A.; Xiong, H.; Persidsky, Y.; Cotter, R.; Niemann, D.; Che, M.; Zeng, Y.C.; Gelbard, H.A.; et al. Intracellular CXCR4 signaling, neuronal apoptosis and neuropathogenic mechanisms of HIV-1-associated dementia. *J. Neuroimmunol.* **1999**, *98*, 185–200. [CrossRef]
92. Maung, R.; Hoefer, M.M.; Sanchez, A.B.; Sejbuk, N.E.; Medders, K.E.; Desai, M.K.; Catalan, I.C.; Dowling, C.C.; de Rozieres, C.M.; Garden, G.A.; et al. CCR5 knockout prevents neuronal injury and behavioral impairment induced in a transgenic mouse model by a CXCR4-using HIV-1 glycoprotein 120. *J. Immunol.* **2014**, *193*, 1895–1910. [CrossRef] [PubMed]

93. Brenneman, D.E.; Westbrook, G.L.; Fitzgerald, S.P.; Ennist, D.L.; Elkins, K.L.; Ruff, M.R.; Pert, C.B. Neuronal cell killing by the envelope protein of HIV and its prevention by vasoactive intestinal peptide. *Nature* **1988**, *335*, 639–642. [CrossRef] [PubMed]
94. Iskander, S.; Walsh, K.A.; Hammond, R.R. Human CNS cultures exposed to HIV-1 gp120 reproduce dendritic injuries of HIV-1-associated dementia. *J. Neuroinflamm.* **2004**, *1*, 7. [CrossRef] [PubMed]
95. Walsh, K.A.; Megyesi, J.F.; Wilson, J.X.; Crukley, J.; Laubach, V.E.; Hammond, R.R. Antioxidant protection from HIV-1 gp120-induced neuroglial toxicity. *J. Neuroinflamm.* **2004**, *1*, 8. [CrossRef] [PubMed]
96. Ohagen, A.; Ghosh, S.; He, J.; Huang, K.; Chen, Y.; Yuan, M.; Osathanondh, R.; Gartner, S.; Shi, B.; Shaw, G.; et al. Apoptosis induced by infection of primary brain cultures with diverse human immunodeficiency virus type 1 isolates: Evidence for a role of the envelope. *J. Virol.* **1999**, *73*, 897–906. [PubMed]
97. Chen, W.; Sulcove, J.; Frank, I.; Jaffer, S.; Ozdener, H.; Kolson, D.L. Development of a human neuronal cell model for human immunodeficiency virus (HIV)-infected macrophage-induced neurotoxicity: Apoptosis induced by HIV type 1 primary isolates and evidence for involvement of the Bcl-2/Bcl-xl-sensitive intrinsic apoptosis pathway. *J. Virol.* **2002**, *76*, 9407–9419. [PubMed]
98. Garden, G.A.; Guo, W.; Jayadev, S.; Tun, C.; Balcaitis, S.; Choi, J.; Montine, T.J.; Moller, T.; Morrison, R.S. HIV associated neurodegeneration requires p53 in neurons and microglia. *FASEB J.* **2004**, *18*, 1141–1143. [CrossRef] [PubMed]
99. Mattson, M.P.; Haughey, N.J.; Nath, A. Cell death in HIV dementia. *Cell Death Differ.* **2005**, *12*, 893–904. [CrossRef] [PubMed]
100. New, D.R.; Ma, M.; Epstein, L.G.; Nath, A.; Gelbard, H.A. Human immunodeficiency virus type 1 tat protein induces death by apoptosis in primary human neuron cultures. *J. Neurovirol.* **1997**, *3*, 168–173. [CrossRef] [PubMed]
101. Adamson, D.C.; Wildemann, B.; Sasaki, M.; Glass, J.D.; McArthur, J.C.; Christov, V.I.; Dawson, T.M.; Dawson, V.L. Immunologic no synthase: Elevation in severe aids dementia and induction by HIV-1 gp41. *Science* **1996**, *274*, 1917–1921. [CrossRef] [PubMed]
102. Piller, S.C.; Jans, P.; Gage, P.W.; Jans, D.A. Extracellular HIV-1 virus protein r causes a large inward current and cell death in cultured hippocampal neurons: Implications for aids pathology. *Proc. Natl. Acad. Sci. USA* **1998**, *95*, 4595–4600. [CrossRef] [PubMed]
103. Koedel, U.; Kohleisen, B.; Sporer, B.; Lahrtz, F.; Ovod, V.; Fontana, A.; Erfle, V.; Pfister, H.W. HIV type 1 nef protein is a viral factor for leukocyte recruitment into the central nervous system. *J. Immunol.* **1999**, *163*, 1237–1245. [PubMed]
104. Ellis, R.; Langford, D.; Masliah, E. HIV and antiretroviral therapy in the brain: Neuronal injury and repair. *Nat. Rev. Neurosci.* **2007**, *8*, 33–44. [CrossRef] [PubMed]
105. Krathwohl, M.D.; Kaiser, J.L. HIV-1 promotes quiescence in human neural progenitor cells. *J. Infect. Dis.* **2004**, *190*, 216–226. [CrossRef] [PubMed]
106. Okamoto, S.; Kang, Y.J.; Brechtel, C.W.; Siviglia, E.; Russo, R.; Clemente, A.; Harrop, A.; McKercher, S.; Kaul, M.; Lipton, S.A. HIV/gp120 decreases adult neural progenitor cell proliferation via checkpoint kinase-mediated cell-cycle withdrawal and G1 arrest. *Cell Stem Cell* **2007**, *1*, 230–236. [CrossRef] [PubMed]
107. Giulian, D.; Vaca, K.; Noonan, C.A. Secretion of neurotoxins by mononuclear phagocytes infected with HIV-1. *Science* **1990**, *250*, 1593–1596. [CrossRef] [PubMed]
108. Genis, P.; Jett, M.; Bernton, E.W.; Boyle, T.; Gelbard, H.A.; Dzenko, K.; Keane, R.W.; Resnick, L.; Mizrachi, Y.; Volsky, D.J.; et al. Cytokines and arachidonic metabolites produced during human immunodeficiency virus (HIV)-infected macrophage-astroglia interactions: Implications for the neuropathogenesis of HIV disease. *J. Exp. Med.* **1992**, *176*, 1703–1718. [CrossRef] [PubMed]
109. Medders, K.E.; Sejbuk, N.E.; Maung, R.; Desai, M.K.; Kaul, M. Activation of p38 mapk is required in monocytic and neuronal cells for HIV glycoprotein 120-induced neurotoxicity. *J. Immunol.* **2010**, *185*, 4883–4895. [CrossRef] [PubMed]
110. Sui, Z.; Fan, S.; Sniderhan, L.; Reisinger, E.; Litzburg, A.; Schifitto, G.; Gelbard, H.A.; Dewhurst, S.; Maggirwar, S.B. Inhibition of mixed lineage kinase 3 prevents HIV-1 tat-mediated neurotoxicity and monocyte activation. *J. Immunol.* **2006**, *177*, 702–711. [CrossRef] [PubMed]
111. Giulian, D.; Wendt, E.; Vaca, K.; Noonan, C.A. The envelope glycoprotein of human immunodeficiency virus type 1 stimulates release of neurotoxins from monocytes. *Proc. Natl. Acad. Sci. USA* **1993**, *90*, 2769–2773. [CrossRef] [PubMed]

112. Dreyer, E.B.; Kaiser, P.K.; Offermann, J.T.; Lipton, S.A. HIV-1 coat protein neurotoxicity prevented by calcium channel antagonists. *Science* **1990**, *248*, 364–367. [CrossRef] [PubMed]
113. O'Donnell, L.A.; Agrawal, A.; Jordan-Sciutto, K.L.; Dichter, M.A.; Lynch, D.R.; Kolson, D.L. Human immunodeficiency virus (HIV)-induced neurotoxicity: Roles for the nmda receptor subtypes. *J. Neurosci.* **2006**, *26*, 981–990. [CrossRef] [PubMed]
114. Olney, J.W.; Labruyere, J.; Wang, G.; Wozniak, D.F.; Price, M.T.; Sesma, M.A. Nmda antagonist neurotoxicity: Mechanism and prevention. *Science* **1991**, *254*, 1515–1518. [CrossRef] [PubMed]
115. Doble, A. The role of excitotoxicity in neurodegenerative disease: Implications for therapy. *Pharmacol. Ther.* **1999**, *81*, 163–221. [CrossRef]
116. Olney, J.W. Brain lesions, obesity, and other disturbances in mice treated with monosodium glutamate. *Science* **1969**, *164*, 719–721. [CrossRef] [PubMed]
117. Tenneti, L.; D'Emilia, D.M.; Troy, C.M.; Lipton, S.A. Role of caspases in *N*-methyl-D-aspartate-induced apoptosis in cerebrocortical neurons. *J. Neurochem.* **1998**, *71*, 946–959. [CrossRef]
118. Garden, G.A.; Budd, S.L.; Tsai, E.; Hanson, L.; Kaul, M.; D'Emilia, D.M.; Friedlander, R.M.; Yuan, J.; Masliah, E.; Lipton, S.A. Caspase cascades in human immunodeficiency virus-associated neurodegeneration. *J. Neurosci.* **2002**, *22*, 4015–4024. [PubMed]
119. Jordan-Sciutto, K.L.; Wang, G.; Murphey-Corb, M.; Wiley, C.A. Cell cycle proteins exhibit altered expression patterns in lentiviral-associated encephalitis. *J. Neurosci.* **2002**, *22*, 2185–2195. [PubMed]
120. Jana, A.; Pahan, K. Human immunodeficiency virus type 1 gp120 induces apoptosis in human primary neurons through redox-regulated activation of neutral sphingomyelinase. *J. Neurosci.* **2004**, *24*, 9531–9540. [CrossRef] [PubMed]
121. Haughey, N.J.; Mattson, M.P. Calcium dysregulation and neuronal apoptosis by the HIV-1 proteins tat and gp120. *J. Acquir. Immune Defic. Syndr.* **2002**, *31* (Suppl. 2), S55–S61. [CrossRef] [PubMed]
122. Haughey, N.J.; Cutler, R.G.; Tamara, A.; McArthur, J.C.; Vargas, D.L.; Pardo, C.A.; Turchan, J.; Nath, A.; Mattson, M.P. Perturbation of sphingolipid metabolism and ceramide production in HIV-dementia. *Ann. Neurol.* **2004**, *55*, 257–267. [CrossRef] [PubMed]
123. Lindl, K.A.; Akay, C.; Wang, Y.; White, M.G.; Jordan-Sciutto, K.L. Expression of the endoplasmic reticulum stress response marker, BiP, in the central nervous system of HIV-positive individuals. *Neuropathol. Appl. Neurobiol.* **2007**, *33*, 658–669. [CrossRef] [PubMed]
124. Federally Approved HIV/AIDS Medical Practice Guidelines. Available online: https://aidsinfo.nih.gov/guidelines (accessed on 2 December 2016).
125. Shah, A.; Gangwani, M.R.; Chaudhari, N.S.; Glazyrin, A.; Bhat, H.K.; Kumar, A. Neurotoxicity in the post-haart era: Caution for the antiretroviral therapeutics. *Neurotox. Res.* **2016**, *30*, 677–697. [CrossRef] [PubMed]
126. Badowski, M.E.; Perez, S.E.; Biagi, M.; Littler, J.A. New antiretroviral treatment for HIV. *Infect. Dis. Ther.* **2016**, *5*, 329–352. [CrossRef] [PubMed]
127. Ciccarelli, N.; Fabbiani, M.; Di, G.S.; Fanti, I.; Baldonero, E.; Bracciale, L.; Tamburrini, E.; Cauda, R.; De, L.A.; Silveri, M.C. Efavirenz associated with cognitive disorders in otherwise asymptomatic HIV-infected patients. *Neurology* **2011**, *76*, 1403–1409. [CrossRef] [PubMed]
128. Canizares, S.; Cherner, M.; Ellis, R.J. HIV and aging: Effects on the central nervous system. *Semin. Neurol.* **2014**, *34*, 27–34. [CrossRef] [PubMed]
129. DeVaughn, S.; Muller-Oehring, E.M.; Markey, B.; Bronte-Stewart, H.M.; Schulte, T. Aging with HIV-1 infection: Motor functions, cognition, and attention—A comparison with parkinson's disease. *Neuropsychol. Rev.* **2015**, *25*, 424–438. [CrossRef] [PubMed]
130. Ma, Q.; Vaida, F.; Wong, J.; Sanders, C.A.; Kao, Y.T.; Croteau, D.; Clifford, D.B.; Collier, A.C.; Gelman, B.B.; Marra, C.M.; et al. Long-term efavirenz use is associated with worse neurocognitive functioning in HIV-infected patients. *J. Neurovirol.* **2016**, *22*, 170–178. [CrossRef] [PubMed]
131. Lewis, W.; Dalakas, M.C. Mitochondrial toxicity of antiviral drugs. *Nat. Med.* **1995**, *1*, 417–422. [CrossRef] [PubMed]
132. Van Dyke, R.B.; Wang, L.; Williams, P.L.; Pediatric AIDS Clinical Trials Group 219C Team. Toxicities associated with dual nucleoside reverse-transcriptase inhibitor regimens in hiv-infected children. *J. Infect. Dis.* **2008**, *198*, 1599–1608. [CrossRef] [PubMed]

133. Apostolova, N.; Blas-Garcia, A.; Esplugues, J.V. Mitochondrial toxicity in haart: An overview of in vitro evidence. *Curr. Pharm. Des.* **2011**, *17*, 2130–2144. [CrossRef] [PubMed]
134. Arnaudo, E.; Dalakas, M.; Shanske, S.; Moraes, C.T.; DiMauro, S.; Schon, E.A. Depletion of muscle mitochondrial DNA in aids patients with zidovudine-induced myopathy. *Lancet* **1991**, *337*, 508–510. [CrossRef]
135. Cherry, C.L.; Gahan, M.E.; McArthur, J.C.; Lewin, S.R.; Hoy, J.F.; Wesselingh, S.L. Exposure to dideoxynucleosides is reflected in lowered mitochondrial DNA in subcutaneous fat. *J. Acquir. Immune Defic. Syndr.* **2002**, *30*, 271–277. [CrossRef] [PubMed]
136. Cote, H.C.; Brumme, Z.L.; Craib, K.J.; Alexander, C.S.; Wynhoven, B.; Ting, L.; Wong, H.; Harris, M.; Harrigan, P.R.; O'Shaughnessy, M.V.; et al. Changes in mitochondrial DNA as a marker of nucleoside toxicity in HIV-infected patients. *N. Engl. J. Med.* **2002**, *346*, 811–820. [CrossRef] [PubMed]
137. Funes, H.A.; Apostolova, N.; Alegre, F.; Blas-Garcia, A.; Alvarez, A.; Marti-Cabrera, M.; Esplugues, J.V. Neuronal bioenergetics and acute mitochondrial dysfunction: A clue to understanding the central nervous system side effects of efavirenz. *J. Infect. Dis.* **2014**, *210*, 1385–1395. [CrossRef] [PubMed]
138. Sun, R.; Eriksson, S.; Wang, L. Down-regulation of mitochondrial thymidine kinase 2 and deoxyguanosine kinase by didanosine: Implication for mitochondrial toxicities of anti-HIV nucleoside analogs. *Biochem. Biophys. Res. Commun.* **2014**, *450*, 1021–1026. [CrossRef] [PubMed]
139. Zhang, Y.; Song, F.; Gao, Z.; Ding, W.; Qiao, L.; Yang, S.; Chen, X.; Jin, R.; Chen, D. Long-term exposure of mice to nucleoside analogues disrupts mitochondrial DNA maintenance in cortical neurons. *PLoS ONE* **2014**, *9*, e85637. [CrossRef] [PubMed]
140. Dragovic, G.; Jevtovic, D. Nucleoside reverse transcriptase inhibitor usage and the incidence of peripheral neuropathy in HIV/AIDS patients. *Antivir. Chem. Chemother.* **2003**, *14*, 281–284. [CrossRef] [PubMed]
141. Dalakas, M.C. Peripheral neuropathy and antiretroviral drugs. *J. Peripher. Nerv. Syst.* **2001**, *6*, 14–20. [CrossRef] [PubMed]
142. Venhoff, N.; Lebrecht, D.; Deveaud, C.; Beauvoit, B.; Bonnet, J.; Muller, K.; Kirschner, J.; Venhoff, A.C.; Walker, U.A. Oral uridine supplementation antagonizes the peripheral neuropathy and encephalopathy induced by antiretroviral nucleoside analogues. *AIDS* **2010**, *24*, 345–352. [CrossRef] [PubMed]
143. Ewings, E.L.; Gerschenson, M.; St Claire, M.C.; Nagashima, K.; Skopets, B.; Harbaugh, S.W.; Harbaugh, J.W.; Poirier, M.C. Genotoxic and functional consequences of transplacental zidovudine exposure in fetal monkey brain mitochondria. *J. Acquir. Immune Defic. Syndr.* **2000**, *24*, 100–105. [CrossRef] [PubMed]
144. Haik, S.; Gauthier, L.R.; Granotier, C.; Peyrin, J.M.; Lages, C.S.; Dormont, D.; Boussin, F.D. Fibroblast growth factor 2 up regulates telomerase activity in neural precursor cells. *Oncogene* **2000**, *19*, 2957–2966. [CrossRef] [PubMed]
145. Sanchez, A.B.; Varano, G.P.; de Rozieres, C.M.; Maung, R.; Catalan, I.C.; Dowling, C.C.; Sejbuk, N.E.; Hoefer, M.M.; Kaul, M. Antiretrovirals, methamphetamine, and HIV-1 envelope protein gp120 compromise neuronal energy homeostasis in association with various degrees of synaptic and neuritic damage. *Antimicrob. Agents Chemother.* **2016**, *60*, 168–179. [CrossRef] [PubMed]
146. Floris-Moore, M.A.; Mollan, K.; Wilkin, A.M.; Johnson, M.A.; Kashuba, A.D.; Wohl, D.A.; Patterson, K.B.; Francis, O.; Kronk, C.; Eron, J.J. Antiretroviral activity and safety of once-daily etravirine in treatment-naive HIV-infected adults: 48-week results. *Antivir. Ther.* **2016**, *21*, 55–64. [CrossRef] [PubMed]
147. Brown, L.A.; Jin, J.; Ferrell, D.; Sadic, E.; Obregon, D.; Smith, A.J.; Tan, J.; Giunta, B. Efavirenz promotes beta-secretase expression and increased abeta1–40,42 via oxidative stress and reduced microglial phagocytosis: Implications for hiv associated neurocognitive disorders (hand). *PLoS ONE* **2014**, *9*, e95500. [CrossRef] [PubMed]
148. Decloedt, E.H.; Maartens, G. Neuronal toxicity of efavirenz: A systematic review. *Expert Opin. Drug Saf.* **2013**, *12*, 841–846. [CrossRef] [PubMed]
149. Purnell, P.R.; Fox, H.S. Efavirenz induces neuronal autophagy and mitochondrial alterations. *J. Pharmacol. Exp. Ther.* **2014**, *351*, 250–258. [CrossRef] [PubMed]
150. Blas-Garcia, A.; Polo, M.; Alegre, F.; Funes, H.A.; Martinez, E.; Apostolova, N.; Esplugues, J.V. Lack of mitochondrial toxicity of darunavir, raltegravir and rilpivirine in neurons and hepatocytes: A comparison with efavirenz. *J. Antimicrob. Chemother.* **2014**, *69*, 2995–3000. [CrossRef] [PubMed]
151. Bertrand, L.; Toborek, M. Dysregulation of endoplasmic reticulum stress and autophagic responses by the antiretroviral drug efavirenz. *Mol. Pharmacol.* **2015**, *88*, 304–315. [CrossRef] [PubMed]

152. Gatanaga, H.; Hayashida, T.; Tsuchiya, K.; Yoshino, M.; Kuwahara, T.; Tsukada, H.; Fujimoto, K.; Sato, I.; Ueda, M.; Horiba, M.; et al. Successful efavirenz dose reduction in HIV type 1-infected individuals with cytochrome p450 2b6 *6 and *26. *Clin. Infect. Dis.* **2007**, *45*, 1230–1237. [CrossRef] [PubMed]
153. Guidelines for the Use of Antiretroviral Agents in HIV-1-Infected Adults and Adolescents. Department of Health and Human Services. Available online: http://aidsinfo.nih.gov/contentfiles/lvguidelines/AdultandAdolescentGL.pdf (accessed on 11 January 2017).
154. Bonfanti, P.; Valsecchi, L.; Parazzini, F.; Carradori, S.; Pusterla, L.; Fortuna, P.; Timillero, L.; Alessi, F.; Ghiselli, G.; Gabbuti, A.; et al. Incidence of adverse reactions in HIV patients treated with protease inhibitors: A cohort study. Coordinamento italiano studio allergia e infezione da HIV (CISAI) group. *J. Acquir. Immune Defic. Syndr.* **2000**, *23*, 236–245. [CrossRef] [PubMed]
155. Ingelman-Sundberg, M. Pharmacogenetics of cytochrome p450 and its applications in drug therapy: The past, present and future. *Trends Pharmacol. Sci.* **2004**, *25*, 193–200. [CrossRef] [PubMed]
156. Gonzalez-Baeza, A.; Carvajal, F.; Bayon, C.; Perez-Valero, I.; Estebanez, M.; Bernardino, J.I.; Monge, S.; Lagarde, M.; Hernando, A.; Arnalich, F.; et al. Pattern of neurocognitive function in patients receiving boosted protease inhibitor monotherapy: A detailed neuropsychological study. *J. Neurovirol.* **2014**, *20*, 362–370. [CrossRef] [PubMed]
157. James, C.W.; McNelis, K.C.; Matalia, M.D.; Cohen, D.M.; Szabo, S. Central nervous system toxicity and amprenavir oral solution. *Ann. Pharmacother.* **2002**, *36*, 174. [CrossRef] [PubMed]
158. Pettersen, J.A.; Jones, G.; Worthington, C.; Krentz, H.B.; Keppler, O.T.; Hoke, A.; Gill, M.J.; Power, C. Sensory neuropathy in human immunodeficiency virus/acquired immunodeficiency syndrome patients: Protease inhibitor-mediated neurotoxicity. *Ann. Neurol.* **2006**, *59*, 816–824. [CrossRef] [PubMed]
159. Vivithanaporn, P.; Asahchop, E.L.; Acharjee, S.; Baker, G.B.; Power, C. HIV protease inhibitors disrupt astrocytic glutamate transporter function and neurobehavioral performance. *AIDS* **2016**, *30*, 543–552. [CrossRef] [PubMed]
160. Gannon, P.J.; Akay-Espinoza, C.; Yee, A.C.; Briand, L.A.; Erickson, M.A.; Gelman, B.B.; Gao, Y.; Haughey, N.J.; Zink, M.C.; Clements, J.E.; et al. HIV protease inhibitors alter amyloid precursor protein processing via beta-site amyloid precursor protein cleaving enzyme-1 translational up-regulation. *Am. J. Pathol.* **2017**, *187*, 91–109. [CrossRef] [PubMed]
161. Cohen, C.; Elion, R.; Ruane, P.; Shamblaw, D.; DeJesus, E.; Rashbaum, B.; Chuck, S.L.; Yale, K.; Liu, H.C.; Warren, D.R.; et al. Randomized, phase 2 evaluation of two single-tablet regimens elvitegravir/cobicistat/emtricitabine/tenofovir disoproxil fumarate versus efavirenz/emtricitabine/tenofovir disoproxil fumarate for the initial treatment of HIV infection. *AIDS* **2011**, *25*, F7–F12. [CrossRef] [PubMed]
162. Harris, M.; Larsen, G.; Montaner, J.S. Exacerbation of depression associated with starting raltegravir: A report of four cases. *AIDS* **2008**, *22*, 1890–1892. [CrossRef] [PubMed]
163. Teppler, H.; Brown, D.D.; Leavitt, R.Y.; Sklar, P.; Wan, H.; Xu, X.; Lievano, F.; Lehman, H.P.; Mast, T.C.; Nguyen, B.Y. Long-term safety from the raltegravir clinical development program. *Curr. HIV Res.* **2011**, *9*, 40–53. [CrossRef] [PubMed]
164. Fung, H.B.; Guo, Y. Enfuvirtide: A fusion inhibitor for the treatment of hiv infection. *Clin. Ther.* **2004**, *26*, 352–378. [CrossRef]
165. Lalezari, J.P.; Henry, K.; O'Hearn, M.; Montaner, J.S.; Piliero, P.J.; Trottier, B.; Walmsley, S.; Cohen, C.; Kuritzkes, D.R.; Eron, J.J., Jr.; et al. Enfuvirtide, an HIV-1 fusion inhibitor, for drug-resistant HIV infection in north and South America. *N. Engl. J. Med.* **2003**, *348*, 2175–2185. [CrossRef] [PubMed]
166. Cherry, C.L.; Duncan, A.J.; Mackie, K.F.; Wesselingh, S.L.; Brew, B.J. A report on the effect of commencing enfuvirtide on peripheral neuropathy. *AIDS Res. Hum. Retrovir.* **2008**, *24*, 1027–1030. [CrossRef] [PubMed]
167. Lazzarin, A.; Clotet, B.; Cooper, D.; Reynes, J.; Arasteh, K.; Nelson, M.; Katlama, C.; Stellbrink, H.J.; Delfraissy, J.F.; Lange, J.; et al. Efficacy of enfuvirtide in patients infected with drug-resistant HIV-1 in europe and australia. *N. Engl. J. Med.* **2003**, *348*, 2186–2195. [CrossRef] [PubMed]
168. Garvey, L.; Nelson, M.; Latch, N.; Erlwein, O.W.; Allsop, J.M.; Mitchell, A.; Kaye, S.; Watson, V.; Back, D.; Taylor-Robinson, S.D.; et al. CNS effects of a CCR5 inhibitor in HIV-infected subjects: A pharmacokinetic and cerebral metabolite study. *J. Antimicrob. Chemother.* **2012**, *67*, 206–212. [CrossRef] [PubMed]
169. Boesecke, C.; Pett, S.L. Clinical studies with chemokine receptor-5 (CCR5)-inhibitors. *Curr. Opin. HIV AIDS* **2012**, *7*, 456–462. [CrossRef] [PubMed]

170. Kelly, K.M.; Beck, S.E.; Pate, K.A.; Queen, S.E.; Dorsey, J.L.; Adams, R.J.; Avery, L.B.; Hubbard, W.; Tarwater, P.M.; Mankowski, J.L. Neuroprotective maraviroc monotherapy in simian immunodeficiency virus-infected macaques: Reduced replicating and latent SIV in the brain. *AIDS* **2013**, *27*, F21–F28. [CrossRef] [PubMed]
171. Murray, K.J.; Grom, A.A.; Thompson, S.D.; Lieuwen, D.; Passo, M.H.; Glass, D.N. Contrasting cytokine profiles in the synovium of different forms of juvenile rheumatoid arthritis and juvenile spondyloarthropathy: Prominence of interleukin 4 in restricted disease. *J. Rheumatol.* **1998**, *25*, 1388–1398. [PubMed]
172. Barr, A.M.; Panenka, W.J.; MacEwan, G.W.; Thornton, A.E.; Lang, D.J.; Honer, W.G.; Lecomte, T. The need for speed: An update on methamphetamine addiction. *J. Psychiatry Neurosci.* **2006**, *31*, 301–313. [PubMed]
173. Kaye, S.; McKetin, R.; Duflou, J.; Darke, S. Methamphetamine and cardiovascular pathology: A review of the evidence. *Addiction* **2007**, *102*, 1204–1211. [CrossRef] [PubMed]
174. Sekine, Y.; Ouchi, Y.; Sugihara, G.; Takei, N.; Yoshikawa, E.; Nakamura, K.; Iwata, Y.; Tsuchiya, K.J.; Suda, S.; Suzuki, K.; et al. Methamphetamine causes microglial activation in the brains of human abusers. *J. Neurosci.* **2008**, *28*, 5756–5761. [CrossRef] [PubMed]
175. Jaehne, E.J.; Salem, A.; Irvine, R.J. Pharmacological and behavioral determinants of cocaine, methamphetamine, 3,4-methylenedioxymethamphetamine, and para-methoxyamphetamine-induced hyperthermia. *Psychopharmacology* **2007**, *194*, 41–52. [CrossRef] [PubMed]
176. Albertson, T.E.; Derlet, R.W.; Van Hoozen, B.E. Methamphetamine and the expanding complications of amphetamines. *West. J. Med.* **1999**, *170*, 214–219. [PubMed]
177. Murray, J.B. Psychophysiological aspects of amphetamine-methamphetamine abuse. *J. Psychol.* **1998**, *132*, 227–237. [CrossRef] [PubMed]
178. Scott, J.C.; Woods, S.P.; Matt, G.E.; Meyer, R.A.; Heaton, R.K.; Atkinson, J.H.; Grant, I. Neurocognitive effects of methamphetamine: A critical review and meta-analysis. *Neuropsychol. Rev.* **2007**, *17*, 275–297. [CrossRef] [PubMed]
179. Theodore, S.; Cass, W.A.; Nath, A.; Maragos, W.F. Progress in understanding basal ganglia dysfunction as a common target for methamphetamine abuse and HIV-1 neurodegeneration. *Curr. HIV Res.* **2007**, *5*, 301–313. [CrossRef] [PubMed]
180. Lynch, J.; House, M.A. Cardiovascular effects of methamphetamine. *J. Cardiovasc. Nurs.* **1992**, *6*, 12–18. [CrossRef] [PubMed]
181. Perez, J.A., Jr.; Arsura, E.L.; Strategos, S. Methamphetamine-related stroke: Four cases. *J. Emerg. Med.* **1999**, *17*, 469–471. [CrossRef]
182. McCann, U.D.; Wong, D.F.; Yokoi, F.; Villemagne, V.; Dannals, R.F.; Ricaurte, G.A. Reduced striatal dopamine transporter density in abstinent methamphetamine and methcathinone users: Evidence from positron emission tomography studies with [11c]win-35,428. *J. Neurosci.* **1998**, *18*, 8417–8422. [PubMed]
183. Wilson, J.M.; Kalasinsky, K.S.; Levey, A.I.; Bergeron, C.; Reiber, G.; Anthony, R.M.; Schmunk, G.A.; Shannak, K.; Haycock, J.W.; Kish, S.J. Striatal dopamine nerve terminal markers in human, chronic methamphetamine users. *Nat. Med.* **1996**, *2*, 699–703. [CrossRef] [PubMed]
184. Volkow, N.D.; Chang, L.; Wang, G.J.; Fowler, J.S.; Ding, Y.S.; Sedler, M.; Logan, J.; Franceschi, D.; Gatley, J.; Hitzemann, R.; et al. Low level of brain dopamine d2 receptors in methamphetamine abusers: Association with metabolism in the orbitofrontal cortex. *Am. J. Psychiatry* **2001**, *158*, 2015–2021. [CrossRef] [PubMed]
185. Sekine, Y.; Ouchi, Y.; Takei, N.; Yoshikawa, E.; Nakamura, K.; Futatsubashi, M.; Okada, H.; Minabe, Y.; Suzuki, K.; Iwata, Y.; et al. Brain serotonin transporter density and aggression in abstinent methamphetamine abusers. *Arch. Gen. Psychiatry* **2006**, *63*, 90–100. [CrossRef] [PubMed]
186. Volkow, N.D.; Chang, L.; Wang, G.J.; Fowler, J.S.; Franceschi, D.; Sedler, M.J.; Gatley, S.J.; Hitzemann, R.; Ding, Y.S.; Wong, C.; et al. Higher cortical and lower subcortical metabolism in detoxified methamphetamine abusers. *Am. J. Psychiatry* **2001**, *158*, 383–389. [CrossRef] [PubMed]
187. Cass, W.A. Decreases in evoked overflow of dopamine in rat striatum after neurotoxic doses of methamphetamine. *J. Pharmacol. Exp. Ther.* **1997**, *280*, 105–113. [PubMed]
188. Thompson, P.M.; Hayashi, K.M.; Simon, S.L.; Geaga, J.A.; Hong, M.S.; Sui, Y.; Lee, J.Y.; Toga, A.W.; Ling, W.; London, E.D. Structural abnormalities in the brains of human subjects who use methamphetamine. *J. Neurosci.* **2004**, *24*, 6028–6036. [CrossRef] [PubMed]
189. Thomas, D.M.; Kuhn, D.M. Attenuated microglial activation mediates tolerance to the neurotoxic effects of methamphetamine. *J. Neurochem.* **2005**, *92*, 790–797. [CrossRef] [PubMed]

190. Ricaurte, G.A.; Guillery, R.W.; Seiden, L.S.; Schuster, C.R.; Moore, R.Y. Dopamine nerve terminal degeneration produced by high doses of methylamphetamine in the rat brain. *Brain Res.* **1982**, *235*, 93–103. [CrossRef]
191. Fukui, K.; Nakajima, T.; Kariyama, H.; Kashiba, A.; Kato, N.; Tohyama, I.; Kimura, H. Selective reduction of serotonin immunoreactivity in some forebrain regions of rats induced by acute methamphetamine treatment; quantitative morphometric analysis by serotonin immunocytochemistry. *Brain Res.* **1989**, *482*, 198–203. [CrossRef]
192. Hotchkiss, A.J.; Gibb, J.W. Long-term effects of multiple doses of methamphetamine on tryptophan hydroxylase and tyrosine hydroxylase activity in rat brain. *J. Pharmacol. Exp. Ther.* **1980**, *214*, 257–262. [PubMed]
193. Wagner, G.C.; Ricaurte, G.A.; Seiden, L.S.; Schuster, C.R.; Miller, R.J.; Westley, J. Long-lasting depletions of striatal dopamine and loss of dopamine uptake sites following repeated administration of methamphetamine. *Brain Res.* **1980**, *181*, 151–160. [CrossRef]
194. Nakayama, M.; Koyama, T.; Yamashita, I. Long-lasting decrease in dopamine uptake sites following repeated administration of methamphetamine in the rat striatum. *Brain Res.* **1993**, *601*, 209–212. [CrossRef]
195. Hirata, H.; Ladenheim, B.; Rothman, R.B.; Epstein, C.; Cadet, J.L. Methamphetamine-induced serotonin neurotoxicity is mediated by superoxide radicals. *Brain Res.* **1995**, *677*, 345–347. [CrossRef]
196. Deng, X.; Cadet, J.L. Methamphetamine administration causes overexpression of nnos in the mouse striatum. *Brain Res.* **1999**, *851*, 254–257. [CrossRef]
197. Frey, K.; Kilbourn, M.; Robinson, T. Reduced striatal vesicular monoamine transporters after neurotoxic but not after behaviorally-sensitizing doses of methamphetamine. *Eur. J. Pharmacol.* **1997**, *334*, 273–279. [CrossRef]
198. Eisch, A.J.; Marshall, J.F. Methamphetamine neurotoxicity: Dissociation of striatal dopamine terminal damage from parietal cortical cell body injury. *Synapse* **1998**, *30*, 433–445. [CrossRef]
199. O'Dell, S.J.; Marshall, J.F. Repeated administration of methamphetamine damages cells in the somatosensory cortex: Overlap with cytochrome oxidase-rich barrels. *Synapse* **2000**, *37*, 32–37. [PubMed]
200. Schmued, L.C.; Bowyer, J.F. Methamphetamine exposure can produce neuronal degeneration in mouse hippocampal remnants. *Brain Res.* **1997**, *759*, 135–140. [CrossRef]
201. Deng, X.; Ladenheim, B.; Jayanthi, S.; Cadet, J.L. Methamphetamine administration causes death of dopaminergic neurons in the mouse olfactory bulb. *Biol. Psychiatry* **2007**, *61*, 1235–1243. [CrossRef] [PubMed]
202. Jayanthi, S.; Deng, X.; Ladenheim, B.; McCoy, M.T.; Cluster, A.; Cai, N.S.; Cadet, J.L. Calcineurin/NFAT-induced up-regulation of the Fas ligand/Fas death pathway is involved in methamphetamine-induced neuronal apoptosis. *Proc. Natl. Acad. Sci. USA* **2005**, *102*, 868–873. [CrossRef] [PubMed]
203. Thiriet, N.; Deng, X.; Solinas, M.; Ladenheim, B.; Curtis, W.; Goldberg, S.R.; Palmiter, R.D.; Cadet, J.L. Neuropeptide y protects against methamphetamine-induced neuronal apoptosis in the mouse striatum. *J. Neurosci.* **2005**, *25*, 5273–5279. [CrossRef] [PubMed]
204. Seiden, L.S.; Sabol, K.E.; Ricaurte, G.A. Amphetamine: Effects on catecholamine systems and behavior. *Annu. Rev. Pharmacol. Toxicol.* **1993**, *33*, 639–677. [CrossRef] [PubMed]
205. Erickson, J.D.; Eiden, L.E. Functional identification and molecular cloning of a human brain vesicle monoamine transporter. *J. Neurochem.* **1993**, *61*, 2314–2317. [CrossRef] [PubMed]
206. Sulzer, D.; Sonders, M.S.; Poulsen, N.W.; Galli, A. Mechanisms of neurotransmitter release by amphetamines: A review. *Prog. Neurobiol.* **2005**, *75*, 406–433. [CrossRef] [PubMed]
207. Nash, J.F.; Yamamoto, B.K. Methamphetamine neurotoxicity and striatal glutamate release: Comparison to 3,4-methylenedioxymethamphetamine. *Brain Res.* **1992**, *581*, 237–243. [CrossRef]
208. Yu, Q.; Zhang, D.; Walston, M.; Zhang, J.; Liu, Y.; Watson, R.R. Chronic methamphetamine exposure alters immune function in normal and retrovirus-infected mice. *Int. Immunopharmacol.* **2002**, *2*, 951–962. [CrossRef]
209. In, S.W.; Son, E.W.; Rhee, D.K.; Pyo, S. Methamphetamine administration produces immunomodulation in mice. *J. Toxicol. Environ. Health A* **2005**, *68*, 2133–2145. [CrossRef] [PubMed]
210. Talloczy, Z.; Martinez, J.; Joset, D.; Ray, Y.; Gacser, A.; Toussi, S.; Mizushima, N.; Nosanchuk, J.; Goldstein, H.; Loike, J.; et al. Methamphetamine inhibits antigen processing, presentation, and phagocytosis. *PLoS Pathog.* **2008**, *4*, e28. [CrossRef]
211. Krasnova, I.N.; Cadet, J.L. Methamphetamine toxicity and messengers of death. *Brain Res. Rev.* **2009**, *60*, 379–407. [CrossRef] [PubMed]

212. Shah, A.; Kumar, S.; Simon, S.D.; Singh, D.P.; Kumar, A. HIV gp120- and methamphetamine-mediated oxidative stress induces astrocyte apoptosis via cytochrome p450 2e1. *Cell Death Dis.* **2013**, *4*, e850. [CrossRef] [PubMed]
213. Carvalho, B.M.; Guadagnini, D.; Tsukumo, D.M.; Schenka, A.A.; Latuf-Filho, P.; Vassallo, J.; Dias, J.C.; Kubota, L.T.; Carvalheira, J.B.; Saad, M.J. Modulation of gut microbiota by antibiotics improves insulin signalling in high-Fat fed mice. *Diabetologia* **2012**, *55*, 2823–2834. [CrossRef] [PubMed]
214. Vearrier, D.; Greenberg, M.I.; Miller, S.N.; Okaneku, J.T.; Haggerty, D.A. Methamphetamine: History, pathophysiology, adverse health effects, current trends, and hazards associated with the clandestine manufacture of methamphetamine. *Dis. Mon.* **2012**, *58*, 38–89. [CrossRef] [PubMed]
215. Kanthasamy, A.; Anantharam, V.; Ali, S.F.; Kanthasamy, A.G. Methamphetamine induces autophagy and apoptosis in a mesencephalic dopaminergic neuronal culture model: Role of cathepsin-D in methamphetamine-induced apoptotic cell death. *Ann. N. Y. Acad. Sci.* **2006**, *1074*, 234–244. [CrossRef] [PubMed]
216. Larsen, K.E.; Fon, E.A.; Hastings, T.G.; Edwards, R.H.; Sulzer, D. Methamphetamine-induced degeneration of dopaminergic neurons involves autophagy and upregulation of dopamine synthesis. *J. Neurosci.* **2002**, *22*, 8951–8960. [PubMed]
217. Pasquali, L.; Lazzeri, G.; Isidoro, C.; Ruggieri, S.; Paparelli, A.; Fornai, F. Role of autophagy during methamphetamine neurotoxicity. *Ann. N. Y. Acad. Sci.* **2008**, *1139*, 191–196. [CrossRef] [PubMed]
218. Yu, S.; Zhu, L.; Shen, Q.; Bai, X.; Di, X. Recent advances in methamphetamine neurotoxicity mechanisms and its molecular pathophysiology. *Behav. Neurol.* **2015**, *2015*, 103969. [CrossRef] [PubMed]
219. Soontornniyomkij, V.; Kesby, J.P.; Morgan, E.E.; Bischoff-Grethe, A.; Minassian, A.; Brown, G.G.; Grant, I.; Translational Methamphetamine AIDS Research Center (TMARC) Group. Effects of hiv and methamphetamine on brain and behavior: Evidence from human studies and animal models. *J. Neuroimmune Pharmacol.* **2016**, *11*, 495–510. [CrossRef] [PubMed]
220. Marquez, C.; Mitchell, S.J.; Hare, C.B.; John, M.; Klausner, J.D. Methamphetamine use, sexual activity, patient-provider communication, and medication adherence among HIV-infected patients in care, San Francisco 2004–2006. *AIDS Care* **2009**, *21*, 575–582. [CrossRef] [PubMed]
221. Langford, D.; Adame, A.; Grigorian, A.; Grant, I.; McCutchan, J.A.; Ellis, R.J.; Marcotte, T.D.; Masliah, E. Patterns of selective neuronal damage in methamphetamine-user AIDS patients. *J. Acquir. Immune Defic. Syndr.* **2003**, *34*, 467–474. [CrossRef] [PubMed]
222. Roberts, A.J.; Maung, R.; Sejbuk, N.E.; Ake, C.; Kaul, M. Alteration of methamphetamine-induced stereotypic behaviour in transgenic mice expressing HIV-1 envelope protein gp120. *J. Neurosci. Methods* **2010**, *186*, 222–225. [CrossRef] [PubMed]
223. Pendyala, G.; Buescher, J.L.; Fox, H.S. Methamphetamine and inflammatory cytokines increase neuronal na+/k+-atpase isoform 3: Relevance for HIV associated neurocognitive disorders. *PLoS ONE* **2012**, *7*, e37604. [CrossRef] [PubMed]
224. Bortell, N.; Morsey, B.; Basova, L.; Fox, H.S.; Marcondes, M.C. Phenotypic changes in the brain of SIV-infected macaques exposed to methamphetamine parallel macrophage activation patterns induced by the common gamma-chain cytokine system. *Front. Microbiol.* **2015**, *6*, 900. [CrossRef] [PubMed]
225. Hoefer, M.M.; Sanchez, A.B.; Maung, R.; de Rozieres, C.M.; Catalan, I.C.; Dowling, C.C.; Thaney, V.E.; Pina-Crespo, J.; Zhang, D.; Roberts, A.J.; et al. Combination of methamphetamine and HIV-1 gp120 causes distinct long-term alterations of behavior, gene expression, and injury in the central nervous system. *Exp. Neurol.* **2015**, *263*, 221–234. [CrossRef] [PubMed]
226. Almeida, A.; Almeida, J.; Bolanos, J.P.; Moncada, S. Different responses of astrocytes and neurons to nitric oxide: The role of glycolytically generated atp in astrocyte protection. *Proc. Natl. Acad. Sci. USA* **2001**, *98*, 15294–15299. [CrossRef] [PubMed]
227. Almeida, A.; Moncada, S.; Bolanos, J.P. Nitric oxide switches on glycolysis through the AMP protein kinase and 6-phosphofructo-2-kinase pathway. *Nat. Cell Biol.* **2004**, *6*, 45–51. [CrossRef] [PubMed]
228. Hung, K.M.; Chen, P.C.; Hsieh, H.C.; Calkins, M.J. Mitochondrial defects arise from nucleoside/nucleotide reverse transcriptase inhibitors in neurons: Potential contribution to HIV-associated neurocognitive disorders. *Biochim. Biophys. Acta* **2017**, *1863*, 406–413. [CrossRef] [PubMed]
229. Wong-Riley, M.T. Cytochrome oxidase: An endogenous metabolic marker for neuronal activity. *Trends Neurosci.* **1989**, *12*, 94–101. [CrossRef]

230. Maday, S.; Twelvetrees, A.E.; Moughamian, A.J.; Holzbaur, E.L. Axonal transport: Cargo-specific mechanisms of motility and regulation. *Neuron* **2014**, *84*, 292–309. [CrossRef] [PubMed]
231. Cai, Q.; Zakaria, H.M.; Simone, A.; Sheng, Z.H. Spatial parkin translocation and degradation of damaged mitochondria via mitophagy in live cortical neurons. *Curr. Biol.* **2012**, *22*, 545–552. [CrossRef] [PubMed]
232. Palikaras, K.; Tavernarakis, N. Mitophagy in neurodegeneration and aging. *Front. Genet.* **2012**, *3*, 297. [CrossRef] [PubMed]
233. Pickrell, A.M.; Youle, R.J. The roles of PINK1, parkin, and mitochondrial fidelity in parkinson's disease. *Neuron* **2015**, *85*, 257–273. [CrossRef] [PubMed]
234. Hardie, D.G. Amp-activated protein kinase: An energy sensor that regulates all aspects of cell function. *Genes Dev.* **2011**, *25*, 1895–1908. [CrossRef] [PubMed]
235. Oakhill, J.S.; Steel, R.; Chen, Z.P.; Scott, J.W.; Ling, N.; Tam, S.; Kemp, B.E. Ampk is a direct adenylate charge-regulated protein kinase. *Science* **2011**, *332*, 1433–1435. [CrossRef] [PubMed]
236. Laplante, M.; Sabatini, D.M. Mtor signaling in growth control and disease. *Cell* **2012**, *149*, 274–293. [CrossRef] [PubMed]
237. Mizushima, N.; Levine, B.; Cuervo, A.M.; Klionsky, D.J. Autophagy fights disease through cellular self-digestion. *Nature* **2008**, *451*, 1069–1075. [CrossRef]
238. Fields, J.; Dumaop, W.; Rockenstein, E.; Mante, M.; Spencer, B.; Grant, I.; Ellis, R.; Letendre, S.; Patrick, C.; Adame, A.; et al. Age-dependent molecular alterations in the autophagy pathway in hive patients and in a gp120 tg mouse model: Reversal with beclin-1 gene transfer. *J. Neurovirol.* **2013**, *19*, 89–101. [CrossRef] [PubMed]
239. Balgi, A.D.; Fonseca, B.D.; Donohue, E.; Tsang, T.C.; Lajoie, P.; Proud, C.G.; Nabi, I.R.; Roberge, M. Screen for chemical modulators of autophagy reveals novel therapeutic inhibitors of mtorc1 signaling. *PLoS ONE* **2009**, *4*, e7124. [CrossRef] [PubMed]
240. Liu, B.; Liu, X.; Tang, S.J. Interactions of opioids and hiv infection in the pathogenesis of chronic pain. *Front. Microbiol.* **2016**, *7*, 103. [CrossRef] [PubMed]
241. Dhillon, N.K.; Williams, R.; Peng, F.; Tsai, Y.J.; Dhillon, S.; Nicolay, B.; Gadgil, M.; Kumar, A.; Buch, S.J. Cocaine-mediated enhancement of virus replication in macrophages: Implications for human immunodeficiency virus-associated dementia. *J. Neurovirol.* **2007**, *13*, 483–495. [CrossRef] [PubMed]
242. Liang, H.; Wang, X.; Chen, H.; Song, L.; Ye, L.; Wang, S.H.; Wang, Y.J.; Zhou, L.; Ho, W.Z. Methamphetamine enhances hiv infection of macrophages. *Am. J. Pathol.* **2008**, *172*, 1617–1624. [CrossRef] [PubMed]
243. Wang, Y.; Wang, X.; Ye, L.; Li, J.; Song, L.; Fulambarkar, N.; Ho, W. Morphine suppresses IFN signaling pathway and enhances AIDS virus infection. *PLoS ONE* **2012**, *7*, e31167. [CrossRef] [PubMed]
244. Rivera-Rivera, L.; Perez-Laspiur, J.; Colon, K.; Melendez, L.M. Inhibition of interferon response by cystatin b: Implication in hiv replication of macrophage reservoirs. *J. Neurovirol.* **2011**, *18*, 20–29. [CrossRef] [PubMed]
245. Purohit, V.; Rapaka, R.S.; Rutter, J.; Shurtleff, D. Do opioids activate latent HIV-1 by down-regulating anti-HIV micrornas? *J. Neuroimmune Pharmacol.* **2012**, *7*, 519–523. [CrossRef] [PubMed]
246. Sampey, G.C.; Meyering, S.S.; Asad, Z.M.; Saifuddin, M.; Hakami, R.M.; Kashanchi, F. Exosomes and their role in CNS viral infections. *J. Neurovirol.* **2014**, *20*, 199–208. [CrossRef] [PubMed]
247. Hu, G.; Yao, H.; Chaudhuri, A.D.; Duan, M.; Yelamanchili, S.V.; Wen, H.; Cheney, P.D.; Fox, H.S.; Buch, S. Exosome-mediated shuttling of microrna-29 regulates HIV tat and morphine-mediated neuronal dysfunction. *Cell Death Dis.* **2012**, *3*, e381. [CrossRef] [PubMed]
248. Rahimian, P.; He, J.J. Exosome-associated release, uptake, and neurotoxicity of HIV-1 tat protein. *J. Neurovirol.* **2016**, *22*, 774–788. [CrossRef] [PubMed]
249. Raymond, A.D.; Diaz, P.; Chevelon, S.; Agudelo, M.; Yndart-Arias, A.; Ding, H.; Kaushik, A.; Jayant, R.D.; Nikkhah-Moshaie, R.; Roy, U.; et al. Microglia-derived hiv NEF+ exosome impairment of the blood-brain barrier is treatable by nanomedicine-based delivery of nef peptides. *J. Neurovirol.* **2016**, *22*, 129–139. [CrossRef] [PubMed]

# 2

# Focus on Clozapine Withdrawal- and Misuse-Related Cases as Reported to the European Medicines Agency (EMA) Pharmacovigilance Database

**Stefania Chiappini [1], Fabrizio Schifano [1,*], John Martin Corkery [1] and Amira Guirguis [2]**

1 Psychopharmacology, Drug Misuse, and Novel Psychoactive Substances Research Unit, School of Life and Medical Sciences, University of Hertfordshire, Hatfield, Hertfordshire AL10 9AB, UK; stefaniachiappini9@gmail.com (S.C.); j.corkery@herts.ac.uk (J.M.C.)

2 Swansea University Medical School, Institute of Life Sciences 2, Swansea University, Singleton Park, Swansea SA2 8PP, UK; amira.guirguis@swansea.ac.uk

* Correspondence: f.schifano@herts.ac.uk

**Abstract:** Background: Clozapine is of high clinical relevance for the management of both treatment-resistant schizophrenia and psychotic disturbances with concurrent drug misuse. Although the molecule presents with a range of well-known side-effects, its discontinuation/withdrawal syndrome has been only anecdotally described. Aims: the 2005–2018 European Medicines Agency (EMA) dataset of Adverse Drug Reactions (ADRs) was analyzed to identify and describe possible clozapine withdrawal- and misuse-/abuse-/dependence-related issues. Method: A descriptive analysis of clozapine-related ADRs was performed when available, data on ADRs' outcome, dosage, and possible concomitant drug(s) were considered. Results: Out of 11,847 clozapine-related ADRs, some 599 (5.05%) were related to misuse/abuse/dependence/withdrawal issues, including 258 withdrawal-related (43.1%); 241 abuse-related (40.2%); and 80 intentional product misuse-related (13.3%) ADRs. A small number of overdose- and suicide-related ADRs were reported as well. Clozapine was typically (69.2%) identified alone, and most (84.7%) fatalities/high-dosage intake instances were reported in association with a history of substance abuse. Conclusions: Previous suggestions about the possibility of a clozapine discontinuation/withdrawal occurrence are here supported, but further studies are needed. However, the misuse/abuse cases here identified might be difficult to interpret, given the lack of studies highlighting the possible recreational use of clozapine. The high-dosage intake, fatal outcomes and clozapine/polydrug abuse issues reported here may, however, be a reason for concern.

**Keywords:** clozapine; adverse drug reactions; misuse; withdrawal; dependence; overdose

---

## 1. Introduction

Clozapine was first synthesized in 1959 [1] and made available on the European market in 1971 for the treatment of schizophrenia [2]. If compared with remaining first-generation antipsychotic agents, clozapine is characterized by a lack of extrapyramidal side-effects [2]. After having been withdrawn from the European market in 1976 due to fatal cases of agranulocytosis, clozapine was approved by the Food and Drug Administration (FDA) in 1989 for treatment-resistant schizophrenia [2,3]. It was then approved in the USA in 2002 for reducing recurrent suicidal behavior in patients with schizophrenia or schizoaffective disorder. Other unlicensed uses include treatment-resistant bipolar disorder, aggression in patients with psychosis, and other brain disorders unresponsive to remaining treatments [4].

### 1.1. *Pharmacodynamic Considerations*

Clozapine is a dibenzodiazepine designated as a Multi-Acting Receptor-Targeted Antipsychotic (MARTA), deriving its therapeutic effects from its action across various neurotransmitter systems [4,5]. In fact, a combination of pharmacological effects is unique to clozapine: (1) although the molecule presents with affinity levels for a range of dopamine/DA receptors (e.g., D1, D2, D3, D4, and D5; [6]), the blockade of dopamine 2 and 4 receptors is particularly relevant, with a preferential affinity for D4 over D2 receptors; this blockade seems to be effective in reducing positive symptoms of psychosis and stabilizing affective symptoms [4]; (2) 5-hydroxytryptamine/5-HT 2A receptor antagonism, causing enhancement of DA release in certain brain regions, and thus reducing motor side-effects and possibly improving cognitive and affective symptoms associated with schizophrenia [4]. Conversely, the clinical effects of the reported interactions at 5HT2C; 5HT1A; 5-HT6; and 5-HT7 receptors [6] might be less clear; (3) α2C-adrenergic receptor blockade; this may contribute to the clozapine-related improvement of cognitive function [7]; (4) significant antimuscarinic and antihistaminergic H1 effects, which may well contribute to the central effect [8]; and (5) possible modulatory actions on a dysfunctional glutamatergic system, improving schizophrenia symptoms and contrasting illness progression [1,4,9–11]. More precisely, clozapine interacts with the N-methyl-D-aspartate (NMDA) receptor complex, affecting either the glycine site of the NMDA receptor or tentatively inhibiting the glycine transporter [12]. Moreover, both clozapine and its major metabolite N-desmethylclozapine behave as: (i) delta-opioid receptor agonists [13–17]; (ii) cannabinoid CB1 receptor agonists [18]; and (iii) antagonists at muscarinic receptors [8]. Indeed, these i-iii pharmacological activities are, per se, typically associated with the occurrence of pleasurable effects [19–22], which could suggest a theoretical potential for clozapine to be misused by vulnerable individuals. Finally, further pharmacological clozapine activities which should be better understood in terms of their clinical effects may include both interaction with GABA-B receptors [22]; and antagonistic actions at D (2)/D (3)/D (4) receptors [23].

The therapeutic response depends on plasma clozapine concentrations, which may be influenced by many factors such as age, gender, and smoking [5], and should normally reach 350 ng/mL [4,5]; levels greater than 700 ng/mL are often not well tolerated [4]. Clozapine is metabolized by CYP450 enzymes, specifically by CYP450 1A2, 2D6 and 3A4 enzymes [5], and its metabolism may be influenced by CYP450 1A2 inhibitors, such as fluvoxamine and ciprofloxacin [14]. Remaining interactions may occur with both strong CYP450 2D6 inhibitors (e.g., bupropion, duloxetine, paroxetine, fluoxetine) and strong CYP450 3A4 (e.g., ketoconazole) inhibitors [4,15].

### 1.2. *Clozapine Abuse Issues and Substance Use Disorders*

Substance use disorders (SUDs), typically involving alcohol, cannabis, and cocaine, commonly occur in patients with schizophrenia, supposedly due to epidemiological and genetic determinants of risk for both psychosis and addiction [1,16]. This co-occurrence ('dual diagnosis') has a negative effect on the course of schizophrenia, due to increased rates of hospitalization, decreased compliance with medication, increased violence and suicide, general deterioration of the patients' condition, and overall increased societal costs [1,17]. In particular, the positive symptoms of schizophrenia are generally exacerbated by the intake of stimulant drugs, such as cocaine, amphetamine derivatives [24], and synthetic cathinones [25]. Due to clozapine's effectiveness, there has been support for considering the molecule in limiting substance use in patients with schizophrenia [26], to achieve both a reduction in substance use [27,28] and an improvement in positive/negative schizophrenia symptoms [29]. Additionally, differently from other antipsychotics, such as quetiapine, which has showed in recent years to be a strong potential for misuse and abuse [30–33], the recreational use of clozapine has not been noted in the literature. Conversely, clozapine withdrawal is a phenomenon which has already been described, even at therapeutic dosages [9]. However, the risk of withdrawal may arguably be significant only when a psychoactive molecule is being misused/ingested at higher dosages. Since SUD patients may be vulnerable to misuse prescribed medications, one could argue that it is relevant to identify and assess any possible clozapine misuse/abuse/withdrawal and dependence issues.

### *1.3. Aims*

We aimed here at identifying and describing the number of European Medicines Agency (EMA) database cases of misuse, abuse, dependence, and withdrawal specifically relating to clozapine; suicide-related cases and fatalities were also considered.

## 2. Methods

### *2.1. Data Source and Acquisition*

EudraVigilance (EV) manages and analyzes information on suspected Adverse Drug Reactions (ADRs) to medicines that have been authorized in the European Economic Area (EEA), according to Directive 2001/83/EC and Regulation (EC) No 726/2004 [34]. In order to investigate the aspects above, EV was specifically requested to provide all Level 2A data [34] comprising case reports of clozapine-related misuse, abuse, dependence, and withdrawal ADRs, which were obtained in the form of line listings, relating to the 2005–June 2018 time-frame. Differently from the publicly available data from the EV website, Level 2A data were presented as Excel sheets divided into information sections reporting in a standardized format according to the Medical Dictionary for Regulatory Activities (MedDRA), which is the internationally agreed list of terms that supports the coding of ADRs [35], which are identified through Preferred Terms (PT). Indeed, MedDRA is a comprehensive and highly standardized medical terminology developed by the International Council for Harmonization of Technical Requirements for Pharmaceuticals for Human Use (ICH) (https://www.meddra.org/) in the late 1990s to facilitate the international sharing of regulatory information for medical products. Such listings showed all information related to the ADR, the patient, the drug, the reporter, and the diagnosis. In line with previous studies from our group [36–39], the ADRs considered here were, per se, voluntary and unsolicited communications [34] reported by both Regulatory Authorities of the EU Member States where the reaction occurred and/or by the Marketing Authorization Holders for those ADRs occurring outside the EEA. Individual Case Safety Reports, such as voluntary reports, refer to the format and content for the reporting of one or several suspected ADRs in relation to a medicinal product that occur in a single patient at a specific point of time [40]. 'Suspect' ADRs were selected, meaning clozapine was considered as 'suspected' for the reaction reported [34]. Within the standardized MedDRA Query (SMQ) 'drug abuse, dependence and withdrawal' section, we identified the following ADRs: dependence, drug abuse, drug abuser, drug dependence, drug diversion, drug withdrawal convulsions, drug withdrawal syndrome, drug withdrawal neonatal syndrome, intentional product misuse, product use issue, substance abuse, and withdrawal syndrome. For the definition of 'abuse'; 'addiction'; 'dependence'; and 'misuse' please refer to references [35–40]. Moreover, in accordance with MedDRA, 'withdrawal' is identified in association with the abrupt cessation or reduction in intake of a drug in a habituated person. A substance-specific syndrome may follow, with withdrawal symptoms varying according to the psychoactive substance used and generally opposite the acute effects of drug. These include nonspecific symptoms e.g., nausea, diarrhea or constipation, profuse sweating, increase in respiratory rate, and tachycardia; remaining common symptoms include anxiety, restlessness, irritability, insomnia, and impaired attention [35].

### *2.2. Data Analysis*

Each case report may refer to one or more reporter; one or more ADR(s); as well as to one or more medicinal product(s). Therefore, a case may be represented by more than one row in the other line listings. All rows of the case have the same 'EV Local Report Number', unequivocally identifying an individual case. Thus, the number of suspected ADRs can be different from the number of case reports as one case report may refer to several suspected ADRs. Moreover, the number of patients can be different from the number of case reports as a patient may have been described in more than one case. Finally, ADRs' numbers differed from those referring to case reports/single patients since different reporters/senders could have independently flagged the same ADR to the EMA.

Patients' data were analyzed using a range of parameters, including: socio-demographic characteristics (age and gender); source/reporter country (EEA or non-EEA) and reporter qualification (i.e., pharmacist, physician); outcomes (fatal, recovered, resolved); clozapine dosage; possible concomitant drug(s); and diagnosis/reporter's comments, if recorded [37]. The analysis included cases of overdoses, suicides, and fatalities.

Suicidal behavior was here defined as 'completed suicide', 'intentional self-injury', 'suicidal behavior', 'suicidal ideation', 'suicide attempt', 'self-injurious ideation', and 'intentional self-injury.' 'Overdose', including 'intentional overdose', was not necessarily interpreted as being a suicidal attempt [35]. The analysis included here both a descriptive study of the dataset and the Confidence Interval (CI) values [41].

### *2.3. Ethics' Issues*

Complying with applicable Personal Data Protection legislation (Regulation (EC) No 45/2001 and Regulation (EC) No 1049/2001 on the protection of privacy and integrity of individuals, certain data elements, including names/identifiers of individuals involved or country-specific information were not disclosed by the EMA to safeguard the identity of individuals [42]. The study was ethically approved in March 2018 by the University of Hertfordshire Ethics' Committee, with reference number LMS/PGR/UH/03234.

## 3. Results

The EMA dataset included a total of 13,596 clozapine-related ADRs. A total of 11,847 ADRs were considered as 'suspect', i.e., as suspected to be related with clozapine. Of those, 599/11,847 (5.05% CI 95% 597–601) related to misuse/abuse/dependence/withdrawal ADRs and were associated with 559 unique subjects. These included: 258 ADRs (258/599 = 43.1% CI 95% 256–260) relating to 'withdrawal syndrome' issues; 241 abuse-related ADRs (241/599 = 40.2% CI 95% 239–242); and 80 ADRs (80/599 = 13.3% CI 95% 76–84) relating to 'intentional product misuse.' A small number of overdose- ($n$ = 29) and suicidal behavior-related ADRs ($n$ = 29) were reported here, resulting in death, respectively, in two and 11 cases (Table 1).

**Table 1.** Analysis of the EudraVigilance (EV) clozapine-related misuse/abuse/dependence and withdrawal ADRs (2005–June 2018).

| EudraVigilance (EV) Clozapine-Related Misuse/Abuse/Dependence and Withdrawal ADRs (2005–June 2018) | $n$ |
|---|---|
| Total "suspect" clozapine-related ADRs | 11,847 |
| Clozapine-related 'abuse, dependence and withdrawal' ADRs | 599 (*CI* 95% 595–603) ($n$ individual cases = 559) |
| Drug abuse | 198 |
| Drug abuser | 1 |
| Substance abuse | 42 |
| Dependence | 7 |
| Drug dependence | 6 |
| Drug diversion | 1 |
| Intentional product misuse | 80 |
| Product use issue | 4 |
| Drug withdrawal convulsions | 1 |
| Drug withdrawal neonatal syndrome | 1 |
| Drug withdrawal syndrome | 91 |
| Withdrawal syndrome | 165 |
| Further issues emerging from the analysis of clozapine ADRs' dataset | |
| Intentional overdose | 12 |
| Overdose | 17 |

**Table 1.** *Cont.*

| EudraVigilance (EV) Clozapine-Related Misuse/Abuse/Dependence and Withdrawal ADRs (2005–June 2018) | *n* |
|---|---|
| Completed suicide | 9 |
| Intentional self-injury | 4 |
| Suicidal behavior | 1 |
| Suicidal ideation | 4 |
| Suicide attempt | 7 |
| Self-injurious ideation | 4 |

Patients were typically males (379/559 = 67.8% CI 95% 378–380), in the 18–65 years age range. Most typical senders were pharmaceutical companies (303/559 = 54.2% CI 95% 301.5–304.5) and regulatory authorities (241/559 = 43.11% CI 95% 239–243) (Table 2).

**Table 2.** Description of clozapine-related misuse, abuse, dependence and withdrawal cases. F: female; M: male; N: no; Y: yes.

| Clozapine-Related Misuse, Abuse, Dependence and Withdrawal Cases | *n* of Unique Patients |
|---|---|
| | 559 |
| **Age range (years)** | 3 neonates,<br>1 child (5 years),<br>2 adolescents (15–16 years),<br>78 adults (18–65 years),<br>1 elderly (67 years),<br>474 Not specified |
| **Gender** | 171 F,<br>379 M,<br>9 Not Specified |
| **Sender** | 241 Regulatory authority,<br>303 Pharmaceutical company,<br>9 Other (distributor, study sponsor, contract research organization),<br>6 Not Specified |
| **Outcome** | |
| Resulted in death | 46 Y, 448 N, 65 Not Specified |
| Life threatening | 35 Y, 447 N, 77 Not Specified |
| Required a prolonged hospitalization | 298 Y, 219 N, 42 Not Specified |
| Disabling | 8 Y, 467 N, 84 Not Specified |

The number of cases increased year by year, with a peak in 2008 (120/559 cases) (Figure 1).

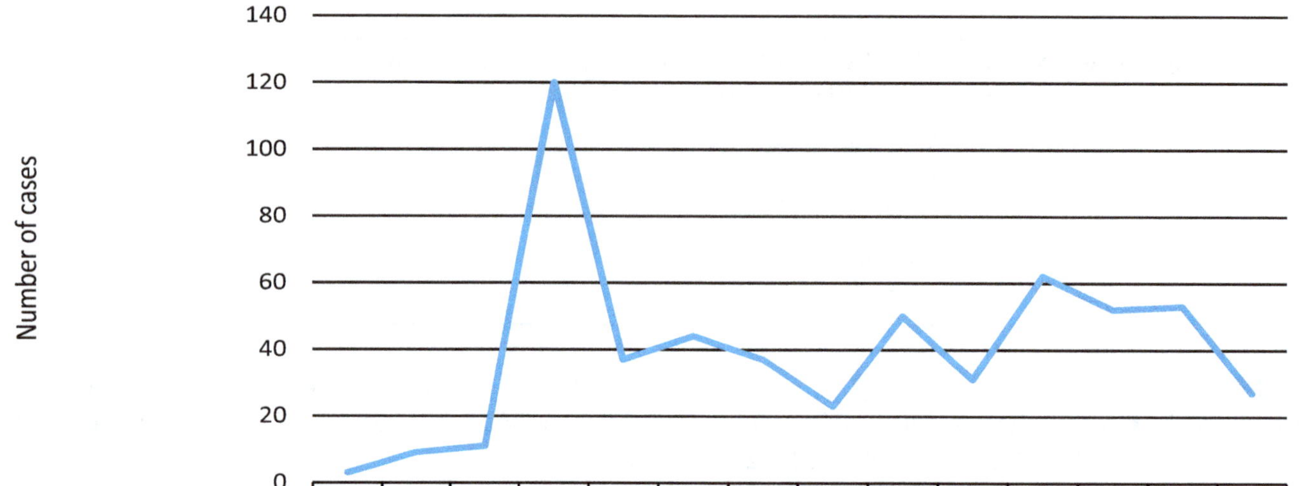


| | 2005 | 2006 | 2007 | 2008 | 2009 | 2010 | 2011 | 2012 | 2013 | 2014 | 2015 | 2016 | 2017 | 2018 (Jun) |
|---|---|---|---|---|---|---|---|---|---|---|---|---|---|---|
| Cases (tot n = 559) | 3 | 9 | 11 | 120 | 37 | 44 | 37 | 23 | 50 | 31 | 62 | 52 | 53 | 27 |

**Figure 1.** Total Number of clozapine-related misuse, abuse, dependence, withdrawal cases reported to EudraVigilance (EV) per year (2005–June 2018).

Oral intake occurred here in 533/559 cases (95.3% CI 95% 532.5–533.5); when recorded, clozapine dosages varied from 12.5 mg/day to high/unlicensed levels (i.e., 2800–5600 mg/day; Figure 2). Only a few cases ($n$ = 7), however, reported high (e.g., >1000 mg) levels. When the relating clinical data were made available, these cases were typically described as 'intentional self-injury', 'completed suicide', and 'drug abuse').

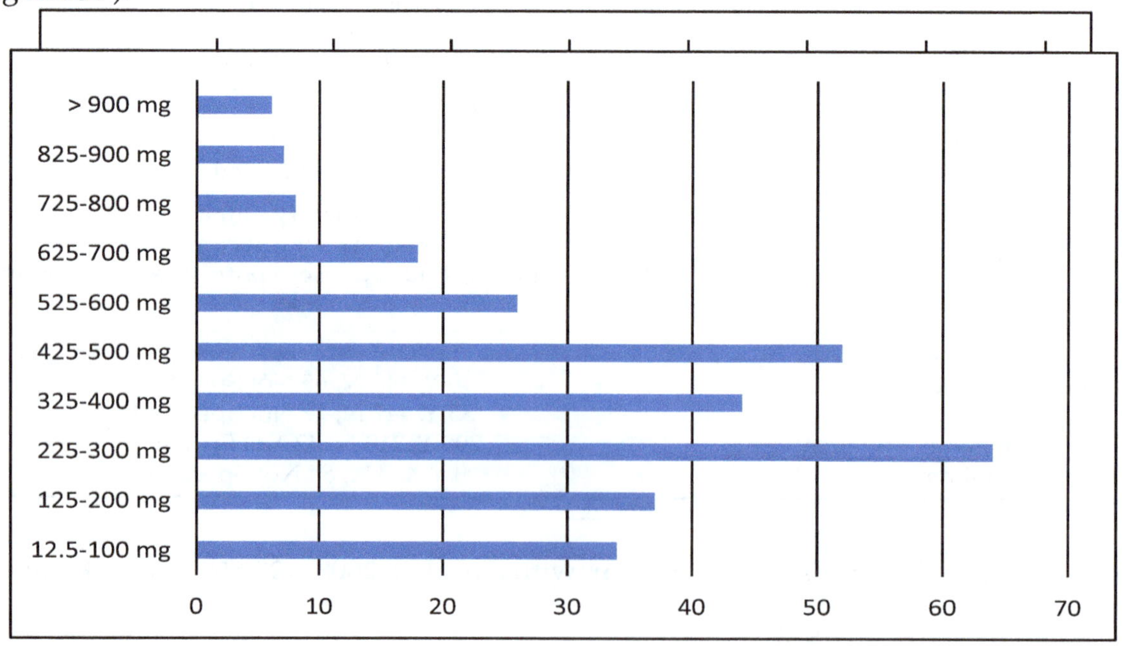


**Figure 2.** Dosages of clozapine reported to the EudraVigilance (EV) dataset of clozapine-related misuse, abuse, dependence, withdrawal ADRs.

Clozapine was the sole molecule reported in 387/559 (69.2% of cases; CI 95% 386–388); remaining drugs included: first/second generation antipsychotics (55/559 cases; 9.8%); benzodiazepines (clonazepam, diazepam, and lorazepam; 54/559 cases; 9.7%); antidepressants (citalopram, escitalopram, sertraline, and venlafaxine; 33/559 cases; 5.9%); and mood stabilizers (valproic acid, carbamazepine, lamotrigine, lithium, and gabapentin; 20/559 cases; 3.6%). Illicit drugs most typically reported here were opioids (15/559 cases), amphetamines (10/559), cannabis, and alcohol (each in seven cases). In 30 cases, two or more prescribed/recreational drugs were recorded in association with clozapine (Table 3).

**Table 3.** Clozapine alone or in combination rates of identification, as recorded by the EudraVigilance (EV) dataset of misuse, abuse, dependence, and withdrawal cases.

| Clozapine-Related Misuse, Abuse, Dependence and Withdrawal Cases Recorded by the EudraVigilance (EV) Dataset | Tot ($n$ = 559) |
|---|---|
| Clozapine ingested as a lone drug | 387 (69.2%) |
| Clozapine identified in combination with remaining drugs | 172 (30.7%) |
| **Prescribing drugs** | |
| Other antipsychotics | 55 |
| Benzodiazepines | 54 |
| Antidepressants | 33 |
| Mood stabilizers | 20 |
| Z-drugs | 4 |
| **Recreational drugs** | |
| Opioids | 15 |
| Amphetamine derivatives | 10 |
| Cannabis | 7 |
| Alcohol | 7 |
| Cocaine | 4 |
| Ketamine | 1 |

The ADRs required in most cases a prolonged hospitalization (298/559 = 53.3% CI 95% 296.5–299.5), while some 46 cases (46/559 = 8.2%) resulted in death (Tables 2 and 4). Of these 46 clozapine-related fatalities, 39 (84.7%) were associated with a previous history of substance abuse (Table 4).

**Table 4.** Description of the clozapine-related fatalities' cases reported to the EudraVigilance (EV) dataset (2005–June 2018). F: female; M: male.

| | | Clozapine Dosage (mg) | Concomitant Drugs | Medical History | Reactions according to the MedDRA Dictionary (Preferred Terms-PT) |
|---|---|---|---|---|---|
| 1 | M, Adult (30 yy) | 200 mg | Benzodiazepines Alcohol | | Intentional product misuse; Antipsychotic drug level increased (clozapine plasmatic 1.1 mg/mL); Blood pressure decreased; Loss of consciousness; Poisoning; Dysarthria; Loss of consciousness; Blood alcohol increased |
| 2 | M, Adult (48 yy) | N/A | Cocaine Opioids Z-drugs | Hypertension; Schizophrenia; Chronic obstructive pulmonary disease; Arteriosclerosis | Substance abuse; Toxicity to various agents |
| 3 | M, Adult (25 yy) | 300 mg | Benzodiazepines Opioids | | Cardiac arrest; Arrhythmia Toxicity to various agents (methadone and clozapine); Drug abuse; Drug level increased (methadone and clozapine) |
| 4 | M, Adult (44 yy) | N/A | Opioids | Hypertension; Alcoholism; Depression; Epigastric discomfort; Anxiety | Pulmonary embolism; Drug abuse |
| 5 | M, Adult | 400 mg | Alcohol | | Liver function test abnormal; Blood alkaline phosphatase increased; Gamma-glutamyl transferase increased; Asphyxia; Alcohol abuse; Drug abuse (heroin) |
| 6 | M, Adult (24yy) | N/A | Alcohol | Anemia | Drug abuse (Clozaril abuse) |

**Table 4.** *Cont.*

| | | Clozapine Dosage (mg) | Concomitant Drugs | Medical History | Reactions according to the MedDRA Dictionary (Preferred Terms-PT) |
|---|---|---|---|---|---|
| 7 | F | 300 mg | | Alcoholism; Mental impairment; Depression; Treatment noncompliance; Deep vein thrombosis | Death; Withdrawal syndrome; Acute psychosis; Cognitive disorder; Amnesia; Speech disorder; Gait disturbance; Chills |
| 8 | F, Adult (54yy) | 350 mg | Benzodiazepines | | Withdrawal syndrome; Insomnia; Completed suicide |
| 9 | M, Adult (66 yy) | N/A | | | Completed suicide; Drug abuse |
| 10 | F, Adult (25yy) | N/A | Antidepressants | | Completed suicide; Drug abuse |
| 11. | M, Adult (31yy) | N/A | | | Completed suicide; Drug abuse |
| 12 | M | N/A | | Obesity; Gastroesophageal reflux; Drug abuse | Drug abuse; Death |
| 13 | F | N/A | Cocaine Benzodiazepines Opioids | Drug dependence | Drug abuse (cocaine, leponex and probably benzodiazepines); Death; Hyperthermia malignant; Cardiac arrest; Circulatory collapse; Delirium |
| 14 | M | N/A | | Hepatitis | Drug abuse (possible use of non-prescribed drugs); Death |
| 15 | M | N/A | | Salivary hypersecretion; Drug abuse (crack cocaine, marijuana, alcohol); Extrapyramidal disorder | Nonspecific reaction; Treatment noncompliance; Drug abuse (mixed polysubstance abuse); Death |
| 16 | F | N/A | Mood stabilizers Antipsychotics | | Drug abuse |
| 17 | M | 1000 mg | | Hypercholesterolemia; Substance abuse; Hypertension; Schizophrenia; Gastro-esophageal reflux disease | Hematemesis; Drug abuse; Cardiac arrest; Completed suicide; Toxicity to various agents; Intentional overdose; Resuscitation; Seizure; Tachycardia |
| 18 | F, Adult (27yy) | N/A | | | Drug abuse |
| 19 | M, Adult (30yy) | N/A | | | Myocardial infarction; Drug abuse; Eye swelling; Glossodynia; Tongue coated; Swollen tongue |
| 20 | F | N/A | | | Intentional self-injury; Meningioma; Drug abuse; Hypoglycemia; Peripheral venous disease; Hepatic steatosis; Scar; Pneumonia; Bronchitis; Arteriosclerosis coronary artery; Purulent discharge; Pulmonary congestion; Death |
| 21 | M, Adult (26yy) | 800 mg | | | Coronary artery disease; Drug abuse; Hallucination, auditory; Epilepsy; Depressed mood |
| 22 | M, Adult (31yy) | N/A | | | Death; Substance abuse |
| 23 | M | N/A | | Surgery; Intentional self-injury; Bipolar disorder | Agitation; Death; Drug abuse; Suicidal ideation; Nasal septum deviation |
| 24 | M, Adult (30yy) | N/A | | | Autonomic nervous system imbalance; Catatonia; Drug withdrawal syndrome; Dyskinesia; Neuroleptic malignant syndrome; Psychotic disorder |

**Table 4.** *Cont.*

| | | Clozapine Dosage (mg) | Concomitant Drugs | Medical History | Reactions according to the MedDRA Dictionary (Preferred Terms-PT) |
|---|---|---|---|---|---|
| 25 | M, Adult (36yy) | N/A | | | Alcohol abuse; Drug abuse; Myocardial infarction; Coronary artery disease |
| 26 | M | 200 mg | | | Drug abuse; Obesity |
| 27 | M, Adult (34yy) | 350 mg | | | Circulatory collapse; Intentional product misuse; Cardiopulmonary failure |
| 28 | M, Adult (33yy) | N/A | Benzodiazepines Opioids | | Death; Drug abuse (heroin, temazepam) |
| 29 | | N/A | | Arm amputation; Drug dependence (including cannabis, benzodiazepines and heroin); Limb reduction defect; Alcohol use | Drug abuse; Loss of consciousness; Hypothermia |
| 30 | M, Adult (31yy) | N/A | | | Abnormal behavior; Myocardial infarction; Drug abuse (heroin, cocaine); Psychomotor hyperactivity; Peripheral coldness; Unresponsive to stimuli; Arteriosclerosis coronary artery; Blood glucose decreased |
| 31. | F, Adult (72yy) | 200 mg | Opioids | Schizophrenia; Depression; Somnolence; Anxiety | Movement disorder; Sudden death; Drug abuse |
| 32. | M, Adult (27yy) | 400 mg | Antipsychotics | Asthma; Nicotine dependence; Drug abuse; Obesity; Substance use; Diabetes mellitus; Mental disorder; Alcohol use | Asphyxia; Substance abuse |
| 33. | M, Adult (50 yy) | 550 mg | | | Hypoxic-ischemic encephalopathy; Drug abuse (cocaine); Pulmonary hemosiderosis; Pulmonary edema; Cardiac arrest; Left ventricular hypertrophy; Arteriosclerosis coronary artery; Aortic arteriosclerosis; Myocardial fibrosis; Hepatic steatosis; Spleen congestion |
| 34. | M, Adult (29yy) | 1000 mg | Opioids | Schizophrenia | Substance abuse (heroin) |
| 35. | F, Adult | N/A | Antidepressants | | Drug abuse |
| 36. | M, Adult (34yy) | 700 mg | | Schizophrenia; Nicotine dependence; Drug abuse | Cardiac arrest; Substance abuse |
| 37. | F, Adult (28yy) | N/A | Antidepressants | | Drug abuse |
| 38. | M | 100 mg | | Blood cholesterol increased; Bipolar disorder; Gastroesophageal reflux; Schizoaffective disorder; Diabetes mellitus | Sudden death; Drug abuse (cocaine and another illicit drug) |
| 39. | F, Adult (50yy) | N/A | Alcohol | Drug abuse; Drug dependence | Completed suicide; Toxicity to various agents; Drug abuse (propofol) |
| 40. | M | N/A | | Product use issue; Psychotic disorder | Product use issue; Drug level increased (clozapine levels in the 600,000 s); Death; Adverse event; Psychotic disorder; Intentional product misuse |

**Table 4.** *Cont.*

| | | Clozapine Dosage (mg) | Concomitant Drugs | Medical History | Reactions according to the MedDRA Dictionary (Preferred Terms-PT) |
|---|---|---|---|---|---|
| 41. | M | N/A | | | Drug withdrawal syndrome; Memory impairment; Disorientation; Completed suicide |
| 42. | F, Adult (28yy) | N/A | Antidepressants | | Toxicity to various agents; Drug abuse |
| 43. | M, Adult (31yy) | 700 mg | | Anxiety; Psychotic disorder; Depression | Completed suicide (suicide due to overdose on clozapine); Intentional product misuse; Overdose; Adverse event |
| 44. | M | N/A | | | Completed suicide (patient jumped to his death); Withdrawal syndrome (periodically he would refrain from taking the medication, thus suffering withdrawal/Initially withdrawal symptoms would consist of disorientation after 2–3 days and memory impairment after 4–7 days) |
| 45. | M | N/A | | | Death; Withdrawal syndrome (withdrawal symptoms from the capsule form of Clozaril antipsychotic medication) |
| 46. | M, Adult (58yy) | 100 mg | | Alcohol use; Hypertension | Drug abuse; Vomiting; Asphyxia; Prescription drug used without a prescription (abuse of clozapine 100 mg tablets) |

In a number of cases, reporters had omitted some relevant details, including diagnosis, drugs involved, and, more importantly, both the white blood cell (WBC) and the absolute neutrophil count (ANC) results. Out of a total of 599 ADRs, referring to 559 individual cases, some 149 ADRs (42 individual cases) mentioned that the WBC count had been carried out. However, the results were reported in only 123 ADRs (32 individual cases). For 68 of these ADRs, the WBC/ANC count was within the normal range; while 42 and 13 ADRs were, respectively, associated with either leukopenia or increased WBC count levels. However, since modifications overtime of WBC count levels were not reported, it would be problematic to unequivocally conclude from here if clozapine had been stopped in association with the occurrence of WBC count abnormalities.

A total of 28 cases reported here catatonia, six of which were specifically described as being associated with clozapine withdrawal issues; further reporters' comments relating to overdose, suicidal behavior, withdrawal, and abuse issues are listed in Table 5.

**Table 5.** Reporter' comments recorded in the line listing; EudraVigilance (EV) clozapine-related misuse/abuse/dependence and withdrawal ADRs (2005-June 2018).

| | Comments in the ADRs Reported in the Dataset |
|---|---|
| **Overdose and suicidal behaviour ADRs** | 1. "Clozapine overdose in suicidal attempt"<br>2. "Patient stopped treatment and then took an overdose of about 2800 mg"<br>3. "Clozapine levels in the 600,000's possible overdose"<br>4. "Clozapine overdose of 3000 mg/took two weeks supply of Clozaril as 4200 mg (300 mg × 14 dd)"<br>5. "Clozapine overdose"<br>6. "Took an overdose of 5600 mg"<br>7. "The patient took 1300 mg for intentional self-injury"<br>8. "Suicide due to overdose on clozapine" |
| **Withdrawal and clozapine discontinuation ADRs** | 1. "Clozaril withdrawal due to non-compliance"<br>2. "Withdrawal reaction cholinergic rebound"<br>3. "Anticholinergic withdrawal syndrome"<br>4. "Withdrawal psychotic episode"<br>5. "Suddcn withdrawal with Clozaril"<br>6. "Clozaril withdrawal psychosis"<br>7. "Psychotic decompensation after clozapine discontinuation"<br>8. "Relapse psychosis"<br>9. "Experiencing extremely negative reactions due to going off this medication"<br>10. "Serotonin syndrome associated with clozapine withdrawal"<br>11. "Withdrawal agitation"<br>12. "Tachycardia and high BP possibly due to Clozaril withdrawal"<br>13. "Acute clozapine withdrawal"<br>14. "Withdrawal symptoms from Clozaril"<br>15. "Compatible with withdrawal effects arising from the abrupt discontinuation of clozapine" |
| **Abuse of clozapine** | 1. "Abusing Clozaril taking more than he needs"<br>2. "Clozaril was prescribed for family members"<br>3. "Took his wife's Clozaril to help him sleep"<br>4. "He depended on clozapine"<br>5. "Died because of clozapine and alcohol"<br>6. "Clozapine as a drug of abuse"<br>7. "Clozaril misuse"<br>8. "Abuse of Leponex"<br>9. "Patient possibly has used Leponex as drug of abuse or he bought Leponex for drug abuse by others" |

## 4. Discussion

To the best of our knowledge, this is the largest collection of literature data relating to clozapine withdrawal and misuse/abuse/dependence cases. Our analysis found 599 ADRs of interest (relating to 559 individuals), representing 5.05% of all 11,847 reports submitted to the EMA EV between 2005 and 2018 and judged as 'suspect.' In contrast with the related knowledge on this topic, mostly focused on small case reports/series [10,43–48], current findings referred to high numbers of patients presenting with clozapine withdrawal and misusing issues.

Clozapine ADRs of interest showed a peak in 2008, but an overall increase was observed between 2010 and 2018. One could argue that this upward trend may have been associated with a range of factors, including the increasing rates of worldwide availability of clozapine due to an overwhelming evidence of its effectiveness [2,49–51] and/or a major awareness of the relevant and significant impact of pharmacovigilance processes and issues, resulting in a rise of spontaneous reporting practices related to safety monitoring of medicinal products in general [52].

Withdrawal cases collected here were recorded according to the related PTs defined in the MedDRA dictionary [35], where withdrawal is described as "the abrupt cessation of a drug use in a habituated person; and a substance specific syndrome following cessation or reduction in intake of a psychoactive substance previously used regularly". Clozapine withdrawal/discontinuation ADRs were the most frequently reported and, as such, current findings confirmed and expanded on previous anecdotal data [6,53,54]. In association with a sudden discontinuation of clozapine, which may be required in cases of blood dyscrasia or suspected myocarditis, instances of withdrawal have already been reported [6,44,54,55]. It is of clear interest that a case of clozapine withdrawal neonatal syndrome was specifically mentioned here as well. The clozapine multi-receptor agonism/antagonism is likely responsible for the occurrence of discontinuation/withdrawal symptoms. Indeed, the clozapine pharmacodynamic profile may well include: (a) a dopaminergic super-sensitivity, with the risk of a dopaminergic psychosis and symptoms such as dystonias, dyskinesias, and catatonia [38,56–59]; (b) a cholinergic rebound, inducing in vulnerable patients a rapid worsening of psychosis, agitation, confusion, insomnia, and symptoms including nausea, vomiting, diarrhea, headache, diaphoresis, and abnormal movements, such as dystonias and dyskinesias [6,54,56,57,60–64]. Consistent with this, symptoms appear to regress rapidly with the help of anti-cholinergic drugs; (c) a serotonergic syndrome, which may occur even without the concomitant use of a serotonergic agent [10,39,61]. In fact, acting as a 5-HT2A antagonist, long-term clozapine use may be associated with receptor downregulation, and thus, its abrupt discontinuation might lead to receptors' upregulation [65,66]; (d) a sudden decrease in gamma-aminobutyric acid (GABA) activity, with the development of catatonic symptoms which may include, mutism, waxy flexibility, staring, posturing, mannerisms, negativism, and also restless, irrelevant speech, and psychomotor agitation [6,67]. The clozapine agonist action on GABA receptors can explain both the drug-drug interaction between clozapine and benzodiazepines, and the flumazenil therapeutic effect in clozapine intoxication cases [6]; and (e) a modification of norepinephrine levels, with clozapine abrupt discontinuation in chronic patients possibly resulting in an increase in suicidal behavior [1,68]. As it may occur with remaining psychotropics, such as antidepressants [69,70], the existence of a discontinuation syndrome following an abrupt stoppage of, or marked reduction in, the dosage of a drug taken on a regular basis does not necessarily mean that a drug causes dependence. Discontinuation should be seen here as distinct from the withdrawal scenario associated with alcohol and other addictive substances, a scenario which commonly presents together with craving, drug seeking behavior, and the inability to stop drug use [71,72]. Thus, if a discontinuation of clozapine is needed, the molecule should be gradually tapered off over several weeks rather than abruptly discontinued, except in cases of emergency (e.g., agranulocytosis), and only with close clinical monitoring [10,67,73]. There are no established guidelines regarding which antipsychotic to choose after withdrawal of clozapine [73], although anticholinergics and olanzapine may be the treatment of choice for preventing withdrawal [53].

The reporters' narrative here formally submitted in a few cases was consistent with both drug seeking and diversion behavior (e.g., " ... clozapine as a drug of abuse ... "; and " ... patient possibly has used Leponex as drug of abuse or he bought Leponex for drug abuse by others ... ".). Considering the current misuse/abuse issues, the number of clozapine related ADRs (e.g., 326 ADRs; referring to: 'drug abuse', 'drug abuser', 'drug diversion', 'intentional product misuse', 'product use issue', and 'substance abuse') here identified may be difficult to interpret. In fact, in comparing quetiapine- and other second-generation antipsychotic-related intentional abuse exposures reported to the US National Poison Data System, Klein et al. [74] suggested that clozapine and olanzapine were significantly associated with frequent instances of severe central effects, including: lethargy/drowsiness/slurred speech; agitation/irritability; confusion and hallucinations. However, no use of clozapine as a recreational drug was reported. One could argue that at least a proportion of these ADRs involved subjects suffering from both schizophrenia and a co-occurring SUD. Furthermore, current findings here did not identify any idiosyncratic intake modalities (e.g., intravenous use) that are typical of a substance misuse behavior. Hypothetically, putative levels of clozapine misuse liability might be tentatively explained considering the range of its pharmacodynamics activities, and the occurrence of rewarding and pleasurable effects due to the agonism at both delta-opioid [13,17,75] and cannabinoid CB1 receptors [18]; and the antagonism at muscarinic receptors [76,77]. Additionally, although clozapine was here ingested on its own in some 69% of cases, remaining antipsychotics and benzodiazepines were the drugs most frequently reported in association. Polypharmacy ingestion may have facilitated the occurrence of synergistic reactions, and hence the EMA ADRs' reporting, due to possible increase in clozapine plasma concentrations associated with metabolism inhibition [14]. Relatively small recreational drugs' numbers were identified here as well, and this may have been associated with complex pharmacological interactions. Indeed, clozapine pre-treatment may increase cocaine concentrations, but significantly reduce subjective responses to cocaine [78].

Regarding the ADRs' outcomes, present figures seem to be a reason for concern, since most cases (298/559 = 53.3%) required a prolonged hospitalization. Furthermore, some 46 (8.2% of 559 subjects) fatalities were here reported, and these mostly occurred in the context of: high dosage clozapine intake; suicidal behavior; and/or polydrug abuse. Although the EMA suggests a maximum clozapine dosage of up to 900 mg/day and warns about side-effects occurring at doses over 450 mg/day [79], cases reported here were at times associated with massive dosages (e.g., in the range of 2800–5600 mg), although most of these cases were associated with overdose/suicide instances. These rates are a reason for concern but seem to be consistent with the suggestion that those subjects diagnosed with treatment-resistant schizophrenia, and hence, who are typically being prescribed with clozapine, present with a higher risk of attempted/completed suicide in comparison to the general population [80]. Clozapine overdose may be lethal due to changes in heart rhythm, respiratory depression, and altered state of consciousness [4,81,82]; clozapine high-dosage ingestion may be associated with a mortality rate of approximately 12% [83], with fatalities most typically being associated with cardiac insufficiency and aspiration pneumonia observed with dosages higher than 2 g [45–48]. Although cases of full recovery after ingestion of either high dosages [46] and/or associated with very high plasma levels (>9000 ng/mL) [45] have been reported, ingestion of 400 mg in a patient not previously treated may be life-threatening [46].

### 4.1. *Limitations*

Overall, pharmacovigilance systems such as the EV in Europe, the Medicines and Healthcare products Regulatory Agency (MHRA) in the United Kingdom and the FDA Adverse Event Reporting System (FAERS) are considered important because the analysis of suspected ADRs may deal with early detection of possible drug safety signals [34]. However, the study of ADRs alone may not be enough to prove causality between a certain suspected reaction and a specific medicine. Any case report should be considered and assessed together with all available data, including case reports worldwide, clinical trials, epidemiological studies, and toxicological investigations.

Unfortunately, the dataset did not typically report here any clinical data, including information on the current/past psychopathology and the medications that were prescribed in association. Furthermore, the study of ADRs may be influenced by the molecule's availability and extent of use, although precise data on the worldwide prescription rates for clozapine were not here identified or available. Moreover, in being voluntarily reported/submitted, the number of ADRs could have been conditioned by both the nature of the reaction and the public awareness of a safety concern, with underreporting possibly having here occurred. Additionally, some data could have been unavailable, invalid or redacted.

### 4.2. *Conclusions*

Current findings focused on a range of clozapine withdrawal and misuse/abuse/dependence issues. It was here confirmed, on a large-scale basis, that, following the abrupt reduction of clozapine dosage a discontinuation/withdrawal syndrome may occur. This may involve possible severe and long-lasting symptoms [10,59,67,84]. Moreover, although this may be an unusual event, it is here suggested that cases of misuse/abuse/dependence could occur in patients with a concomitant SUD and this is despite clozapine being of clinical value for the treatment of dual diagnosis. Conversely, current findings emphasized a range of severe and fatal health consequences associated with clozapine high-dosage intake, and patients taking clozapine should be educated thoroughly about the risks associated with polydrug intake. In being a prescribed drug of highly significant clinical value [85], increased awareness is essential towards prevention, diagnosis, and treatment of cases of clozapine abuse/recreational use in patients diagnosed with schizophrenia [86].

**Author Contributions:** S.C. conceived the paper, the main conceptual ideas, proof outline and designed the study. S.C. wrote the first draft and led on the analysis of the results with the support of A.G. and J.M.C. under the supervision of F.S. All authors have read and agreed to the published version of the manuscript.

## References

1. Khokhar, J.; Henricks, A.M.; Sullivan, E.D.; Green, A.I. Unique Effects of Clozapine: A Pharmacological Perspective. *Adv. Pharmacol.* **2018**, *82*, 137–162.
2. Warnez, S.; Alessi-Severini, S. Clozapine: A review of clinical practice guidelines and prescribing trends. *BMC Psychiatry* **2014**, *14*, 102. [CrossRef]
3. ArrayExpress—A database of functional genomics experiments. Available online: http://www.ebi.ac.uk/arrayexpress/ (accessed on 12 November 2012).
4. Stahl, S.M. *Stahl's Essential Psychopharmacology-Prescriber's Guide*, 6th ed.; Cambridge University Press: Cambridge, UK, 2017.
5. Mauri, M.C.; Paletta, S.; Maffini, M.; Colasanti, A.; Dragogna, F.; Di Pace, C.; Altamura, A. Clinical pharmacology of atypical antipsychotics: An update. *EXCLI J.* **2014**, *13*, 1163–1191.
6. Lawrence, R.E.; First, M.B.; Lieberman, J.A. *Schizophrenia and Other Psychoses*; Wiley: Hoboken, NJ, USA, 2015; Volume 1, pp. 791–856.
7. O Kalkman, H.; Loetscher, E. alpha2C-Adrenoceptor blockade by clozapine and other antipsychotic drugs. *Eur. J. Pharmacol.* **2003**, *462*, 33–40. [CrossRef]
8. Fjalland, B.; Boeck, V. Neuroleptic Blockade of the Effect of Various Neurotransmitter Substances. *Acta Pharmacol. Toxicol.* **1978**, *42*, 206–211. [CrossRef] [PubMed]
9. Bilbily, J.; Mccollum, B.; De Leon, J. Catatonia Secondary to Sudden Clozapine Withdrawal: A Case with Three Repeated Episodes and a Literature Review. *Case Rep. Psychiatry* **2017**, *2017*, 1–11. [CrossRef] [PubMed]
10. Stevenson, E.; Schembri, F.; Green, D.M.; Burns, J. Serotonin Syndrome Associated with Clozapine Withdrawal. *JAMA Neurol.* **2013**, *70*, 1054. [CrossRef]
11. Meltzer, H.Y. An overview of the mechanism of action of clozapine. *J. Clin. Psychiatry* **1994**, *55*.
12. Schwieler, L.; Engberg, G.; Erhardt, S. Clozapine modulates midbrain dopamine neuron firing via interaction with the NMDA receptor complex. *Synapse* **2004**, *52*, 114–122. [CrossRef]
13. Kobayashi, T.; Ikeda, K.; Kumanishi, T. Effects of clozapine on the delta- and kappa- opioid receptors and the G-protein-activated K+ (GIRK) channel expressed in Xenopus oocytes. *Br. J. Pharmacol.* **1998**, *123*, 421–426. [CrossRef]
14. Aronson, J.K. Clozapine. In *Meyler's Side Effects of Drugs (Sixteenth Edition): The International Encyclopedia of Adverse Drug Reactions and Interactions*; Elsevier: Kidlington, UK, 2016; pp. 443–477.
15. Trenton, A.J.; Currier, G.W.; Zwemer, F.L. Fatalities associated with therapeutic use and overdose of atypical antipsychotics. *CNS Drugs* **2003**, *17*, 307–324. [CrossRef] [PubMed]
16. Khokhar, J.; Dwiel, L.L.; Henricks, A.M.; Doucette, W.T.; Green, A.I. The link between schizophrenia and substance use disorder: A unifying hypothesis. *Schizophr. Res.* **2018**, *194*, 78–85. [CrossRef] [PubMed]

17. Olianas, M.C.; Dedoni, S.; Ambu, R.; Onali, P.L. Agonist activity of N-desmethylclozapine at δ-opioid receptors of human frontal cortex. *Eur. J. Pharmacol.* **2009**, *607*, 96–101. [CrossRef] [PubMed]
18. Sundram, S.; Copolov, D.; Dean, B. Clozapine decreases [3H] CP 55940 binding to the cannabinoid1 receptor in the rat nucleus accumbens. *Naunyn-Schmiedeberg's Arch. Pharmacol.* **2005**, *371*, 428–433. [CrossRef]
19. Chung, P.C.S.; Kieffer, B.L. Delta opioid receptors in brain function and diseases. *Pharmacol. Ther.* **2013**, *140*, 112–120. [CrossRef]
20. Schifano, F.; Chiappini, S.; Corkery, J.M.; Guirguis, A. Abuse of Prescription Drugs in the Context of Novel Psychoactive Substances (NPS): A Systematic Review. *Brain Sci.* **2018**, *8*, 73. [CrossRef]
21. Bersani, F.S.; Corazza, O.; Simonato, P.; Mylokosta, A.; Levari, E.; Lovaste, R.; Schifano, F. Drops of madness? Recreational misuse of tropicamide collyrium; early warning alerts from Russia and Italy. *Gen. Hosp. Psychiatry* **2013**, *35*, 571–573. [CrossRef]
22. Wu, Y.; Blichowski, M.; Daskalakis, Z.J.; Wu, Z.; Liu, C.C.; Cortez, M.A.; Snead, O.C. Evidence that clozapine directly interacts on the GABAB receptor. *NeuroReport* **2011**, *22*, 637–641. [CrossRef]
23. López-Gil, X.; Artigas, F.; Adell, A. Unraveling monoamine receptors involved in the action of typical and atypical antipsychotics on glutamatergic and serotonergic transmission in prefrontal cortex. *Curr. Pharm. Des.* **2010**, *16*, 502–515. [CrossRef]
24. Schifano, F.; Orsolini, L.; Papanti, G.D.; Corkery, J.M. Novel psychoactive substances of interest for psychiatry. *World Psychiatry* **2015**, *14*, 15–26. [CrossRef]
25. Schifano, F.; Napoletano, F.; Arillotta, D.; Zangani, C.; Gilgar, L.; Guirguis, A.; Corkery, J.M.; Vento, A. The clinical challenges of synthetic cathinones. *Br. J. Clin. Pharmacol.* **2019**. [CrossRef] [PubMed]
26. Zimmet, S.V.; Strous, R.D.; Burgess, E.S.; Kohnstamm, S.; Green, A.I. Effects of clozapine on substance use in patients with schizophrenia and schizoaffective disorder: A retrospective survey. *J. Clin. Psychopharmacol.* **2000**, *20*, 94–98. [CrossRef] [PubMed]
27. Krause, M.; Huhn, M.; Schneider-Thoma, J.; Bighelli, I.; Gutsmiedl, K.; Leucht, S. Efficacy, acceptability and tolerability of antipsychotics in patients with schizophrenia and comorbid substance use. A systematic review and meta-analysis. *Eur. Neuropsychopharmacol.* **2019**, *29*, 32–45. [CrossRef] [PubMed]
28. Brunette, M.F.; Drake, R.E.; Xie, H.; McHugo, G.J.; Green, A.I. Clozapine Use and Relapses of Substance Use Disorder Among Patients with Co-occurring Schizophrenia and Substance Use Disorders. *Schizophr. Bull.* **2006**, *32*, 637–643. [CrossRef]
29. Okhuijsen-Pfeifer, C.; Sterk, A.Y.; Horn, I.M.; Terstappen, J.; Kahn, R.S.; Luykx, J.J. Demographic and clinical features as predictors of clozapine response in patients with schizophrenia spectrum disorders: A systematic review and meta-analysis. *Neurosci. Biobehav. Rev.* **2020**, *111*, 246–252. [CrossRef]
30. Chang, J.; Kim, S.; Lee, G.; Kim, E.; Jung, H. Quetiapine misuse and abuse: Is it an atypical paradigm of drug seeking behavior? *J. Res. Pharm. Pr.* **2017**, *6*, 12–15. [CrossRef]
31. Chiappini, S.; Schifano, F. Is There a Potential of Misuse for Quetiapine? Literature Review and Analysis of the European Medicines Agency/European Medicines Agency Adverse Drug Reactions' Database. *J. Clin. Psychopharmacol.* **2018**, *38*, 72–79. [CrossRef]
32. Evoy, K.; Teng, C.; Encarnacion, V.G.; Frescas, B.; Hakim, J.; Saklad, S.; Frei, C.R. Comparison of Quetiapine Abuse and Misuse Reports to the FDA Adverse Event Reporting System with Other Second-Generation Antipsychotics. *Subst. Abus. Res. Treat.* **2019**, *13*. [CrossRef]
33. Vento, A.E.; Kotzalidis, G.D.; Cacciotti, M.; Papanti, G.D.; Orsolini, L.; Rapinesi, C.; Savoja, V.; Calabrò, G.; Del Casale, A.; Piacentino, D.; et al. Quetiapine Abuse Fourteen Years Later: Where Are We Now? A Systematic Review. *Subst. Use Misuse* **2019**, *55*, 304–313. [CrossRef]
34. European Medicines Agency (EMA). Guideline on good pharmacovigilance practices, Module VI—Collection, management and submission of reports of suspected adverse reactions to medicinal products (Rev 2). Available online: http://www.ema.europa.eu/docs/en_GB/document_library/Regulatory_and_procedural_guideline/2017/08/WC500232767.pdf (accessed on 25 July 2019).
35. MedDRA. Version 21. 2018. Available online: https://www.meddra.org/sites/default/files/guidance/file/smq_intguide_21_0_english.pdf (accessed on 25 July 2019).
36. Schifano, F.; Chiappini, S.; Corkery, J.M.; Guirguis, A. Assessing the 2004–2018 Fentanyl Misusing Issues Reported to an International Range of Adverse Reporting Systems. *Front. Pharmacol.* **2019**, *10*, 46. [CrossRef]

37. Schifano, F.; Chiappini, S.; Corkery, J.M.; Guirguis, A. An Insight into Z-Drug Abuse and Dependence: An Examination of Reports to the European Medicines Agency Database of Suspected Adverse Drug Reactions. *Int. J. Neuropsychopharmacol.* **2019**, *22*, 270–277. [CrossRef] [PubMed]
38. Schifano, F.; Chiappini, S. Is there such a thing as a 'lope' dope? Analysis of loperamide-related European Medicines Agency (EMA) pharmacovigilance database reports. *PLoS ONE* **2018**, *13*, e0204443. [CrossRef] [PubMed]
39. Schifano, F.; Chiappini, S. Is There a Potential of Misuse for Venlafaxine and Bupropion? *Front. Pharmacol.* **2018**, *9*. [CrossRef] [PubMed]
40. European Medicines Agency (EMA). Note for Guidance—EudraVigilance Human—Processing of Safety Messages and Individual Case Safety Reports (ICSRs) (EMA/H/20665/04/Final Rev. 2). Available online: https://www.ema.europa.eu/en/documents/regulatory-procedural-guideline/note-guidance-eudravigilance-human-processing-safety-messages-individual-case-safety-reports-icsrs_en.pdf (accessed on 25 July 2019).
41. European Medicines Agency (EMA). EudraVigilance Working Group (EV-EWG). Guideline on the Use of Statistical Signal Detection Methods in the EudraVigilance Data Analysis System. Available online: https://www.ema.europa.eu/en/documents/regulatory-procedural-guideline/draft-guideline-use-statistical-signal-detection-methods-eudravigilance-data-analysis-system_en.pdf (accessed on 25 July 2019).
42. European Medicines Agency (EMA). ICH Guideline E2B (R3) on Electronic Transmission of Individual Case Safety Reports (ICSRs)—Data Elements and Message Specification—Implementation Guide. Available online: https://www.ema.europa.eu/en/documents/scientific-guideline/international-conference-harmonisation-technical-requirements-registration-pharmaceuticals-human-use_en-4.pdf (accessed on 25 July 2019).
43. Bastiampillai, T.; Forooziya, F.; Dhillon, R. Clozapine-withdrawal catatonia. *Aust. N. Z. J. Psychiatry* **2013**, *43*, 283–284.
44. Goudie, A.J.; Smith, J.A.; Robertson, A.; Cavanagh, C. Clozapine as a drug of dependence. *Psychopharmacology* **1999**, *142*, 369–374. [CrossRef]
45. Ines, S.; Mahal, A.; Hoss, J.; Gaertner, H.J. Intoxication with clozapine: Plasma levels above 9000 ng/mL. Typical clinical picture diagnostic confusion (abstract). *Neuropsychopharmacology* **1994**, *10*, 122S.
46. Le Blaye, I.; Donatini, B.; Hall, M. Acute over dosage with clozapine: A review of the available clinical experience. *Pharm. Med.* **1992**, *6*, 169–178.
47. Piccini, G.; Ceroni, P.; Marchesi, C.; Maggini, C.; Maestri, G. Acute clozapine overdosage. *Br. J. Psychiatry* **1997**, *170*, 290. [CrossRef]
48. Worm, K.; Kringsholm, B.; Steentoft, A. Clozapine cases with fatal, toxic or therapeutic concentrations. *Int. J. Leg. Med.* **1993**, *106*, 115–118. [CrossRef]
49. Niehues, G.D.; Balan, A.B.; Prá, V.B.; Pellizzaro, R.S.; Da Silva, P.R.A.; Schwarzbold, M.L.; Diaz, A.P.; Costa, A.P. Trends in the prescription of clozapine in a psychiatric hospital: A 5-year observational study. *Trends Psychiatry Psychother.* **2017**, *39*, 158–164. [CrossRef]
50. Nielsen, J.; Røge, R.; Schjerning, O.; Sørensen, H.J.; Taylor, D. Geographical and temporal variations in clozapine prescription for schizophrenia. *Eur. Neuropsychopharmacol.* **2012**, *22*, 818–824. [CrossRef] [PubMed]
51. Verdoux, H.; Pambrun, E.; Cortaredona, S.; Coldefy, M.; Le Neindre, C.; Tournier, M.; Verger, P. Geographical disparities in prescription practices of lithium and clozapine: A community-based study. *Acta Psychiatr. Scand.* **2016**, *133*, 470–480. [CrossRef] [PubMed]
52. Santoro, A.; Genov, G.; Spooner, A.; Raine, J.; Arlett, P. Promoting and Protecting Public Health: How the European Union Pharmacovigilance System Works. *Drug Saf.* **2017**, *40*, 855–869. [CrossRef] [PubMed]
53. Galova, A.; Berney, P.; Desmeules, J.; Sergentanis, I.; Besson, M. A case report of cholinergic rebound syndrome following abrupt low-dose clozapine discontinuation in a patient with type I bipolar affective disorder. *BMC Psychiatry* **2019**, *19*, 73. [CrossRef] [PubMed]
54. Lander, M.; Bastiampillai, T.; Sareen, J. Review of withdrawal catatonia: What does this reveal about clozapine? *Transl. Psychiatry* **2018**, *8*, 139. [CrossRef] [PubMed]
55. Koychev, I.; Hadjiphilippou, S.; Lynch, J.; Whelan, P.; MacCabe, J. Sudden-Onset Catatonia Following Clozapine Withdrawal: A Case Report. *J. Clin. Psychiatry* **2016**, *77*, e899. [CrossRef]

56. Moncrieff, J. Does antipsychotic withdrawal provoke psychosis? Review of the literature on rapid onset psychosis (supersensitivity psychosis) and withdrawal-related relapse. *Acta Psychiatr. Scand.* **2006**, *114*, 3–13. [CrossRef]
57. Sarma, S.; Chetia, D.; Raha, B.; Agarwal, G. Clozapine withdrawal emergent dystonia, oculogyric crisis and rebound psychosis in a single patient. *Ther. Adv. Psychopharmacol.* **2015**, *6*, 145–146. [CrossRef]
58. Shore, D.; Matthews, S.; Cott, J.; Lieberman, J.A. Clinical implications of clozapine discontinuation: Report of a NIMH workshop. *Schizophr Bull.* **1995**, *21*, 333–338. [CrossRef]
59. Wang, B.Z.; Gupta, A.; Bastiampillai, T.; Sani, F. Recurrent clozapine and lorazepam withdrawal psychosis with catatonia. *Aust. New Zealand J. Psychiatry* **2012**, *46*, 795–796. [CrossRef]
60. Breen, E.G. Clozapine withdrawal syndrome. *BJPsych Bull.* **2017**, *41*, 366. [CrossRef] [PubMed]
61. Kumar, S.; Sur, S.; Singh, A. Catatonia Following Abrupt Stoppage of Clozapine. *Aust. New Zealand J. Psychiatry* **2011**, *45*, 499. [CrossRef] [PubMed]
62. Shiovitz, T.M.; Welke, T.L.; Tigel, P.D.; Anand, R.; Hartman, R.D.; Sramek, J.J.; Kurtz, N.M.; Cutler, N.R. Cholinergic Rebound and Rapid Onset Psychosis Following Abrupt Clozapine Withdrawal. *Schizophr. Bull.* **1996**, *22*, 591–595. [CrossRef]
63. Yeh, A.W.-C.; Lee, J.W.Y.; Cheng, T.-C.; Wen, J.-K.; Chen, W.-H. Clozapine withdrawal catatonia associated with cholinergic and serotonergic rebound hyperactivity: A case report. *Clin. Neuropharmacol.* **2004**, *27*. [CrossRef] [PubMed]
64. Wadekar, M.; Syed, S. Clozapine-Withdrawal Catatonia. *Psychosomatics* **2010**, *51*, 355. [CrossRef]
65. Zerjav-Lacombe, S.; Dewan, V. Possible serotonin syndrome associated with clomipramine after withdrawal of clozapine. *Ann. Pharmacother.* **2001**, *35*. [CrossRef] [PubMed]
66. Huang, X.F.; Tan, Y.Y.; Huang, X.; Wang, Q. Effect of chronic treatment with clozapine and haloperidol on 5-HT2A and 2C receptor mRNA expression in the rat brain. *Neurosci. Res.* **2007**, *59*, 314–321. [CrossRef]
67. Shields, M.K.; Bastiampillai, T.; Mohan, T. Managing clozapine discontinuation—Acute and chronic maintenance strategies. *Aust. New Zealand J. Psychiatry* **2012**, *46*, 1104–1105. [CrossRef]
68. Meltzer, H.Y.; Alphs, L.; Green, A.I.; Altamura, A.C.; Anand, R.; Bertoldi, A.; Bourgeois, M.; Chouinard, G.; Islam, M.Z.; Kane, J.; et al. International Suicide Prevention Trial Study Group. Clozapine treatment for suicidality in schizophrenia: International Suicide Prevention Trial (InterSePT). *Arch. Gen. Psychiatry.* **2003**, *60*, 82–91. [CrossRef]
69. Fava, G.A.; Gatti, A.; Belaise, C.; Guidi, J.; Offidani, E. Withdrawal Symptoms after Selective Serotonin Reuptake Inhibitor Discontinuation: A Systematic Review. *Psychother. Psychosom.* **2015**, *84*, 72–81. [CrossRef]
70. Gabriel, M.; Sharma, V. Antidepressant discontinuation syndrome. *CMAJ* **2017**, *189*, E747. [CrossRef] [PubMed]
71. Schatzberg, A.F.; Haddad, P.; Kaplan, E.M.; Lejoyeux, M.; Rosenbaum, J.F.; Young, A.H.; Zajecka, J. Serotonin reuptake inhibitor discontinuation syndrome: A hypothetical definition. Discontinuation Consensus panel. *J. Clin. Psychiatry* **1997**, *58*, 5–10. [PubMed]
72. Shelton, R. The nature of the discontinuation syndrome associated with antidepressant drugs. *J. Clin. Psychiatry* **2006**, *67*, 3–7. [PubMed]
73. Szafrański, T.; Gmurkowski, K. Clozapine withdrawal. *Psychiatr. Pol.* **1999**, *33*, 51–67.
74. Klein, L.; Bangh, S.; Cole, J.B. Intentional Recreational Abuse of Quetiapine Compared to Other Second-generation Antipsychotics. *West. J. Emerg. Med.* **2016**, *18*, 243–250. [CrossRef]
75. Pradhan, A.A.; Befort, K.; Nozaki, C.; Gavériaux, C.; Kieffer, B.L. The delta opioid receptor: An evolving target for the treatment of brain disorders. *Trends Pharmacol. Sci.* **2011**, *32*, 581–590. [CrossRef]
76. Solismaa, A.; Kampman, O.; Lyytikäinen, L.-P.; Seppälä, N.; Viikki, M.; Mononen, N.; Lehtimaki, T.; Leinonen, E. Genetic Polymorphisms Associated with Constipation and Anticholinergic Symptoms in Patients Receiving Clozapine. *J. Clin. Psychopharmacol.* **2018**, *38*, 193–199. [CrossRef]
77. Torrents, R.; Ferré, J.F.; Konareff, A.; Hemery, P.; Sherwin, K.; Lassalle, C.; Simon, N.; Scerra, S. Misuse of Trihexyphenidyl (Artane) on Réunion Island. *J. Clin. Psychopharmacol.* **2018**, *38*, 250–253. [CrossRef]
78. Farren, C.; Hameedi, F.A.; Rosen, M.A.; Woods, S.; Jatlow, P.; Kosten, T.R. Significant interaction between clozapine and cocaine in cocaine addicts. *Drug Alcohol Depend.* **2000**, *59*, 153–163. [CrossRef]

79. European Medicines Agency (EMA); Committee for Proprietary Medicinal Products (CPMP). Summary information on referral opinion following arbitration pursuant to Article 30 of Council Directive 2001/83/EC for Leponex and associated names. Available online: https://www.ema.europa.eu/en/medicines/human/referrals/leponex (accessed on 24 July 2019).
80. Kasckow, J.; Felmet, K.; Zisook, S. Managing suicide risk in patients with schizophrenia. *CNS Drugs* **2011**, *25*, 129–143. [CrossRef]
81. He, J.-L.; Xiang, Y.-T.; Li, W.-B.; Cai, Z.-J.; Ungvari, G.S. Hemoperfusion in the Treatment of Acute Clozapine Intoxication in China. *J. Clin. Psychopharmacol.* **2007**, *27*, 667–671. [CrossRef] [PubMed]
82. Broich, K.; Heinrich, S.; Marneros, A. Acute Clozapine Overdose: Plasma Concentration and Outcome. *Pharmacopsychiatry* **1998**, *31*, 149–151. [CrossRef] [PubMed]
83. Kramer, I.; Rauber-Lüthy, C.; Kupferschmidt, H. Minimal dose for severe poisoning and influence factors in acute human clozapine intoxication: A 13-year retrospective study. *Clin. Neuropharm.* **2011**, *33*, 230–234. [CrossRef] [PubMed]
84. Ulrich, S.; Baumann, B.; Wolf, R.; Lehmann, D.; Peters, B.; Bogerts, B.; Meyer, F. Therapeutic drug monitoring of clozapine and relapse—A retrospective study of routine clinical data. *Int. J. Clin. Pharmacol. Ther.* **2003**, *41*, 3–13. [CrossRef]
85. Cipriani, A.; Boso, M.; Barbui, C. Clozapine combined with different antipsychotic drugs for treatment resistant schizophrenia. *Cochrane Database Syst. Rev.* **2009**, CD006324.
86. Pandarakalam, J.P. The art of clozapine therapy and "clozaphobia". *BMJ* **2019**, *364*, l484. [CrossRef]

# 3

# Exploring the Baseline Knowledge and Experience of Healthcare Professionals in the United Kingdom on Novel Psychoactive Substances

**Camille Ramos [1], Amira Guirguis [1,2,*], Nigel Smeeton [1], Hadar Zaman [3], Anna-Marie Felice [4], Stephanie Bancroft [5], Rosalind Gittins [6], Gill Hawksworth [7], John Martin Corkery [1] and Fabrizio Schifano [1]**

1 Psychopharmacology, Drug Misuse and Novel Psychoactive Substances Research Unit, School of Life and Medical Sciences, University of Hertfordshire, Hatfield AL10 9AB, UK; camille27ramos@gmail.com (C.R.); n.smeeton@herts.ac.uk (N.S.); j.corkery@herts.ac.uk (J.M.C.); f.schifano@herts.ac.uk (F.S.)

2 Swansea University Medical School, Institute of Life Sciences 2, Swansea University, Swansea SA2 8PP, UK

3 Bradford School of Pharmacy & Medical Sciences, Faculty of Life Sciences, University of Bradford, Horton Road, Bradford BD7 1DP, UK; H.Zaman4@bradford.ac.uk

4 CGL, St Martins House, 14 The Common, Hatfield AL10 0UR, UK; annamarie.felice@cgl.org.uk

5 London North West Local Pharmacy Forum (LNWLPF) of the Royal Pharmaceutical Society, Pinner, Middlesex HA5 3EP, UK; steph_bancroft@hotmail.com

6 Humankind, Inspiration House, Unit 22 Bowburn North Industrial Estate, Durham DH6 5PF, UK; rgittins1@nhs.net

7 Royal Pharmaceutical Society, 66-68 E Smithfield, Whitechapel, London E1W 1AW, UK; gill.hawksworth@virgin.net

* Correspondence: amira.guirguis@swansea.ac.uk

**Abstract: Objective**: This survey aimed to explore knowledge and experience on novel psychoactive substances (NPS) of healthcare professionals (HCPs). The study also aimed to assess how HCPs would like to improve their knowledge of NPS. **Methods**: Seventy paper questionnaires were disseminated in 2017 within continuing education events to pharmacists, nurses and general practitioners (GPs). Additionally, 127 online surveys were completed using the Qualtrics platform by other HCPs and mental health nurses in six United Kingdom (UK) independent mental health hospitals long-stay in-patient rehabilitation services. Two educational sessions involving pharmacists and GPs were also held in late 2017 and mid-2018. Knowledge of NPS by HCPs was evaluated prior to the start of the educational events. Evaluation forms were handed out post-sessions to garner feedback, especially on areas for improvement for future sessions. Statistical analysis of data was undertaken using SPSS (V.25). **Results**: Most HCPs reported only 'basic' to 'intermediate' NPS knowledge. Substance misuse service staff felt more informed, were more often consulted and had greater confidence regarding NPS compared to hospital and primary care professionals. A negative association was found between the age of the HCP and knowledge of NPS. Most participants expressed a need for regular training and updates as insufficient NPS-related information is currently received. **Conclusions**: An improvement within the self-reported knowledge of HCPs on NPS is evident in comparison to previous studies. Continued education of HCPs on NPS is fundamental for the provision of improved harm reduction services, which can enhance overall care for NPS service users.

**Keywords:** novel psychoactive substances; NPS; healthcare professionals; drug education; substance misuse; harm reduction

## 1. Background

Numerous definitions of novel psychoactive substances (NPS) are currently used, most of which highlight their negative impact upon public health. The United Nations (UN) stated that NPS are "substances of abuse, either in a pure form or a preparation, that are not controlled by the 1961 Single Convention on Narcotic Drugs or the 1971 Convention on Psychotropic Substances, but which may pose a public health threat" [1]. The European Council's definition places an emphasis on the threats posed by NPS and describes such a substance as "a new narcotic or psychotropic drug, in pure form or in preparation, that is not controlled by the United Nations drug conventions, but which may pose a public health threat comparable to that posed by substances listed in these conventions" [2]. The Advisory Council on the Misuse of Drugs (ACMD) in the United Kingdom (UK) uses a definition which incorporates both international and UK drug legislation: "Psychoactive drugs which are not prohibited by the United Nations Single Convention on Narcotic Drugs or by the Misuse of Drugs Act 1971, and which people in the UK are seeking for intoxicant use" [3]. The UK Psychoactive Substances Act (PSA) (2016) opted for a broader definition of NPS and defined them as "any substance, which is capable of producing a psychoactive effect" [4]. The term 'new' does not necessarily mean new inventions but instead addresses how such substances were recently made available, including failed pharmaceuticals or old patents which have been 'rediscovered' as 'recreational' molecules [5]. In addition, Corkery et al. [6] proposed that the term 'new' may correspond to an NPS molecule that has a 'novelty' appeal due to their innovative or unusual way of consumption. Ultimately, definitions of NPS vary according to the context(s) in which they are discussed [7].

Presently in the UK, NPS are regulated by the PSA 2016, which prohibits NPS production, sale, possession in custodial institutions or possession with intention to supply. This legislation introduced offences for the production, distribution, sale and supply of psychoactive substances in the UK for human consumption; it "builds on and complements" the Misuse of Drugs Act 1971 (MDA 1971) for the regulation of "dangerous or otherwise harmful" substances [4]. In accordance with the UK's 2017 drug strategy, the PSA underwent a review by the Home Office in November 2018 to measure any changes in outcomes before and after the implementation of the Act [8]. The review showed that PSA enforcement led to the ban of NPS sale through headshops, has limited the sales and availability of NPS and reduced use, and as a result, there is evidence of reduction in health and social harms [8]. Deligianni and colleagues [9] evaluated the impact and effectiveness of the PSA 2016 through an updated survey in 2017 regarding NPS awareness, use, experiences and risk awareness and concluded that this regulation has not impacted on health risk awareness and motivations for NPS use in the UK.

The United Nations Office on Drugs and Crime (UNODC) classifies NPS into six categories: synthetic cannabinoid receptor agonists (SCRAs; e.g., AB-PINACA), stimulants (e.g., 4-fluoroamphetamine), classic hallucinogens (e.g., 2C-I), dissociatives (e.g., deschloroketamine), sedatives/hypnotics (e.g., etizolam) and opioids (e.g., furanyl fentanyl) [10]. Additionally, the 'plant-based' category includes substances such as 'khat'.

From 2009 to December 2018, almost 900 different NPS from 119 countries and territories were reported to the UNODC Early Warning Advisory, most of which have been associated with unpredictable adverse effects [11]. According to the Global Drug Survey 2019, highly potent hallucinogen compounds including NBOMes and potent amphetamine analogues such as 4-fluoro-amphetamine have been associated with deaths in recent years and have remained increasingly problematic across Europe and Australia [12,13]. Furthermore, Poland ranked first as the country with the highest 12-month rates of NPS use by country globally, with England ranking seventh [13]. According to the Office for National Statistics (ONS) [14], a 29% reduction in the number of NPS-related poisoning deaths registered (as opposed to occurring) was recorded for both England and Wales following the introduction of the PSA 2016. However, the number of such events registered in 2018 showed a return to 2016 levels [14]. More importantly, the numbers of NPS-related poisoning deaths registered in Scotland have increased by 525% in the last four years, accounting for 45% of all drug-related poisoning deaths registered in 2018 [15]. Webb et al. [16] suggest that the total acute

NPS toxicity presentations to a single emergency department (ED) in central London did not change significantly in the year after the introduction of the PSA 2016. Henshall et al. [17] recommended that government campaigns should cater for older individuals to help reduce the potential burden to the National Health Service arising from NPS-related hospital presentations.

### 1.1. *Current NPS Drug Scenes, Related Implications and Responses within the Healthcare System*

The European Monitoring Centre for Drugs and Drug Addiction (EMCDDA) has advised that the proliferation of highly potent substances including new synthetic opioids (NSOs), for example, carfentanil, pose life-threatening poisoning risks which has overwhelmed law enforcement and healthcare systems [18]. Carfentanil is one of the most potent derivatives of fentanyl, being approximately 10,000 times more potent than morphine [19,20]. Limited research has been conducted to explore the toxicological profiles of newly emerging fentanyl derivatives, and this highlights the risks to humans who may be unaware of the presence of these active adulterants and other NSO when taking heroin or counterfeit pain medications [21]. Schifano et al. [22] identified 26,500 fentanyl misuse/abuse/dependence/withdrawal cases over 2004-2018 from pharmacovigilance databases including the European Medicines Agency (EMA), the UK Yellow Card Scheme and the United States Food and Drug Administration Adverse Event Reporting System. They recommended that fatalities associated with NSOs, especially fentanyls, should be thoroughly investigated using combined toxicological analyses.

Evidence presented by the Home Office [8] suggests that the potency of SCRAs has increased despite the introduction of the PSA 2016. Martinotti et al. [23] reported that patients admitted to a psychiatric ward in a nightlife resort following the use of psychoactive substances, particularly those who reported recent use of SCRAs as their main substance, often presented with aggression on their arrival. Furthermore, violence during pre-admission and during admission to acute mental health services is more prevalent in NPS users compared to non-NPS users; thus, more education and support in the management of NPS users has been requested by HCPs who experienced an increasing risk of violence within their workplace [24]. Synthetic cathinones (SC) were the second most frequently seized group of NPS in 2016, where symptoms of intoxication can be long-lasting compared to SCRAs and may potentially be fatal [25,26]. Furthermore, SC such as mephedrone are commonly used during 'chemsex' [27,28]. Chemsex is associated with high-risk injection (known as 'slamming') and sexual risk-taking behaviour (e.g., unprotected sex), both of which may facilitate the transmission of sexually transmitted infections (STIs) or blood-borne viruses (BBVs) including hepatitis C virus (HCV) and human immunodeficiency virus (HIV) [29].

Diversion of prescription-only medicines (POMs) within an NPS context has been assessed by Chiappini and Schifano [30]. They evaluated the EMA's EudraVigilance (EV) database on POM misuse-related adverse drug reactions (ADRs) over the last decade. A total of 7639 and 4301 ADR reports of misuse/abuse/dependence were respectively associated with the gabapentinoids pregabalin and gabapentin. They recommended that combined intake of opioids and sedatives leads to enhanced psychoactive effects, which has been shown to result in fatalities [31,32].

In the UK, stricter prescribing measures have possibly prompted the emergence of 'designer' benzodiazepines, which were not originally controlled drugs, such as the NPS phenazepam and etizolam [33–35]. Etizolam overtook diazepam as the benzodiazepine most frequently reported in drug-related deaths registered in Scotland in 2016 and again in 2017 [15,36,37]. The above shows the dramatic changes in the drug scene and the limited knowledge available to inform HCPs on adequate responses to these unknown substances.

### *1.2. Studies Exploring NPS Knowledge Among Healthcare Professionals (HCPs)*

Previous studies have addressed the inadequacy in essential knowledge and skills required by HCPs on NPS to inform various interventions and highlighted the need for education on these novel molecules [38–43]. However, several studies only focused on specific professions and geographical locations in the UK [40–43]. The deficit in general knowledge on NPS may lead to inappropriate medical diagnoses and potentially the provision of inappropriate medical advice or interventions. Guirguis et al. [40] distributed a revised 'ReDNet' survey utilised initially by Simonato et al. [44]. This was an anonymous questionnaire that was part of a project funded by the European Commission to provide updates about NPS-related information [45,46]. London pharmacists in community settings were involved and most had poor knowledge of the 38 relatively well-known NPS listed in the survey, and few ($n$ = 20; 37%) considered NPS as having 'little' work-related significance. Likewise, Campbell and colleagues [38] addressed how over 50% of HCPs did not have 'adequate knowledge' on drug interactions involving NPS, which is alarming and should be treated urgently through the delivery of appropriate training. Wood et al. [43] concluded that greater confidence was reported by both physicians and nurses on managing acute toxicity due to classical recreational drugs compared to NPS. Similarly, Owie et al. [42] found that most psychiatrists had inadequate overall knowledge of NPS. Lastly, Gittins et al. [39] utilised semi-structured interviews to gather detailed information from clients regarding their NPS use and concluded there is a need for further education and training for HCPs, who encounter NPS service users by adopting multi-agency and multi-disciplinary approaches to gauge awareness of changing trends in NPS use. When and where appropriate, referral to drug and alcohol treatment services or other professionals, such as psychiatry, sexual health or social services can be offered to individuals [47]. Additionally, Tracy and colleagues [48] listed the different NPS-related resources that are accessible to HCPs, including the UK National Poisons Information Service and its clinical toxicology database TOXBASE, NEPTUNE (novel psychoactive treatment UK network) and an NPS resource pack for informal educators and frontline practitioners. None of the above studies indicated an effective educational tool or strategy for HCPs on NPS.

Against the ever-changing backdrop of NPS, in the UK and elsewhere, and the demonstrable lack of awareness and need for education of HCPs concerning the phenomenon and how they can deal with the consequences of NPS use, the main aim of our study was to scope the perceptions of HCPs from various sectors and regions within the UK of these issues. Although the authors are cautious about the generalisability of the findings, the results provide an insight about the self-reported baseline knowledge of HCPs on NPS. This work aimed to build on what was already known with the inclusion of a wider range of HCPs from different health sectors. It is hoped that the findings may seek the views of HCPs on improvements required for education/training and public health intervention research by reviewing existing knowledge of NPS use.

## 2. Methods

### *2.1. Survey Design*

Both online and paper-copy surveys were utilised (Figure 1). The survey consisted of 31 questions, adapted from the 'ReDNet' survey, used initially by Simonato et al. [44], which was revised by Guirguis et al. [40], and updated with more recent NPS compounds. The survey questions included respondents' demographic information (gender, age, health sector, profession, working town and country). Participants were then asked if they have heard of 93 compounds under six categories: POMs ($n$ = 16), benzodiazepines ($n$ = 8), SCRAs ($n$ = 21), opioids ($n$ = 16), SC ($n$ = 17) and 'others' ($n$ = 15). Participants could respond with a "yes", "no" or "know of customers/patients who have abused it" for each compound.

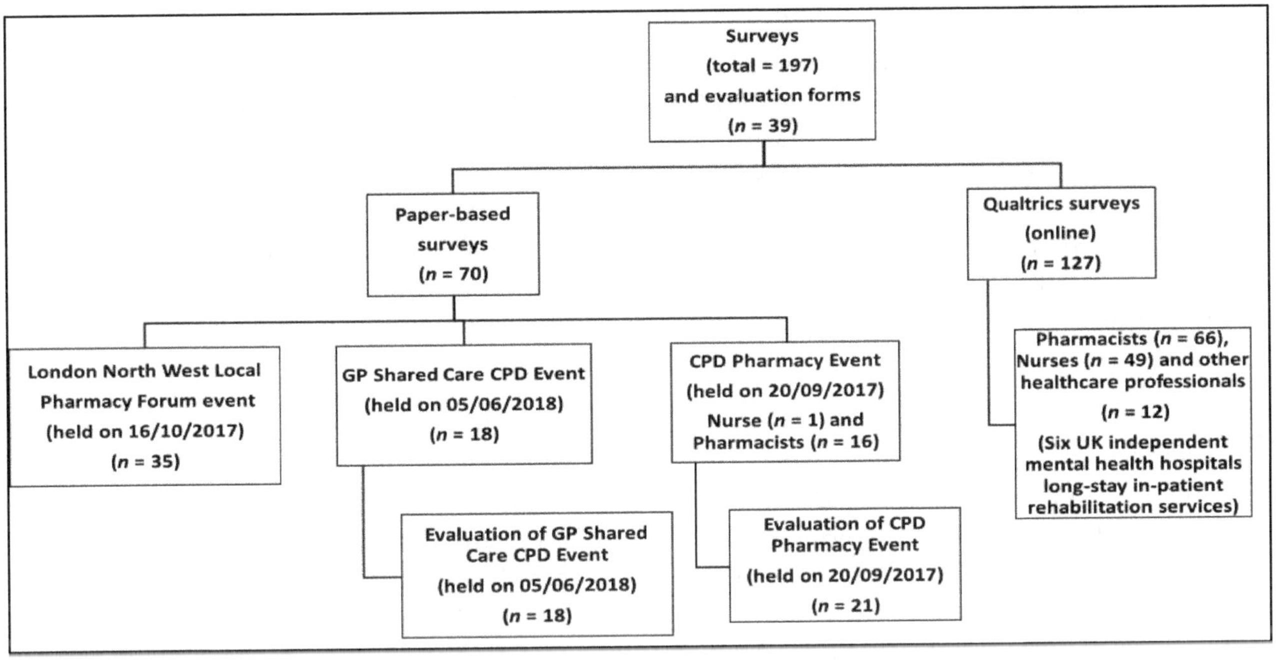


**Figure 1.** Survey distribution flow chart.

The choice of NPS compounds was based upon formal reporting to the EMCDDA by its early warning system on NPS and lists contained in its European Database on New Drugs (EDND) [49]. NPSs included in the survey were associated with the highest number of fatalities prior to data collection.

Likert scales were also used in the survey, including one where respondents were asked to rate their level of knowledge about NPS/'legal highs', with 1 being "poor" and 5 being "very good". Such scales are easier to read and complete, and offer a range of opinions that respondents can choose from [50]. Lastly, open-ended questions were utilised in the evaluation forms of the educational workshops, such as listing up to three aspects that were learnt from the session as well as a dedicated section for suggestions or any additional comments. This was advantageous as improvements for future sessions could be sought from respondents and gaps in knowledge about commonly abused/misused drugs could be identified.

### 2.2. Survey Distribution

There were no pilot studies for this survey as it was adapted with a few minor amendments, such as updating the list of NPS (Table S1), from the same survey instrument used by Guirguis et al. [40]. The study targeted all pharmacists in the UK who are members of both the Royal Pharmaceutical Society (RPS) and the College of Mental Health Pharmacy (CMHP), as well as other healthcare professionals within substance misuse and mental health services. Purposive sampling was implemented, which involved adult HCPs (18 years and older) completing paper-based surveys distributed by the individuals leading the educational events for pharmacists, nurses and general practitioners (GPs).

As illustrated in Figure 1, the online survey (File S1) was delivered via the Qualtrics platform (https://www.qualtrics.com/). Survey links were sent to mental health nurses working across six independent mental health hospitals (non-National Health Service (NHS) hospitals) to mental health pharmacy professionals via CMHP. Likewise, the RPS Science educational lead sent links to all RPS London local practices for community pharmacists. Responses were received by Qualtrics up to 15 October 2017.

Leaders in charge of the LNWLPF event on 16 October 2017 and the 'Change, Grow, Live' (CGL) charity events disseminated paper-based surveys on premises. Lastly, at the end of each of the two educational workshops (both for the Pharmacy and GP Shared Care Continuing Professional Development (CPD) events), feedback forms were provided.

### 2.3. *Data Extraction, Cleaning and Analysis*

Statistical analysis for both datasets from paper-based and online surveys was carried out using the statistics software package SPSS V.25 (IBM Corporation, Armonk, NY, USA). The single continuous variable—age—was checked for normality. Basic summary statistics were obtained as means or percentages. Qualitative variables were analysed using the chi-squared test, with the exact $p$-value being reported for contingency tables having more than 20% of cells with an expected value of less than 5. Where appropriate, Spearman's correlation coefficient was used to assess associations for ordered and continuous variables. Text from open-ended questions was analysed according to emerging themes.

## 3. Results

### 3.1. *Participants*

There was sufficient data from 197 responses for inclusion in the analyses: 127 (64.5%) respondents fully completed the online surveys and 70 (35.5%) paper-based surveys were fully completed. Forty-four of the online responses could not be used (e.g., partially completed). The majority of respondents were females ($n$ = 138; 70.4%). Age had an approximate normal distribution with a mean of 41.79 years ($SD$ = 12.4). Most respondents qualified between the years 2000-2009 ($n$ = 51; 27.1%) and 2010 and later ($n$ = 58; 30.9%). The mean number of years qualified was 17.66 ± 12.1 (range: 1-48) years. Most respondents were from England ($n$ = 183; 95.9%), with four (2.1%) from Wales and four (2.1%) from outside the UK. The most represented Government Office Region was the North (n = 55; 28.8%), followed by Greater London and the South East ($n$ = 49; 25.7%), the East of England ($n$ = 45; 23.6%), the Midlands ($n$ = 19; 9.9%), and the South West ($n$ = 15; 7.9%). From the respondents who stated their profession ($n$ = 186), the largest group of HCPs were pharmacists ($n$ = 107; 57.5%), of whom 30 were community pharmacists (16.1%), 38 (20.4%) were from hospitals and 5 (2.7%) worked in substance misuse services. Additionally, 50 nurses (26.9%) were involved, where 22 (11.8%) had a mental health background, 11 (5.9%) worked in a substance misuse setting, 2 (1.1%) were non-medical prescribers and 15 (8.1%) belonged to other health sectors. General practitioners comprised the third largest group of HCPs ($n$ = 17; 9.1%). Figures 2 and 3 provide further specifics relating to professions and health sectors.

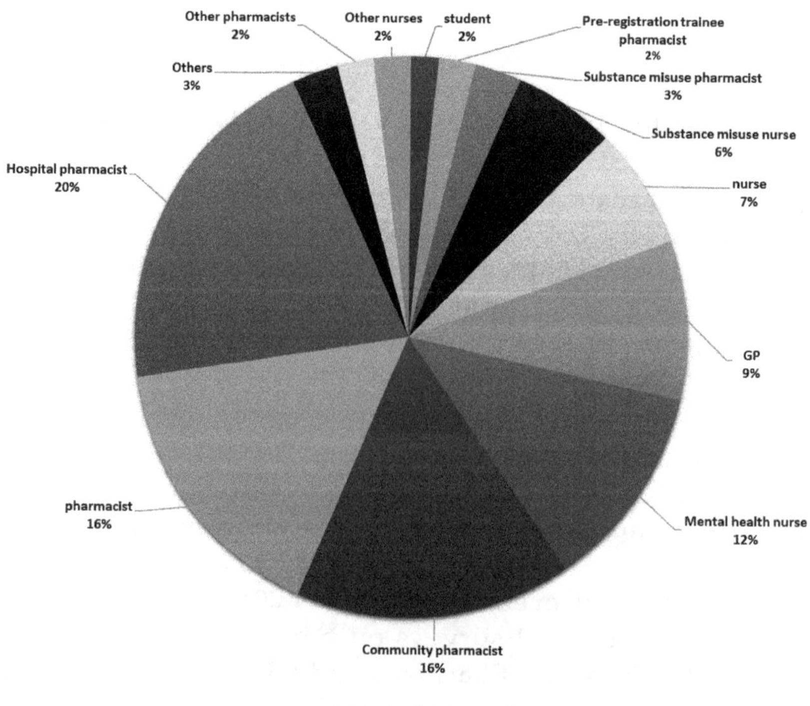


**Figure 2.** Profession types ($n$ = 186).

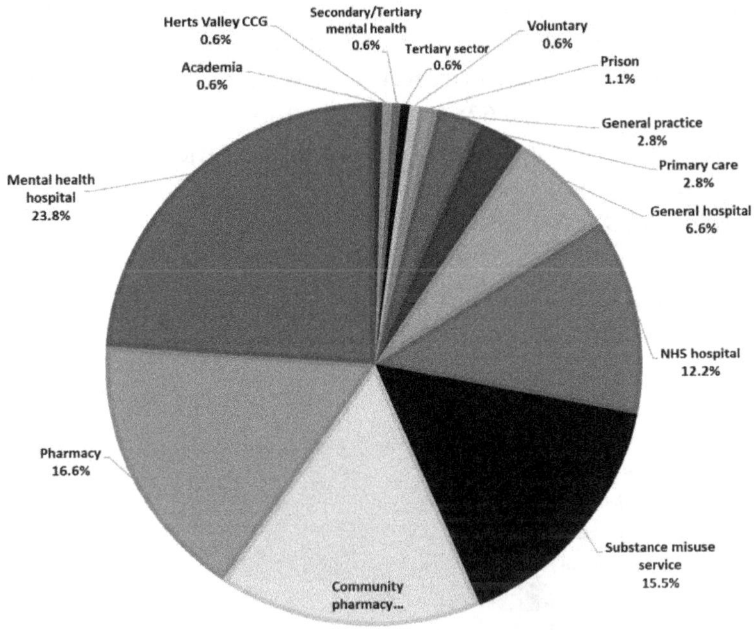


**Figure 3.** Health sectors ($n$ = 181).

Also includes other pharmacists (advanced specialist pharmacist, prison pharmacist, clinical pharmacist, general practitioner (GP) pharmacist), other nurses (learning disabilities nurse, drug and alcohol liaison nurse, non-medical prescriber nurses) and others (family safeguard worker, substance misuse manager, pharmacy technician, university lecturer).

### 3.2. *Knowledge of NPS*

When asked about their expertise/knowledge of NPS (Figure 4), most perceived themselves as having a 'basic' ($n$ = 76; 39.2%) or an 'intermediate' level ($n$ = 73; 37.6%) of knowledge. By contrast, 14 HCPs (7.2%) regarded themselves as having 'poor' NPS knowledge, followed by 'good' ($n$ = 25; 12.9%) and 'very good' ($n$ = 6; 3.1%). A negative association was found between the age of the HCP and knowledge of NPS (Spearman's correlation = – 0.176, $p$ = 0.015).

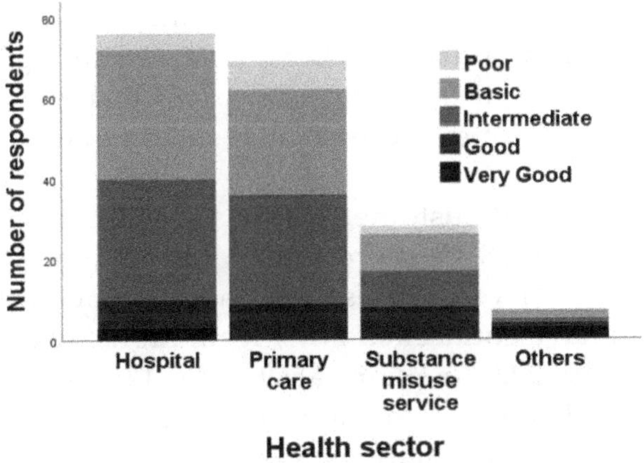


**Figure 4.** Self-reported level of knowledge on novel psychoactive substances (NPS) among different health sectors.

For the 16 listed POMs, zopiclone was the most recognised ($n$ = 109; 64.1%), followed by gabapentin ($n$ = 106; 62.7%) and pregabalin ($n$ = 103; 60.2%). The top three POMs that HCPs claimed to be misused by customers/patients were pregabalin ($n$ = 48; 28.1%), zopiclone ($n$ = 47; 27.6%) and gabapentin

($n$ = 41; 24.3%). Of the opioids ($n$ = 16) included, carfentanil ($n$ = 41; 29.3%) was the most recognised, followed by benzoyl fentanyl ($n$ = 39; 28.3%), furanyl fentanyl ($n$ = 32; 23.4%) and then 3-fluorofentanyl ($n$ = 31; 22.6%). Six (4.4%) claimed that 3-fluorofentanyl was used by customers/patients.

Of the 17 listed SC, mephedrone ($n$ = 62; 44.9%) was the most recognised, where 15 HCPs (10.9%) were also aware of its use by customers/patients. The most commonly known benzodiazepines ($n$ = 8) were 4-chlorodizepam ($n$ = 46; 32.9%), phenazepam ($n$ = 19; 13.8%) and bromazolam ($n$ = 18; 13.2%).

For the 21 listed SCRAs, MDMB-CHMICA ($n$ = 6; 4.6%) and MDMB-FUBINACA ($n$ = 6, 4.6%) were the most commonly known. Lastly, for NPS that were classified as 'others' ($n$ = 15), the most recognised compounds included methoxetamine ($n$ = 17; 13.3%), diphenidine ($n$ = 16; 12.5%) and PMA/PMMA ($n$ = 15; 12.0%). The most commonly known NPS are shown in Figure 5.

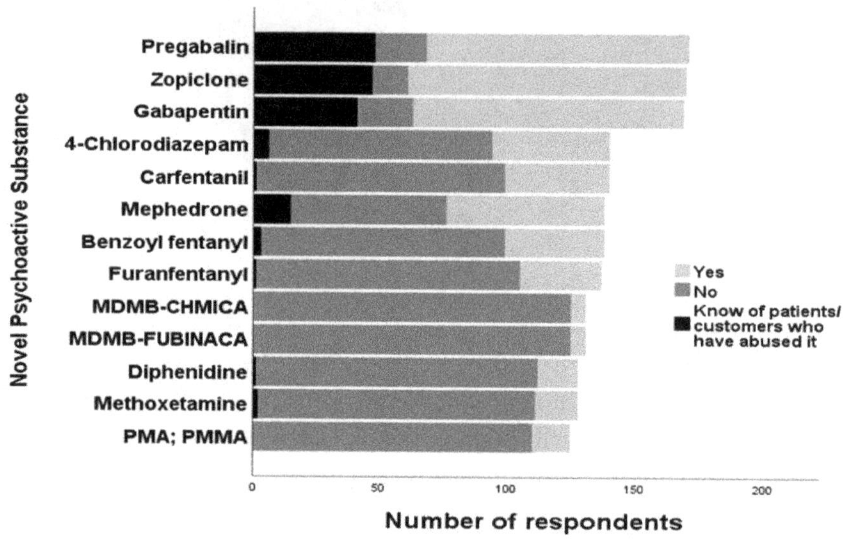


**Figure 5.** Most commonly known NPS by healthcare professionals (HCPs).

Several respondents also stated the names of the NPS they were aware of. 'Spice' was mentioned 26 times (53.1%), followed by 'Black Mamba' ($n$ = 4; 8.2%), 'synthetic cannabinoids' ($n$ = 4; 8.2%), 'poppers' ($n$ = 2; 4.1%) and even 'vapes' ($n$ = 1; 2.0%) were stated.

In terms of NPS route of administration, 155 HCPs (78.7%) were aware of oral, followed by smoking ($n$ = 148; 75.1%), inhaling ($n$ = 136; 69.0%), snorting ($n$ = 131; 66.5%) and through the vaginal route ($n$ = 28; 14.2%). Other administration routes include vaping ($n$ = 94; 47.7%), 'bombing' ($n$ = 61; 31.0%), rectal administration ($n$ = 47; 23.9%) and 'slamming' ($n$ = 27; 13.7%). 'Bombing' involves grounding and wrapping the drug in a cigarette paper then swallowed, whereas 'slamming' is the injection of psychostimulants (e.g., mephedrone) in a sexual context to improve mood and facilitate sexual disinhibition [51,52].

Of those HCPs who encountered customer/patients seeking advice about the management of adverse effects from NPS ($n$ = 49), 18.4% were nurses ($n$ = 9) and 20.4% ($n$ = 10) were hospital pharmacists. Likewise, 22.4% ($n$ = 11) were nurses with similar encounters in substance misuse services. Eighty-three HCPs claimed to have counselled NPS/'legal highs' users, where HCPs from hospital settings including nurses ($n$ = 19; 22.9%), pharmacists ($n$ = 14; 16.9%) and GPs ($n$ = 3; 3.6%) were involved. GPs in primary care also provided counselling ($n$ = 5; 6.0%). The majority of those who provided counselling in substance misuse settings were nurses ($n$ = 17; 20.5%). In contrast, the HCPs who did not counsel customers/patients who use NPS ($n$ = 78) were mainly pharmacists in primary care ($n$ = 29; 37.2%). Counselling may involve the provision of advice on the safe management of adverse effects or about the safe use of NPS (i.e., safer injecting techniques or through needle and syringe exchange programs). However, the authors could not identify from the collected data whether the counselling was simple advice, or part of a brief intervention or structured counselling.

Moreover, participants were then asked to elaborate any ADRs they had encountered, resulting from NPS use. Physical- and mental health-related symptoms were frequently experienced by NPS service users, where hallucinations and paranoia were commonly reported. Most HCPs were 'not confident' in providing advice about safe use of NPS/'legal highs' ($n = 97$; 50.3%). Furthermore, most HCPs ($n = 109$; 60.6%) assessed themselves as 'not confident' about the provision of advice regarding the safe management of ADRs resulting from NPS use. Among the 43 HCPs who were 'fairly confident' on this aspect, 16 were from hospitals (37.2%), whilst 14 were from substance misuse services (32.6%).

### 3.3. *Relevance of NPS to HCPs*

Grouping respondents by health sector (Table 1) and profession (Table 2) demonstrated important differences. Reported knowledge regarding NPS was somewhat greater for nurses compared to GPs and pharmacists. Nurses were more likely to be asked for advice regarding NPS use and felt more knowledgeable and confident about giving such advice.

**Table 1.** Comparison of type of practitioner by aspects of NPS use between health sectors.

| | **Positive Response: Number Out of Total (%)** | | | | |
|---|---|---|---|---|---|
| | **Hospital** | **Primary Care** | **Substance Misuse Service** | **Others** | ***p*-Value** |
| Good/very good level of knowledge | 11/77 (14.3) | 8/68 (11.8) | 8/28 (28.6) | 4/7 (57.1) | 0.008 * |
| Provide advice/counselling | 40/72 (55.6) | 20/55 (36.4) | 19/26 (73.1) | 4/4 (100.0) | 0.002 * |
| Fairly/very confident about providing advice | 34/77 (44.2) | 21/68 (30.9) | 15/28 (53.6) | 5/7 (71.4) | 0.051 * |
| Encounter customers/patients seeking advice | 22/76 (28.9) | 8/68 (11.8) | 13/28 (46.4) | 5/7 (71.4) | < 0.001 |
| Fairly/very confident about providing advice on adverse effects | 17/72 (23.6) | 11/63 (17.5) | 14/28 (50.0) | 4/7 (57.1) | 0.003 |
| Knowledge on NPS/legal highs fairly/very significant in work | 58/68 (85.3) | 40/57 (70.2) | 24/26 (92.3) | 5/6 (83.3) | 0.058 * |

* Exact $p$-value.

**Table 2.** Comparison of type of practitioner by aspects of NPS use between professions.

| | **Positive Response: Number Out of Total (%)** | | | | |
|---|---|---|---|---|---|
| | **GP** | **Nurse** | **Pharmacist** | **Others** | ***p*-Value** |
| Good/very good level of knowledge | 0/17 (0.0) | 10/50 (20.0) | 16/106 (15.1) | 4/12 (33.3) | 0.086 * |
| Provide advice/counselling | 8/16 (50.0) | 38/48 (79.2) | 31/90 (34.4) | 5/6 (83.3) | <0.001 * |
| Fairly/very confident about providing advice | 4/17 (23.5) | 28/50 (56.0) | 35/105 (33.3) | 6/12 (50.0) | 0.021 |
| Encounter customers/patients seeking advice | 5/17 (29.4) | 21/50 (42.0) | 19/104 (18.3) | 4/12 (33.3) | 0.018 * |
| Fairly/very confident about providing advice on adverse effects | 3/16 (18.8) | 21/49 (42.9) | 18/97 (18.6) | 2/10 (20.0) | 0.013 * |
| Knowledge on NPS/legal highs fairly/very significant in work | 10/17 (58.8) | 41/46 (89.1) | 69/87 (79.3) | 8/9 (88.9) | 0.052 * |

* Exact $p$-value.

Substance misuse service staff reported greater knowledge regarding NPS relative to hospital and primary care professionals. Substance misuse service professionals were also more likely to receive requests for advice and counselling regarding NPS and felt more confident about giving advice than professionals working in hospitals or primary care.

Most respondents believed that having knowledge about NPS is 'fairly' significant ($n$ = 69; 41.8%) for their work. However, many were unaware of websites or videos promoting NPS use ($n$ = 150; 84.7%). Although 120 HCPs (68.2%) were aware of illegitimate online 'pharmacies' selling medicinal products, most of the respondents were unaware of the existence of Report Illicit Drug Reactions (RIDR), the Public Health England/MHRA reporting system (https://report-illicit-drug-reaction.phe.gov.uk/) for NPS ($n$ = 134; 73.2%). The RIDR database officially closed down in January 2020 due to lack of reporting by HCPs. Moreover, 118 HCPs (67.0%) claimed a lack of awareness about NPS use for improvement of physical/mental performance. Additionally, the average age range of customers/patients using NPS was 20-29 years old, as claimed by 108 HCPs (65.9%).

Furthermore, 164 HCPs (92.1%) stated that they do not receive enough information about NPS to safely care for their patients. As indicated in Table 3, several HCPs mentioned the invaluable impact of education on NPS to keep pace with the constantly changing drug scenes. Nonetheless, most received NPS information from colleagues ($n$ = 100; 50.8%), media (e.g., TV; $n$ = 99; 50.3%), specific websites (e.g., www.novelpsychoactivesubstances.com; $n$ = 73; 37.1%), followed by email ($n$ = 59; 29.9%), service users ($n$ = 57; 28.9%), scientific literature ($n$ = 56; 28.4%), other websites (e.g., for a; $n$ = 48; 24.4%), conferences/seminars/workshops ($n$ = 44; 22.3%), online courses ($n$ = 25; 12.7%), others ($n$ = 12; 6.1 %) and short message services (SMS; $n$ = 5; 2.5%).

**Table 3.** Free text responses regarding other comments and suggestions.

| Participant | Response |
|---|---|
| Nurse, mental health hospital | "It is an issue that still has elements of being unclear as what is legal and what is now illigel [sic], however the increase and potency of the drug on the street makes it an issue that affects all aspects of society." |
| Pharmacist, substance misuse service | "NPS are not going away—and if anything, are going to get more designer and specific—we need to have understanding of their basics so we can formulate a base line approach as names and formulas change." |
| General practitioner, general practice | "should be taught in schools about dangers of these. Use in universities seems very high" |
| Family safeguard worker, substance misuse service | "Please implement training as soon as possible. It is much needed to keep abreast of information and dangers on current legal highs." |
| Pharmacist, community | "We have a significant problem with customers wanting to purchase codeine products in excess. These people are addicted to it but the only place to refer them to is the RISE addiction team who are overworked already." |

Lastly, some participants also emphasised the growing complexity surrounding NPS, which "*still has elements of being unclear of what is legal*" (nurse, mental health hospital). Perhaps, the potency of such substances may be increased as they "get more designer and specific"; thus, requiring a basic understanding on NPS is crucial to "*formulate a baseline approach as names and formulas change*" (pharmacist, substance misuse service). Several HCPs mentioned the invaluable impact of education on NPS to keep pace with the constantly changing drug scenes. Consequently, it has been addressed how education on NPS should be introduced early on and "be taught in schools about their dangers" (general practitioner, general practice). A sense of urgency was highlighted to "*implement training as soon as possible . . . to keep abreast of information and dangers on current legal highs*" (family safeguard worker, substance misuse service). Lastly, the increasing pressure that drug treatment and recovery services experience was mentioned, who appear to be "*overworked*" (pharmacist, community).

### 3.4. Feedback from Educational Training and Future Learning Needs

Of the 175 participants who gave information regarding their CPD in the previous 12 months, 152 (86.9%) included NPS/'legal highs' as part of their training and 167 (95.4%) believed that NPS should be integrated into undergraduate curricula. When HCPs were asked about their desired area for improvement (Figure 6), 'overview about product' was most frequently ranked first ($n$ = 70; 35.5%), 'clinical warnings' was most frequently ranked second ($n$ = 49, 24.9%) and 'legal status' was most frequently ranked third ($n$ = 48, 24.4%). Regarding available updates on NPS, 155 HCPs wanted to be informed regularly. Of these participants, preferred types of communication were emails ($n$ = 136; 87.7%), online course ($n$ = 77, 49.7%), specific websites ($n$ = 75; 48.4%), followed by social networks (e.g., Facebook, Twitter; $n$ = 19; 12.3%), SMS ($n$ = 10; 6.5%) and 'others' (e.g., alcohol/drug misuse training; $n$ = 8; 5.2%).

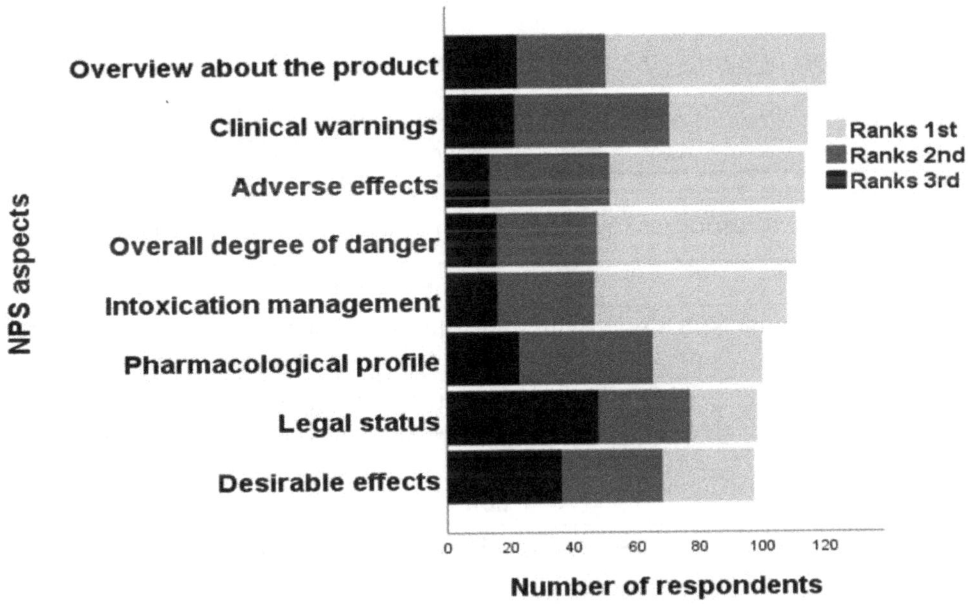


**Figure 6.** Ranking of various NPS aspects fundamental for improvement.

There were 168 HCPs who were willing to partake in further training on NPS. Preferences for mode of delivery were online ($n$ = 108; 64.3%), via workshops ($n$ = 99; 58.9%) and lectures ($n$ = 99; 58.9%), followed by blended learning ($n$ = 46; 27.4%), webinars ($n$ = 42; 25.0%) and 'others' (e.g., written information sent to practices; $n$ = 2; 1.0%).

Both the Pharmacy and GP Shared Care CPD Events addressed work-related premature mortality/intoxications related to NPS use (multi-drug use incorporating NPS) in different user groups. Feedback was obtained from the attendees ($n$ = 18) of the GP Shared Care Event (Table 4). Most believed that the issue of NPS was 'most certainly' relevant to their work area ($n$ = 12; 66.7%). Similarly, 12 GPs stated that it was 'most certainly' relevant to be aware of the risks of pregabalin and gabapentin in their daily work. There was an equal proportion of GPs that believed the event was either 'excellent' ($n$ = 9; 50.0%) or 'good' ($n$ = 9; 50.0%). Many GPs valued the topics discussed particularly about the pharmacokinetic and pharmacodynamic pathways of commonly abused drugs (Table 5). The lack of awareness amongst many GPs about the misuse potential of many POMs (e.g., pregabalin and fentanyl) was also highlighted (Table 6). Likewise, the CPD Pharmacy Event collected feedback from 21 attendees; the overall rating of the event was considered as 'excellent' by the majority ($n$ = 20; 95.2%) (Table 5). Lastly, several participants from both events (Table 6) addressed the importance of being updated regularly about drugs of abuse and addiction in general.

**Table 4.** Free text responses regarding learning from the GP Shared Care Continuing Professional Development (CPD) Event.

| Participant | Response |
|---|---|
| GP 1 | "Abuse of medications I didn't realise had abuse potential; pharmacokinetics of Gaba meds/opiates & withdrawal of Benzos." |
| GP 2 | "misuse of prescriber drugs such as tramadol & fentanyl patch." |
| GP 3 | "Pregabalin/Gabapentin have high abuse potential." |
| GP 4 | "Massive growth in NPS. Actually feel helpless against this! I ran an EMIS search immediately. We have 5 ppl (out of 14000) on repeat for fentanyl patches. I'll write to all regarding safe disposal." |
| GP 5 | "The pharmacodynamic pathways were really well explained & all makes a lot more sense again!; The number of potency of NPS's -very scary.; The prevalence of NPS in herbal/food supps." |
| GP 6 | "Lots of things about NPS; RIDR; how various drugs are abused and dangers of withdrawal." |
| GP 7 | "The pharmacodynamic pathways were really well explained & it all makes a lot more sense again!" |

**Table 5.** Free text responses regarding learning from the CPD Pharmacy Event.

| Participant | Response |
|---|---|
| Ph 1 | "Naloxone isn't always suitable antagonist for NPS; Drug wars and NPS are very prevalent; Drug tests miss a lot of drugs of abuse . . . " |
| Ph 2 | "Different classes of NPS; New substances being introduced all the time-not always detected; Rx drugs misused—gabapentin, pregabalin, venlafaxine." |
| Ph 3 | "How to educate patients on NPS; Different types of NPS; Potential drugs that can be abused (e.g., POMs)." |
| Ph 5 | "NPS market, NPS user groups; What can we do? Harm reduction, awareness . . . " |
| Ph 6 | "What NPS drugs; How dangerous NPS drugs are and the harm they can cause; Didn't know before the presentation: Buscopan, Gabapentin, Pregabalin can be abused . . . " |
| Ph 8 | "Challenges re using NPS-adverse reactions/toxicity/fatalities; Scale of the problem—in terms of use/difficulty monitoring; How quickly NPS are changing/its limitations in research . . . " |

**Table 6.** Free text responses regarding future sessions and additional comments in the evaluation of GP Shared Care Event and CPD Pharmacy Event.

| Participant | Response |
|---|---|
| Ph 4 | "more updates . . . . .. on new drugs of abuse both legal POMs Ps etc . . . and illicit" |
| Ph 9 | "Extremely informative & interesting session" |
| Ph 10 | "Regular talks to update us on them!" |
| Ph 20 | "To have more trainings, talks, workshops & to include also recovery workers; perhaps an NPS representative/head?" |
| GP 8 | "Discussion/evidence on why people abuse meds. Discussion about . . . . . . drug addiction" |
| GP 9 | "update on alcohol abuse" |
| GP 10 | "Would be nice to have back to basic update + local services again some point" |
| GP 11 | "How to identify and treat drug overdose /withdrawal." |

## 4. Discussion

### 4.1. Characteristics of HCPs

Previously, Schifano et al. [53] stressed the need for HCPs to be continuously updated with regards to the constantly changing drug scenarios to identify new, emerging trends that can help with the provision of immediate interventions. Results (Figure 4) suggested improvements where self-reported levels of knowledge on NPS were mostly 'basic' ($n$ = 76; 39.2%) and 'intermediate' ($n$ = 73; 37.6%), which is in contrast to other studies that have reported inadequate HCP knowledge [40–42]. Nurses and pharmacists, predominantly working in hospitals and substance misuse services, had the most encounters with NPS use. Hence, this is an intervention opportunity to make individuals more aware of the health-related consequences of using drugs with misuse potential when they access hospitals or substance misuse services. Provision of counselling about NPS use was less frequently done, as claimed by pharmacists in primary care who completed our survey. However, this must be treated with some caution given that purposive sampling was utilised, which comprised a small group of HCPs and therefore cannot be representative of the above-mentioned cohort of HCPs in the UK. Lack of knowledge about NPS can lead to misdiagnoses and under-recognition of potential physical and psychological repercussions of NPS use; stigma attached to seeking help for substance misuse may lead to non-engagement by NPS service users [42,54]. Hence, the topics for future educational sessions should be tailored according to the type of HCP and/or their role(s) as the context or their work area, as well as the type of clientele, may have an influence on the type of response/intervention that can be conducted by HCPs.

Both negative associations between age and ability to use electronic tools, and between age and level of NPS knowledge corroborate with the findings of Guirguis et al. [40]—the lower the age, the higher the number of NPS they were aware of. Given that most of the available educational resources on NPS are accessed online (e.g., NEPTUNE clinical guidelines or RIDR for reporting NPS adverse events), perhaps older HCPs may have less exposure to NPS-related information given their reduced use of electronic platforms.

### 4.2. NPS Types

Prescribed medications zopiclone, gabapentin and pregabalin were the most commonly known compounds listed in our survey, perhaps not unexpectedly. Feedback from the GP Shared Care CPD Event addressed a recurring theme of uncertainty about the misuse potential and proper use of medications like fentanyl and gabapentinoids. The analyses of databases provided by the EMA identified zopiclone as the most frequently reported 'Z-drug' involved in overdose and ADRs [55]. The findings also suggest caution be exercised when prescribing 'Z-drugs' to patients with psychiatric illness and/or history of drug abuse [55]. Moreover, benzodiazepines can enhance the effect of co-consumed opioids, but such co-use increases the risk of overdose through respiratory depression [33,56]. Similarly, pregabalin has been reported to cause central nervous system (CNS) depression when misused in combination with sedatives such as benzodiazepines, alcohol and opiates/opioids [57–59]. Our results suggest a high awareness of the NSO carfentanil; yet, most respondents were unaware of its misuse potential (Figure 5). The Global Drug Survey (2018) [60] stated that new opioids including acetyl fentanyl and carfentanil have caused numerous fatalities in the UK, Canada and the United States, thus requiring more awareness and greater vigilance [61]. Consequently, as a public health response, the NEPTUNE clinical guidelines about the harms and clinical management of NSOs were issued [62].

Amongst the SC, respondents were most aware of mephedrone. From the misuse of traditional substances such as ecstasy and cocaine, a shift towards injecting mephedrone is known to be popular in the 'chemsex' scene involving Men having sex with Men [63,64]. Among the miscellaneous NPS that were categorised as 'other', methoxetamine ($n$ = 17; 13.3%) and PMA/PMMA ($n$ = 15; 12.0%) were commonly known, whereas PMA/PMMA was sold as ecstasy in 'superman' tablets, which caused fatalities of party-goers on Christmas Eve 2015 [65]. Clearly, purity of sold substances is compromised where contamination often occurs with one or more controlled and uncontrolled substances [66]. Additionally, our data highlighted a poor awareness of SCRAs (e.g., MDMB-CHMICA, MDMB-FUBINACA) compared to other NPS groups (Figure 5). This is concerning as SCRAs are the largest group of NPS monitored by the EMCDDA [18]. Nonetheless, the 'spice' brand was frequently stated in the survey when asked to list what NPS were known to them. Using the street name 'spice' is inaccurate as it has become a generic term for SCRAs. Most NPS cannot be fully quantified where ingredients listed on the package are generally incomplete or false, with high variability between packages [67,68]. Further ingredients within 'spice' have been known to include the β2-mimetic clenbuterol, which potentially causes tachycardia and hypokalaemia, and tocopherol (vitamin E) possibly as a vehicle to improve intake via vaping [69].

### *4.3. Educational Sessions' Feedback*

Most HCPs expressed their need to learn more about NPS products, clinical warnings associated with them and their legal status. Although they expressed that their current source of knowledge is via peer support, media-style videos, websites, direct emails and scientific literature, they expressed their preference for online-based platforms on NPS updates, including emails, websites and online courses. However, resources must be cost-effective, regularly updated and widen the participation of most HCPs, including those who are not confident with electronic platforms. Furthermore, HCPs are often overloaded by various online training opportunities to aid their professional development. Attending a conference in which accreditation points can be collected would seem more feasible to improve their knowledge. Likewise, sending monthly newsletters to GP practices or having talks by specialists on NPS may cater to these HCPs. Overall, lectures, online and workshops were the most preferred methods of training. The World Health Organization (WHO) has recommended some effective educational strategies for HCPs [70]. These include targeted educational undergraduate and postgraduate programmes, the use of practical approaches such as artificial intelligence and point-of-care testing, evaluating effectiveness of educational methods, using indicators to monitor outcomes, developing trainers and educational resources and widening the range of HCPs being trained [70]. Further training provision for HCPs on NPS and the establishment of knowledge platforms for clinicians, health workers and social workers both locally and nationally is required [49]. This would enable the rapid dissemination of information about emerging NPS and the appropriate responses on the harms associated with them. Equally, implementation of multidisciplinary approaches by health providers in different settings (including sexual health clinics, custodial settings and drug treatment centres) can potentially improve referral pathways for NPS service users [71]. To our knowledge, evaluation of educational pedagogies for NPS have not been undertaken to date.

### *4.4. Conceptualisation of an Evidence-Informed Public Health Approach to NPS use in the UK*

Having an evidenced-based public health approach is fundamental to tackling NPS use. Uncertainties associated with the current and future public health burden of NPS suggests the importance of synthesising available data to inform national and international responses including interventions [72]. Certain NPS have transient life cycles, as 60 NPS seem to have disappeared from the market since 2013, whereas over 80 NPS became established on the global market between 2009 and 2015 [73]. Therefore, it may be inappropriate to employ evidence-based responses and regulation similar to those used for alcohol, tobacco and illicit drugs, due to the complex life cycles of NPS, along with the limited information available on their pharmacology and toxicology [74–76]. Challenges in identification and regulation are not only problematic for the legal system but also to HCPs who encounter NPS users. HCPs should have adequate knowledge about NPS classifications, user groups, NPS symptoms/effects and harm reduction strategies. In most cases, psychosocial interventions are employed in order to influence positive behavioural changes [77]. Front-line HCPs should be familiar with the PHE (Public Health England)/MHRA (Medicines and Healthcare products

Regulatory Agency) initiatives such as RIDR and the MHRA Yellow Card Scheme, which allows HCPs to report cases of suspected and actual harm from illicit substance use and ADRs from medications, respectively. HCPs can refer to the NEPTUNE clinical guidance [27,62], along with online e-learning modules, which cover the clinical management of acute and chronic harm from NPS. Similarly, a quick reference guide and factsheet on NPS [51,78,79] and a section on the PSA (2016) can be found within one of the undergraduate and postgraduate essential resources for pharmacists and pharmacy students *"RPS Medicines, Ethics and Practice (MEP)"* [69], all of which have been co-developed by the corresponding author of this manuscript and are accessible via the RPS website for pharmacy professionals [79].

### *4.5. Implications and Recommendations for Policy-making and Clinical Practice*

Specific treatment recommendations for ADRs associated with NPS is limited. Hence, PHE's preliminary advice is to focus on individuals' presenting symptoms rather than substance identification [43,77]. With the continuous growth of this market and increasing research, it became clear that identification of NPS through the classification of subcategories/subfamilies/derivatives with similar substructure or chemical backbone may assist HCPs in tailoring appropriate treatment for a patient [74]. In addition, chemical analyses of NPS voluntarily submitted by service users suggest that NPS were frequently consumed with other substances rather than in isolation [79]. In the era of digital healthcare, drug checking within a substance misuse service has been trialled by pharmacists and has enabled the provision of tailored harm reduction advice on the basis of a holistic multi-disciplinary approach [80]. Combining NPS with other substances may be intentionally used as a means to self-medicate to counteract side-effects of illicit substances [81]. However, users may unintentionally be consuming NPS mixtures with unclaimed ingredients [66]. Adulterants and bulking agents including benzocaine, caffeine, lidocaine, phenacetin and procaine were found to be commonly combined with NPS, especially in SC mixtures [81–83]. Their presence may produce synergistic, additive, supra-additive effects, and hence potentiate the effects of controlled drugs of abuse [84]. Similarly, involuntary contamination or presence of by-products from incomplete chemical reactions during the illicit manufacture of NPS may lead to inadvertent intoxication [85].

It is therefore recommended that GPs and non-medical prescribers should be vigilant when reviewing vulnerable individuals, especially those that are prescribed medicines that are particularly liable to misuse: gabapentinoids, antidepressants, antipsychotics and opioid analgesics [57]. Community pharmacists in primary care can provide harm reduction services including needle and syringe exchange/provision and advice on safer injecting techniques [79]. Additionally, during medicine reconciliations, NPS use may be identified by pharmacists, which may prompt appropriate advice to be given and/or referrals to be made [86]. Schifano and Chiappini [87] identified 1085 cardiovascular-related loperamide adverse drug reactions from the EMA's EV during 2005-2017. Given that community pharmacists are potentially the first point-of-contact able to identify a repeat supply issue, their links with prescribers/clinicians should be enhanced for appropriate referrals to be made, thus allowing individuals to have more access to treatment services [88].

HCPs in hospitals, particularly nurses, pharmacists and doctors, should receive educational resources that are tailored to the clinical management of NPS-related adverse acute toxicity. Other HCPs including paramedics, first-responders, ambulance staff and first-aid responders should also access optimal and up-to-date NPS-related information about managing suspected toxicity arising from NPS use from the National Poisons Information Service (NPIS) through its telephone service and TOXBASE database. Care bundles can help in the management of acute intoxication and overdose (e.g., NEPTUNE care bundle on the harms of synthetic cannabinoid receptor agonists), particularly where individuals may have taken more than one substance [89,90]. Hence, treatment can be delivered safely and consistently within routine clinical practice. Similarly, the 'Drugs Wheel' designed by Mark Adley [91] can be utilised by HCPs, as it provides a simpler method of learning drugs by their category.

Referrals to sexual health services can help educate individuals about the repercussions of partaking in high-risk sexual activities (e.g., 'chemsex') and address the prevention and treatment of sexually transmitted infections. Equally, it is also important to highlight the issue of emerging styles of alcohol consumption such as 'binge' drinking in future educational sessions for HCPs, as this has been reported by various studies as concurrent with poly-NPS abuse, which can potentially worsen a patient's clinical presentation [92–94].

The private sectors providing drug treatment services should have access to evidence-based psychosocial and pharmacological approaches in order to increase an individual's likelihood of recovery, as recommended by the 'Orange Guidelines' [95]. Ralphs and Gray [54] also recommended clearer referral pathways and strengthened links between existing drug treatment services, where more innovative strategies should be implemented to increase the engagement from NPS service users.

Perhaps it may be more beneficial to provide objective regular assessments for HCPs, which test their awareness of NPS (e.g., clinical management, presenting symptoms, NPS classification). Wood et al. [43] recommended the utilisation of objective measures through simulation studies or objective structured clinical examinations (OSCEs) to ascertain knowledge. Potentially, this provides a more detailed measure of a HCP's areas of strength or weakness and whether this is determined by how much exposure to NPS they obtain in their workplace.

Lastly, databases, such as the EMA's EV, which is considered worldwide as an exemplar, should be maintained to capture NPS-related adverse effects along with data about accident and emergency admissions [96]. Moreover, information-sharing should be improved at national, European and global levels to enable more prompt responses when highly toxic NPS are identified.

### *4.6. Limitations of Research and Suggestions for Future Research*

Purposive sampling via the distribution of the paper-based surveys to the respondents present in the events described above may have introduced a possible bias because it only gathered the views of a limited number of HCPs who may have genuine interest in knowing more about NPS. Additionally, it may be open to selection bias due to lack of random sampling [97]. Likewise, the Qualtrics survey may be limited to those who were only confident in answering the survey online. Given the cross-sectional nature of the survey, generalisability of our results should be treated with caution given that we have made inferences from a group of purposively sampled HCPs at one point in time. Indeed, our results provide a perception of their current baseline knowledge, but it should be emphasised that NPS consumption fluctuates regionally and over time [98]. Future studies should involve more data from these geographical regions as well as from Wales, Scotland and Northern Ireland and should include more representation of specialist doctors (e.g., general and addiction psychiatrists) and emergency service personnel (e.g., paramedics) to obtain an even distribution of HCPs, including private sectors, across the UK and in different settings, and to make the data more generalisable across the UK. Further research is needed in order to evaluate the pedagogic strategies employed to improve HCP's knowledge of NPS.

## 5. Conclusions

Despite the overall evidence of lack/poor knowledge of HCPs of NPS, the provision of educational CPD workshops showed an improvement within the self-reported knowledge of HCPs on NPS in comparison to previous studies. The health sector may have a considerable impact on NPS knowledge that HCPs can acquire.

Continual education about NPS is indeed fundamental for the provision of improved harm reduction interventions, better referral pathways, effective dissemination of information and sharing of best practice to help NPS service users achieve full recovery and enhance their care throughout their treatment journey. Through this research, we recommend adopting innovative approaches for drug identification such as novel point-of-care testing that can be undertaken on-site, especially at emergency settings, by HCPs. We also recommend inclusion of integrated NPS toxicology/pharmacology/psychopathology education in undergraduate and postgraduate national healthcare curricula. The provision of regular updates through accredited quality-assured sector- and specialty-specific online platforms coupled with targeted and tailored educational tools. Connecting educators through peer-support to enhance the impact of these educational resources is also recommended. This is especially important, as NPS of varying types continue to emerge, and drug scenarios are ever-changing.

**Author Contributions:** A.G. conceived the paper, the main conceptual ideas and proof outline, and designed the study. C.R. wrote the first draft and led the analysis of the results under the supervision of A.G. A.G., J.M.C. and H.Z. were involved in the development of the questionnaire. J.M.C. advised on the NPS to be included. A.G. and F.S. delivered the educational sessions. N.S. advised and reviewed the statistical work. A.-M.F., G.H., H.Z., R.G. and S.B. collected the information from various sources. All authors reviewed and contributed to the writing of the paper. All authors have read and agreed to the published version of the manuscript.

**Acknowledgments:** The authors would like to acknowledge the support of the RPS and Gareth Kitson (RPS), the University of Hertfordshire, CGL, CMHP, Addaction and the independent mental health hospitals that assisted in disseminating the survey.

**Ethics Statement:** Ethics approval was granted by the Health, Science, Engineering and Technology Ethics Committee with Delegated Authority, University of Hertfordshire, Hatfield, UK (16 August 2017; protocol number LMS/SF/UH/02951;PHAEC/1042-Recreational Drugs' European Network: an ICT prevention service addressing the use of a novel compound in vulnerable individuals).

## References

1. UNODC. *The Challenge of New Psychoactive Substances*; United Nation Office on Drugs and Crime: Vienna, Austria, 2013. Available online: https://www.unodc.org/documents/scientific/NPS_2013_SMART.pdf (accessed on 19 September 2019).
2. EMCDDA-Europol. *The state of the drugs problem in Europe—Annual report 2012*; Publications Office of the European Union: Luxembourg; Available online: http://www.emcdda.europa.eu/attachements.cfm/att_190854_EN_TDAC12001ENC_.pdf (accessed on 19 September 2019).
3. ACMD. *Consideration of the Novel Psychoactive Substances ('Legal Highs')*; Advisory Council on the Misuse of Drugs, Home Office: London, UK, 2011. Available online: https://assets.publishing.service.gov.uk/government/uploads/system/uploads/attachment_data/file/119139/acmdnps2011.pdf (accessed on 19 September 2019).
4. *Psychoactive Substances Act 2016*; The Stationary Office Limited, 2016. Available online: https://www.legislation.gov.uk/ukpga/2016/2/pdfs/ukpga_20160002_en.pdf (accessed on 19 September 2019).
5. Schifano, F. Recent Changes in Drug Abuse Scenarios: The New/Novel Psychoactive Substances (NPS) Phenomenon. *Brain Sci.* **2018**, *8*, 221. [CrossRef] [PubMed]
6. Corkery, J.; Orsolini, L.; Papanti, D.; Schifano, F. Novel psychoactive substances (NPS) and recent scenarios: Epidemiological, anthropological and clinical pharmacological issues. In *Light in Forensic Science: Issues and Applications*; Royal Society of Chemistry: London, UK, 2018; Chapter 8; pp. 207–256.
7. Goodair, C.M.; Corkery, J.; Claridge, H. Legal highs: A problem of definitions? *Lett. Lancet* **2014**, *383*, 1715. [CrossRef]
8. Home Office. *Review of the Psychoactive Substances Act 2016*; Home Office: London, UK, 2018. Available online: https://www.gov.uk/government/publications/review-of-the-psychoactive-substances-act-2016 (accessed on 26 February 2020).
9. Deligianni, E.; Daniel, O.J.; Corkery, J.M.; Schifano, F.; Lione, L. Impact of the UK Psychoactive Substances Act on awareness, use, experiences and knowledge of potential associated health risks of Novel Psychoactive Substances. *Br. J. Clin. Pharmacol.* **2019**. [CrossRef] [PubMed]

10. UNODC. *UNODC World Drug Report*; United Nations Office on Drugs and Crime: Vienna, Austria, 2018. Available online: https://www.unodc.org/LSS/announcement/Details/fa879924-6bdf-4ba2-a8eb-a87185d26439 (accessed on 19 September 2019).
11. UNODC. *UNODC-SMART: Almost 900 NPS Reported to UNODC from 119 countries and territories*; United Nations Office on Drugs and Crime: Vienna, Austria, 2019. Available online: https://www.unodc.org/LSS/Announcement/Details/eff8dc38-7ab0-42b0-8cd9-753b89953fcc (accessed on 19 September 2019).
12. Dignam, G.; Bigham, C. Novel psychoactive substances: A practical approach to dealing with toxicity from legal highs. *BJA Educ.* **2017**, *17*, 172–177. [CrossRef]
13. Winstock, A.; Barratt, M.; Maier, L.; Aldridge, A.; Zhuparis, A.; Davies, E.; Ferris, J. Global Drug Survey (GDS) 2019 Key Findings Report. 2019. Available online: https://www.globaldrugsurvey.com/gds-2019/ (accessed on 26 February 2020).
14. ONS. *Deaths related to drug poisoning in England and Wales: 2018 registrations*; Office for National Statistics: Newport, Gwent, 2019. Available online: https://www.ons.gov.uk/peoplepopulationandcommunity/birthsdeathsandmarriages/deaths/bulletins/deathsrelatedtodrugpoisoninginenglandandwales/2018registrations/pdf (accessed on 19 September 2019).
15. NRS. *Drug-related Deaths in Scotland in 2018*; National Records of Scotland: Edinburgh, Scotland, 2019. Available online: https://www.nrscotland.gov.uk/files//statistics/drug-related-deaths/2018/drug-related-deaths-18-pub.pdf (accessed on 19 September 2019).
16. Webb, N.E.; Wood, D.M.; Greene, S.L.; Hunter, L.J.; Archer, J.R.H.; Dines, A.M.; Dargan, P.I. Change in the new psychoactive substances associated with Emergency Department acute toxicity presentations associated with the introduction of the UK 2016 Psychoactive Substances Act. *Clin. Toxicol.* **2019**, *57*, 36–41. [CrossRef]
17. Henshall, D.E.; Innes, C.W.; Morrison, S.R.; Wilson, B.; Brown, R.A.; McAllister, S.M.; Reda, E. A prospective observational study of emergency department presentations following novel psychoactive substance use. *Scott. Med. J.* **2018**, *63*, 39–44. [CrossRef]
18. EMCDDA. *Fentanils and Synthetic Cannabinoids: Driving Greater Complexity into the Drug Situation*; European Monitoring Centre for Drugs and Drug Addiction: Lisbon, Portugal, 2018. Available online: http://www.emcdda.europa.eu/system/files/publications/8870/2018-2489-td0118414enn.pdf (accessed on 19 September 2019).
19. Janssen, P.A. Potent, new analgesics, tailor-made for different purposes. *Acta Anaesthesiol. Scand.* **1982**, *26*, 262–268. [CrossRef]
20. WHO. *Carfentanil Critical Review Report Agenda Item 4.8 Expert Committee*; World Health Organisation: Geneva, Switzerland, 2017; Available online: https://www.who.int/medicines/access/controlled-substances/Critical_Review_Carfentanil.pdf (accessed on 26 February 2020).
21. Baumann, M.H.; Majumdar, S.; Le Rouzic, V.; Hunkele, A.; Uprety, R.; Huang, X.P.; Pasternak, G.W. Pharmacological characterization of novel synthetic opioids (NSO) found in the recreational drug marketplace. *Neuropharmacology* **2018**, *134*, 101–107. [CrossRef]
22. Schifano, F.; Chiappini, S.; Corkery, J.M.; Guirguis, A. Assessing the 2004–2018 Fentanyl Misusing Issues Reported to an International Range of Adverse Reporting Systems. *Front. Pharmacol.* **2019**, *10*, 1–10. [CrossRef]
23. Martinotti, G.; Cinosi, E.; Santacroce, R.; Papanti, D.; Pasquini, A.; Mancini, V.; erino del Villar, C. Substance-related psychopathology and aggressiveness in a nightlife holiday resort: Results from a pilot study in a psychiatric inpatient unit in Ibiza. *Hum. Psychopharmacol.* **2017**, *32*, 2586. [CrossRef]
24. Shafi, A.; Gallagher, P.; Stewart, N.; Martinotti, G.; Corazza, O. The risk of violence associated with novel psychoactive substance misuse in patients presenting to acute mental health services. *Hum. Psychopharmacol. Clin. Exp.* **2017**, *32*, e2606. [CrossRef] [PubMed]
25. EMCDDA. *European Drug Report Trends and Developments*; European Monitoring Centre for Drugs and Drug Addiction: Lisbon, Portugal, 2018. Available online: http://www.emcdda.europa.eu/system/files/publications/8585/20181816_TDAT18001ENN_PDF.pdf (accessed on 19 September 2019).
26. Fujita, Y.; Koeda, A.; Fujino, Y.; Onodera, M.; Kikuchi, S.; Niitsu, H.; Inoue, Y. Clinical and toxicological findings of acute intoxication with synthetic cannabinoids and cathinones. *Acute Med. Surg.* **2016**, *3*, 230–236. [CrossRef] [PubMed]

27. Abdulrahim, D.; Bowden-Jones, O.; On behalf of the NEPTUNE Group. *Guidance on the Clinical Management of Acute and Chronic Harms of Club Drugs and Novel Psychoactive Substances*; The Health Foundation: London, UK, 2015; Available online: http://neptune-clinical-guidance.co.uk/wp-content/uploads/2015/03/NEPTUNE-Guidance-March-2015.pdf (accessed on 19 September 2019).
28. Bourne, A.; Reid, D.; Hickson, F.; Torres-Rueda, S.; Weatherburn, P. Illicit drug use in sexual settings ('chemsex') and HIV/STI transmission risk behaviour among gay men in South London: Findings from a qualitative study. *Sex. Transm. Infect.* **2015**, *91*, 564–568. [CrossRef] [PubMed]
29. Bourne, A.; Reid, D.; Hickson, F.; Torres-Rueda, S.; Steinberg, P.; Weatherburn, P. "Chemsex" and harm reduction need among gay men in South London. *Int. J. Drug Policy* **2015**, *26*, 1171–1176. [CrossRef] [PubMed]
30. Chiappini, S.; Schifano, F. A Decade of Gabapentinoid Misuse: An Analysis of the European Medicines Agency's 'Suspected Adverse Drug Reactions' Database. *CNS Drugs* **2016**, *30*, 647–654. [CrossRef]
31. Daly, C.; Griffin, E.; Ashcroft, D.M.; Webb, R.T.; Perry, I.J.; Arensman, E. Intentional Drug Overdose Involving Pregabalin and Gabapentin: Findings from the National Self-Harm Registry Ireland, 2007–2015. *Clin. Drug Investig.* **2018**, *38*, 373–380. [CrossRef]
32. Reeves, R.R.; Ladner, M.E. Potentiation of the Effect of Buprenorphine/Naloxone With Gabapentin or Quetiapine. *Am. J. Psychiatry* **2014**, *171*, 691. [CrossRef]
33. EMCDDA. *The misuse of benzodiazepines among high-risk opioid users in Europe*; European Monitoring Centre for Drugs and Drug Addiction: Lisbon, Portugal, 2018. Available online: http://www.emcdda.europa.eu/system/files/publications/2733/Misuse%20of%20benzos_POD2015.pdf (accessed on 26 February 2020).
34. Johnson, C.F.; Barnsdale, L.R.; McAuley, A. Investigating the role of benzodiazepines in drug-related mortality: A systematic review undertaken on behalf of The Scottish National Forum on Drug-Related Deaths. 2016. Available online: https://dspace.stir.ac.uk/handle/1893/23220#.XCtFKlz7TtQ (accessed on 19 September 2019).
35. Manchester, K.R.; Lomas, E.C.; Waters, L.; Dempsey, F.C.; Maskell, P.D. The emergence of new psychoactive substance (NPS) benzodiazepines: A review. *Drug Test. Anal.* **2018**, *10*, 37–53. [CrossRef]
36. NRS. *Drug-related deaths in Scotland 2016*; National Records of Scotland: Edinburgh, Scotland, 2017. Available online: https://www.nrscotland.gov.uk/files//statistics/drug-related-deaths/drd2016/drug-related-deaths-16-pub.pdf (accessed on 19 September 2019).
37. NRS. *Drug-related deaths in Scotland in 2017*; National Records of Scotland: Edinburgh, Scotland, 2018. Available online: https://www.nrscotland.gov.uk/files/statistics/drug-related-deaths/17/drug-related-deaths-17-pub.pdf (accessed on 19 September 2019).
38. Campbell, A.; O Neill, N.; Higgins, K. Health and Social Care workers' perceptions of NPS use in Northern Ireland. *Int. J. Drug Policy* **2017**, *40*, 93–101. [CrossRef]
39. Gittins, R.; Guirguis, A.; Schifano, F.; Maidment, I. Exploration of the use of new psychoactive substances by individuals in treatment for substance misuse in the UK. *Brain Sci.* **2018**, *8*, 58. [CrossRef]
40. Guirguis, A.; Corkery, J.M.; Stair, J.L.; Kirton, S.; Zloh, M.; Goodair, C.M.; Davidson, C. Survey of knowledge of legal highs (novel psychoactive substances) amongst London pharmacists. *Drugs Alcohol Today* **2015**, *15*, 93–99. [CrossRef]
41. Hughes, E.; Bressington, D.; Sharratt, K.; Gray, R. Novel psychoactive substance use by mental health service consumers: An online survey of inpatient health professionals' views and experiences. *Adv. Dual Diagn.* **2018**, *11*, 30–39. [CrossRef]
42. Owie, R.E.; Gosney, P.; Roney, A.; O'brien, A. Psychiatrists' knowledge of novel psychoactive substances. *Drugs Alcohol Today* **2017**, *17*, 178–185. [CrossRef]
43. Wood, D.M.; Ceronie, B.; Dargan, P.I. Healthcare professionals are less confident in managing acute toxicity related to the use of new psychoactive substances (NPS) compared with classical recreational drugs. *QJM* **2016**, *109*, 527–529. [CrossRef] [PubMed]
44. Simonato, P.; Corazza, O.; Santonastaso, P.; Corkery, J.; Deluca, P.; Davey, Z.; Schifano, F. Novel psychoactive substances as a novel challenge for health professionals: Results from an Italian survey. *Hum. Psychopharmacol. Clin. Exp.* **2013**, *28*, 324–331. [CrossRef] [PubMed]
45. Corazza, O.; Assi, S.; Trincas, G.; Simonato, G.; Corkery, J.; Davey, Z.; Deluca, P. Novel Drugs, Novel Solutions: Exploring the potential of technological tools for prevention of drug abuse. *Ital. J. Addict.* **2011**, *1*, 25–30.

46. ReDNet Research Group. Le nuove potenzialità della prevenzione digitale in materia di nuove droghe—Research Database—University of Hertfordshire. Dipendenze Patologiche. 2010. Available online: http://researchprofiles.herts.ac.uk/portal/en/publications/le-nuove-potenzialita-della-prevenzione-digitale-in-materia-di-nuove-droghe(e4511105-5c1d-479f-b9ea-e6bea4e489c7)/export.html (accessed on 19 September 2019).
47. Tracy, D.K.; Wood, D.M.; Baumeister, D. Novel psychoactive substances: Identifying and managing acute and chronic harmful use. *BMJ (Clin. Res. Ed.)* **2017**, *356*, 6814. [CrossRef]
48. Tracy, D.K.; Wood, D.M.; Baumeister, D. Novel psychoactive substances: Types, mechanisms of action, and effects. *BMJ (Clin. Res. Ed.)* **2017**, *356*, 6848. [CrossRef]
49. EMCDDA-Europol. *EMCDDA–Europol 2017 Annual Report on the implementation of Council Decision 2005/387/JHA*; European Monitoring Centre for Drugs and Drug Addiction: Lisbon, Portugal, 2017. Available online: http://www.emcdda.europa.eu/system/files/publications/9282/20183924_TDAN18001ENN_PDF.pdf (accessed on 19 September 2019).
50. Macleod, S. Likert Scale. Simply Psychology. 2008. Available online: https://www.simplypsychology.org/likert-scale.html (accessed on 19 September 2019).
51. Guirguis, A.; Hawksworth, G.; Bond, C.; Lawrence, J.; Martini, L.G. *New Psychoactive Substances: A Guide for Pharmacists*; Royal Pharmaceutical Society: London, UK, 2018; Available online: https://www.rpharms.com/Portals/0/RPS%20document%20library/Open%20access/Science/RPS%20NPS%20Fact%20sheet.pdf?ver=2018-06-18-141822-160 (accessed on 19 September 2019).
52. Batisse, A.; Grégoire, M.; Marillier, M.; Fortias, M.; Djezzar, S. Usage de cathinones à Paris. *L'Encéphale* **2016**, *42*, 354–360. [CrossRef]
53. Schifano, F.; Leoni, M.; Martinotti, G.; Rawaf, S.; Rovetto, F. Importance of cyberspace for the assessment of the drug abuse market: Preliminary results from the Psychonaut 2002 project. *Cyberpsychology Behav.* **2003**, *6*, 405–410. [CrossRef]
54. Ralphs, R.; Gray, P. New psychoactive substances: New service provider challenges. *Drugs Educ. Prev. Policy* **2018**, *25*, 301–312. [CrossRef]
55. Schifano, F.; Chiappini, S.; Corkery, J.M.; Guirguis, A. An Insight into Z-Drug Abuse and Dependence: An Examination of Reports to the European Medicines Agency Database of Suspected Adverse Drug Reactions. *Int. J. Neuropsychopharmacol.* **2019**, *22*, 270–277. [CrossRef] [PubMed]
56. White, J.M.; Irvine, R.J. Mechanisms of fatal opioid overdose. *Addiction (Abingdon Engl.)* **1999**, *94*, 961–972. [CrossRef]
57. Schifano, F.; Chiappini, S.; Corkery, J.M.; Guirguis, A. Abuse of prescription drugs in the context of novel psychoactive substances (NPS): A systematic review. *Brain Sci.* **2018**, *8*, 73. [CrossRef] [PubMed]
58. Cairns, R.; Schaffer, A.L.; Ryan, N.; Pearson, S.; Buckley, N.A. Rising pregabalin use and misuse in Australia: Trends in utilization and intentional poisonings. *Addiction* **2019**, *114*, 1026–1034. [CrossRef] [PubMed]
59. Schifano, F.; Chiappini, S. Pregabalin: A range of misuse-related unanswered questions. *CNS Neurosci. Ther.* **2019**, *25*, 659–660. [CrossRef]
60. Winstock, A.; Barratt, M.; Maier, L.; Aldridge, A.; Zhuparis, A.; Davies, E.; Ferris, J. Global Drug Survey (GDS) 2018 Key Findings Report. 2018. Available online: https://www.globaldrugsurvey.com/gds-2018/ (accessed on 26 February 2020).
61. Hikin, L.; Smith, P.R.; Ringland, E.; Hudson, S.; Morley, S.R. Multiple fatalities in the North of England associated with synthetic fentanyl analogue exposure: Detection and quantitation a case series from early 2017. *Forensic Sci. Int.* **2018**, *282*, 179–183. [CrossRef]
62. Abdulrahim, D.; Bowden-Jones, O. *The Misuse of Synthetic Opioids: Harms and Clinical Management of Fentanyl, Fentanyl Analogues and Other Novel Synthetic Opioids Information for Clinicians*; The Health Foundation: London, UK, 2018; Available online: http://neptune-clinical-guidance.co.uk/wp-content/uploads/2018/03/The-misuse-of-synthetic-opioids.pdf (accessed on 19 September 2019).
63. Bourne, A.; Reid, D.; Hickson, F.; Torres, S.; Weatherburn, R.P. *The Chemsex Study: Drug Use in Sexual Settings Among Gay and Bisexual Men in Lambeth, Southwark and Lewisham*; Sigma Research, London School of Hygiene & Tropical Medicine, 2014. Available online: https://www.lambeth.gov.uk/sites/default/files/ssh-chemsex-study-final-main-report.pdf (accessed on 19 September 2019).

64. Keogh, P.; Reid, D.; Bourne, A.; Weatherburn, P.; Hickson, F.; Jessup, K.; Hammond, G. *Wasted Opportunities: Problematic Alcohol and Drug Use among Gay Men and Bisexual Men*; Sigma Research, London School of Hygiene & Tropical Medicine, 2009; Available online: http://researchonline.lshtm.ac.uk/1408/ (accessed on 19 September 2019).
65. Sample, I. 'Superman' pill deaths spark calls for dangerous-drugs alert system. *The Guardian*. 2015. Available online: https://www.theguardian.com/society/2015/jan/16/superman-pill-deaths-dangerous-drugs-alert-system (accessed on 19 September 2019).
66. Guirguis, A.; Corkery, J.M.; Stair, J.L.; Zloh, M.; Kirton, S.B.; Schifano, F. Intended and unintended use of cathinone mixtures. *J. Hum. Psychopharmacol. Clin. Exp.* **2017**, *32*. [CrossRef]
67. Hillebrand, J.; Olszewski, D.; Sedefov, R. Legal Highs on the Internet. *Subst. Use Misuse* **2010**, *45*, 330–340. [CrossRef]
68. Simolka, K.; Lindigkeit, R.; Schiebel, H.-M.; Papke, U.; Ernst, L.; Beuerle, T. Analysis of synthetic cannabinoids in "spice-like" herbal highs: Snapshot of the German market in summer 2011. *Anal. Bioanal. Chem.* **2012**, *404*, 157–171. [CrossRef]
69. Guirguis, A.; Hawksworth, G.; Bond, C.; Lawrence, J.M.; Martini, L.G. New psychoactive substances. In *Quick Reference Guides*; Royal Pharmaceutical Society: London, UK, 2018; Available online: https://www.rpharms.com/resources/quick-reference-guides/new-psychoactive-substances (accessed on 19 September 2019).
70. World Health Organization. *Technical Series on Safer Primary Care. Education and Training: Technical Series on Safer Primary Care*; World Health Organization: Geneva, Switzerland, 2016; ISBN 978-92-4-151160-5.
71. EMCDDA. *Health Responses to New Psychoactive Substances*; European Monitoring Centre for Drugs and Drug Addiction: Lisbon, Portugal, 2016. Available online: http://www.emcdda.europa.eu/system/files/publications/2812/TD0216555ENN.pdf (accessed on 19 September 2019).
72. Meader, N.; Mdege, N.; McCambridge, J. The public health evidence-base on novel psychoactive substance use: Scoping review with narrative synthesis of selected bodies of evidence. *J. Public Health (Oxf. Engl.)* **2018**, *40*, e303–e319. [CrossRef] [PubMed]
73. UNODC. *Market Analysis of Synthetic Drugs. Amphetamine-Type Stimulants, New Psychoactive Substances. World Drug Report 2017*; United Nations Office on Drugs and Crime: Vienna, Austria, 2017. Available online: http://www.unodc.org/documents/scientific/Booklet_4_Market_Analysis_of_Synthetic_Drugs_ATS_NPS.pdf (accessed on 19 September 2019).
74. Guirguis, A. New psychoactive substances: A public health issue. *Int. J. Pharm. Pract.* **2017**, *25*, 323–325. [CrossRef] [PubMed]
75. EMCDDA. *Health and Social Responses to Drug Problems. A European Guide*; European Monitoring Centre for Drugs and Drug Addiction: Lisbon, Portugal, 2017. Available online: https://publications.europa.eu/en/publication-detail/-/publication/d8574d27-ae31-11e7-837e-01aa75ed71a1/language-en (accessed on 19 September 2019).
76. Strang, J.; Babor, T.; Caulkins, J.; Fischer, B.; Foxcroft, D.; Humphreys, K. Drug policy and the public good: Evidence for effective interventions. *Lancet* **2012**, *379*, 71–83. [CrossRef]
77. PHE. *New Psychoactive Substances (A toolkit for Substance Misuse Commissioners)*; Public Health England: London, UK, 2014. Available online: https://assets.publishing.service.gov.uk/government/uploads/system/uploads/attachment_data/file/669429/nps-a-toolkit-for-substance-misuse-commissioners.pdf (accessed on 19 September 2019).
78. Guirguis, A.; Lawrence, M.J. New Psychoactive Substances (NPS). In *Medicines, Ethics and Practice. The Professional Guide for Pharmacists*, 41st ed.; Tang, W., Ed.; Royal Pharmaceutical Society: London, UK, 2017; pp. 90–91.
79. Royal Pharmaceutical Society. Medicines, Ethics and Practice (MEP) 43. 2019. Available online: https://www.rpharms.com/resources/publications/medicines-ethics-and-practice-mep (accessed on 19 September 2019).
80. Helander, A.; Beck, O.; Hägerkvist, R.; Hultén, P. Identification of novel psychoactive drug use in Sweden based on laboratory analysis—Initial experiences from the STRIDA project. *Scand. J. Clin. Lab. Investig.* **2013**, *73*, 400–406. [CrossRef] [PubMed]
81. Burns, C. First Home Office-licensed street drug-testing clinic opens. *Pharm. J.* **2019**, *302*, 7923.
82. Chary, M.; Yi, D.; Manini, A.F. Candyflipping and Other Combinations: Identifying Drug-Drug Combinations from an Online Forum. *Front. Psychiatry* **2018**, *9*, 135–144. [CrossRef]

83. Alotaibi, M.R.; Husbands, S.M.; Blagbrough, I.S. 1H, 13C, 15N HMBC, and 19F NMR spectroscopic characterisation of seized flephedrone, cut with benzocaine. *J. Pharm. Biomed. Anal.* **2015**, *107*, 535–538. [CrossRef]
84. Kavanagh, P.; O'Brien, J.; Fox, J.; O'Donnell, C.; Christie, R.; Power, J.D.; McDermott, S.D. The analysis of substituted cathinones. Part 3. Synthesis and characterisation of 2,3-methylenedioxy substituted cathinones. *Forensic Sci. Int.* **2012**, *216*, 19–28. [CrossRef]
85. Zuba, D.; Byrska, B. Prevalence and co-existence of active components of "legal highs.". *Drug Test. Anal* **2013**, *5*, 420–429. [CrossRef]
86. Zamengo, L.; Frison, G.; Bettin, C.; Sciarrone, R. Understanding the risks associated with the use of new psychoactive substances (NPS): High variability of active ingredients concentration, mislabelled preparations, multiple psychoactive substances in single products. *Toxicol. Lett.* **2014**, *229*, 220–228. [CrossRef]
87. Guirguis, A. Novel psychoactive substances: Understanding the new illegal drug market. *Clin. Pharm.* **2018**, *10*, 1116. [CrossRef]
88. Schifano, F.; Chiappini, S. Is there such a thing as a "lope" dope? Analysis of loperamide-related European Medicines Agency (EMA) pharmacovigilance database reports. *PLoS ONE* **2018**, *13*, 1–12. [CrossRef] [PubMed]
89. Schifano, F.; Papanti, G.D.; Orsolini, L.; Corkery, J.M. The consequences of drug misuse on post-marketing surveillance. *Expert Rev. Clin. Pharmacol.* **2016**, *9*, 867–871. [CrossRef]
90. Lavallée, J.F.; Gray, T.A.; Dumville, J.; Russell, W.; Cullum, N. The effects of care bundles on patient outcomes: A systematic review and meta-analysis. *Implement. Sci.* **2017**, *12*, 142. [CrossRef] [PubMed]
91. Abdulrahim, D.; Bowden-Jones, O. *Harms of Synthetic Cannabinoid Receptor Agonists (SCRAs) and Their Management*; The Health Foundation: London, UK, 2016; Available online: http://neptune-clinical-guidance.co.uk/wp-content/uploads/2016/07/Synthetic-Cannabinoid-Receptor-Agonists.pdf (accessed on 19 September 2019).
92. Adley, M. The Drugs Wheel. Version 2.0.6. 2018. Available online: http://www.thedrugswheel.com/ (accessed on 16 April 2019).
93. Bersani, F.S.; Corazza, O.; Albano, G.; Valeriani, G.; Santacroce, R.; Bolzan Mariotti Posocco, F.; Schifano, F. 25C-NBOMe: Preliminary data on pharmacology, psychoactive effects, and toxicity of a new potent and dangerous hallucinogenic drug. *Biomed Res. Int.* **2014**, *2014*, 734749. [CrossRef] [PubMed]
94. Martinotti, G.; Lupi, M.; Acciavatti, T.; Cinosi, E.; Santacroce, R.; Signorelli, M.S.; Alvin di Giannantonio, M. Novel psychoactive substances in young adults with and without psychiatric comorbidities. *Biomed Res. Int.* **2014**, *2014*, 815424. [CrossRef]
95. Vento, A.E.; Martinotti, G.; Cinosi, E.; Lupi, M.; Acciavatti, T.; Carrus, D.; Schifano, F. Substance Use in the Club Scene of Rome: A Pilot Study. *Biomed Res. Int.* **2014**, *2014*, 617546. [CrossRef]
96. Independent Expert Working Group. *Drug Misuse and Dependence: UK Guidelines on Clinical Management*; Department of Health: London, UK, 2017. Available online: https://assets.publishing.service.gov.uk/government/uploads/system/uploads/attachment_data/file/673978/clinical_guidelines_2017.pdf (accessed on 19 September 2019).
97. Schifano, F.; Chiappini, S. Is there a potential of misuse for venlafaxine and bupropion? *Front. Pharmacol.* **2018**, *9*, 239. [CrossRef]
98. Etikan, I.; Musa, S.A.; Alkassim, R.S. Comparison of Convenience Sampling and Purposive Sampling. *Am. J. Theor. Appl. Stat.* **2016**, *5*, 1. [CrossRef]

# 4

# Exploration of the Use of New Psychoactive Substances by Individuals in Treatment for Substance Misuse in the UK

**Rosalind Gittins [1,*], Amira Guirguis [2,*], Fabrizio Schifano [2] and Ian Maidment [3]**

1 Addaction, 67-69 Cowcross St., London EC1M 6PU, UK
2 Psychopharmacology, Drug Misuse and Novel Psychoactive Substances Research Unit, University of Hertfordshire, Hatfield AL10 9AB, UK; f.schifano@herts.ac.uk
3 Pharmacy Department, School of Life and Health Sciences, Aston University, Birmingham B4 7ET, UK; i.maidment@aston.ac.uk
* Correspondence: Roz.Gittins@addaction.org.uk (R.G.); a.guirguis2@herts.ac.uk (A.G.)

**Abstract:** Substance misuse services need to meet the growing demand and needs of individuals using new psychoactive substances (NPS). A review of the literature identified a paucity of research regarding NPS use by these individuals and UK guidelines outline the need for locally tailored strategies. The purpose of this qualitative study was to identify and explore key themes in relation to the use of NPS by individuals receiving community treatment for their substance use. Electronic records identified demographics and semi-structured interviews were undertaken. A thematic analysis of transcripts identified a variety of substance use histories; 50% were prescribed opiate substitutes and 25% used NPS as a primary substance. All were males, age range 26–59 years (SD = 9), who predominantly smoked cannabinoids and snorted/injected stimulant NPS. The type of NPS used was determined by affordability, availability, side-effect profile and desired effects (physical and psychological: 25% reported weight loss as motivation for their use). Poly-pharmacy, supplementation and displacement of other drugs were prevalent. In conclusion, NPS use and associated experiences vary widely among people receiving substance use treatment. Development of effective recovery pathways should be tailored to individuals, and include harm reduction strategies, psychosocial interventions, and effective signposting. Services should be vigilant for NPS use, "on top" use and diversion of prescriptions.

**Keywords:** new psychoactive substances; substance use; cannabinoids; stimulants; substance misuse services; substance use treatment; psychosocial interventions; harm reduction

---

## 1. Introduction

"New Psychoactive Substances" (NPS) is "a generic term for ... substances produced to mimic the effects of traditional illicit drugs" [1]. Formerly known as "legal highs", NPS have dramatically changed the UK drug scene and introduced a new challenge for healthcare professionals (HCPs) [2]. The internet and the media may have had a significant impact on the proliferation of this market. A study by Bright et al. (2013) showed that the media played a significant role in increasing the public's awareness of new NPS, which sparked curiosity and increased use. This, in turn, created a media "moral panic", resulting in legislative reactions, which led to the emergence of more harmful substances [3]. At a global level, NPS are unregulated products with unpredictable effects and clandestine chemists continuously and rapidly produce newly modified compounds [4]. The analysis of NPS products have found controlled substances, mixtures of active substances and different constituents even from the same supplier and using the same "brand" name [1,4,5]. People who use NPS present with unpredictable adverse effects, creating a dilemma for HCPs [6]. Previously, NPS were often labelled as "not for human consumption", so that under the Medicines Act 1968, manufacturers of NPS were not legally required to list their ingredients or determine their safety [1,4,7,8]. The UK Government subsequently introduced the Psychoactive Substances Act (UK PSA) in May 2016, to prohibit NPS sale, supply, production, possession with intention to supply or possession in a custodial institution, with an aim to reduce use [9,10].

Owing to their continuous emergence and sheer numbers (increased from 166 substances in 2009 to over 740 in 2016) [11], NPS are categorized based on their chemical class [12], legal status [13] or chemical structure [14]. However, in clinical practice, NPS are more commonly considered in the context of their pharmacological effects and the substances they have been designed to replicate. Public Health England (PHE) [15] therefore categorizes NPS as: sedating, stimulating, hallucinogenic, cannabinoids, dissociative and "other" (not otherwise specified). Consequently, these PHE categories [15] are used by substance misuse services (SMSs) to record information on the National Drug Treatment Monitoring System (NDTMS) [16], which enables the monitoring of people receiving treatment and national comparisons.

There are a variety of guidelines available to support HCPs working in mental health and SMSs, such as those produced by the Department of Health [17] and the Novel Psychoactive Treatment UK Network (NEPTUNE) [4]; however, none cover specific details for all NPS categories. Due to their "novelty", there is a lack of clinical data to support an evidence-based approach to the management of individuals who use NPS [1]. Recent studies have shown that HCP baseline knowledge of NPS is poor and that they are less confident in managing acute toxicities related to the use of NPS compared with traditional illicit drugs [18,19]. Reports by both the Care Quality Commission and the HM Inspectorate of Probation showed that SMSs did not offer NPS-specific interventions and that people who use NPS poorly engaged [20]. Similarly, in Europe, HCPs in Italy within addiction, psychiatry, pediatrics and A&E services also reported a lack of knowledge and confidence with regards to NPS. They also affirmed that no questions are asked when taking drug histories during admission [2].

To understand the motivation for using NPS by individuals registered within SMSs, a detailed electronic search of NHS evidence was undertaken using the Allied and Complementary Medicine (AMED), Excerpta Medica Database (EMBASE), Health Management Information Consortium (HMIC), British Nursing Index (BNI), Cumulative Index to Nursing and Allied Health Literature (CINAHL), Medline, PsycInfo and Health Business Elite databases. This identified that the rapid proliferation of NPS use may be changing drug taking habits (by displacing or supplementing pre-existing drug repertoires), and may be affected by availability, price, purity and legal status [1,7,21,22]. In Ireland, in depth interviews found people switching from illicit substances to "legal" NPS, due to perceptions regarding improved effects, safety profile and overall higher quality for a lower price; however, the individuals were aged 18–33 years [23] and adult SMSs frequently treat people who are older than this. Another group of Irish interviewees were found to transition from nasal administration to injecting and binged excessively for long durations on stimulant NPS, but after they became controlled substances, their use reduced following headshop closures, increased prices and concerns about contamination [24]. Qualitative case reports of people using stimulant NPS in the UK, prior to the introduction of the UK PSA 2016, suggested their euphoric effects may lead to "more persistent patterns of drug use" due to their perceived legal status and poor quality of their illicit equivalents [21]. The analysis of cryptomarkets such as Alpha Bay, Valhalla, Agora and Evolution Market Place has also allowed the exploration of views and perspectives of vendors and customers on a large scale [25–28]. A study by Van Hout and Hearne (2017) has identified that cryptomarket customers prefer the sequential and concurrent use of psychedelics as well as NPSs, in particular, GABA ($\gamma$-aminobutyric acid)-activating NPSs [29]. The study showed that research of these market place forums can provide an insight on novel trends of NPS use. Similarly, in their study, Bright et al. (2013) utilized Google Trends as a data collection tool of NPS-specific news and employed it to generate media links related to "Kronic"—a Canadian brand known to contain cannabis. Interviewees stated that they are mainly motivated by the poor detectability of this substance at workplaces, which outweigh the unknown harms associated with this substance [3].

In contrast, a field study of people attending "gay dance clubs" in London, who may be considered early adopters of new substances, found they were not deterred by changes in legislation and that stimulant NPS were more popular than any other substance [30]. The same survey found their addition to existing drug repertoires to supplement more established "club drugs" (e.g., ecstasy and cocaine), rather than replacing or displacing them [30]; however, use was affected by availability and purity [22]. A survey of experienced users in Holland also found that people who preferred stimulant NPS were undeterred by legal status and did not displace other illicit substances [31].

Perhaps the reasons for these conflicting findings is that individuals may not always be open or honest about their substance use behaviors when questioned, and NPS packaging may not always contain the expected substance [1,5,32]. Therefore, some novel approaches have been utilized, such as surveying websites and online forums such as Facebook and Twitter [29,33]. The former study found that NPS were used for pleasure, out of curiosity, alongside or as an alternative to other substances [33], whereas, the latter highlighted the diverted use of prescription medicines and poly-drug use due to "high level of social media engagement" [29]; however this methodology requires individuals to have internet access, which may not always be possible for or desired by people who have problems with substances, for example, if they are leading particularly chaotic lives or are homeless. Analyzing samples in isolation also does not allow for exploration of confounding factors or perhaps more importantly, discussion with individuals regarding their reasons for use, experiences with them or any treatment needs.

Historically, SMSs have focused on provision of services for people using crack-cocaine and opiates because these substances previously dominated the UK drug market [15]. Currently, people using NPS are increasingly presenting to SMSs with physical and psychological problems, including dependency [4,8,21]. Researchers working at the Camden and Islington NHS Foundation Trust studied 442 people who were engaging in substance use admitted to a mental health unit. The sample comprised 58 people who use NPS among which, 32 initially presented to A&E, 29 involved the police, 30 were sectioned under the Mental Health Act, and 46 presented with violence before and during admission; most of them were poly-substance users [34]. SMSs therefore need to adapt and change to meet the growing demand from people using NPS [8,35]. Once engaged, limited treatment data suggests that individuals often respond well, with high rates of successful treatment completion when compared to other substances [15]; however, concerns about poor engagement of high-risk people who engage in risky NPS use (e.g., MSM (men who have sex with men)) with SMSs remain [36]. They may present elsewhere such as sexual health services; therefore, this data may not be captured by NDTMS [37]. On general adult inpatient wards of a Scottish psychiatric hospital, NPS use was found to be prevalent among 22% of young male inpatients, in particular those with drug-induced psychosis and often used with other drugs including cannabis and prescribed opiate substitutes [38]. In Hungary, a study by Kapitány-Fövény et al. (2017) also outlined stimulant NPS prevalence among individuals receiving opiate substitution therapy. The main reasons for NPS use were curiosity and practical reasons (including availability) rather than psychopharmacological preferences [39].

Further research is required into the use of NPS by those attending SMSs as highlighted in the 2014 Home Office review [1]. For example, a large Hungarian needle exchange program study found that high risk drug users switched from injecting predominantly illicit amphetamine to NPS and the study recommended further exploration of purity, price and availability [40]. In depth interviews of eleven Irish high-risk stimulant NPS injectors recommended further investigation into their adverse health effects and displacement of other drugs [24]. Some people in SMSs use non-stimulant NPS and do not always inject, so further research is required, which should include all NPS types used via different routes of administration. UK research is particularly lacking, and more is required because SMSs, legislation and illicit drug supply chains can be very different to other countries.

As described above, published research, which definitively outlines the use of NPS by individuals, who engage with specialist adult SMSs in the UK was lacking. Due to the paucity of research, this study will consequently have national and international resonance, contributing to existing knowledge of how NPS may be changing drug taking habits and consequently positively impact upon current practice.

The aim of the study was to explore NPS use by individuals receiving treatment for substance use by exploring their type and pattern of NPS use and associated positive and negative experiences.

## 2. Materials and Methods

In the South West Peninsula of England, the charities RISE (Recovery and Integration Service) in Devon (excluding Plymouth and Torbay) and Addaction in Cornwall have been commissioned to provide integrated specialist SMSs (where RISE is a subsidiary of Addaction, a national organization). RISE and Addaction work with people regardless of which substance(s) they have a problem with. They cover predominantly rural areas, where national data suggests that NPS use may be more common [1,15], although the reasons for this are poorly understood. The use of NPS by the population who engage with these services has not been investigated. This is required because, in accordance with PHE guidance [15], an improved, local understanding of NPS use is important to enable the development of an effective recovery pathway, which appropriately supports the needs of those requiring treatment. There is limited information on international, national or local recovery pathways, to which these SMSs can refer. Ethics approval was obtained from Aston University's Life and Health Sciences Ethics Committee on the 20 January 2015 (Project Identification Code No. 726). The study was reviewed and approved by Addaction/RISE internal governance processes on 13 February 2015. Time was then taken to undertake the study and to seek approval for its publication.

### *2.1. Study Design: Methodological Orientation and Theory*

This was an explorative, qualitative study using thematic analysis [41–44]. Purposive sampling [41,42], where all eligible individuals (as outlined by the inclusion and exclusion criteria below) were identified by their Recovery Co-ordinators (RC) and invited to participate in face-to-face in depth semi-structured interviews [41,42], enabled a range of relevant views to be obtained. This methodology was chosen because it is suited to exploring knowledge in poorly understood areas such as an individual's use of NPS [41–44]. Such methodology has been shown to be successful in obtaining detailed information from individuals regarding their NPS use [42–44]. This study has been reviewed and approved by Addaction's internal governance processes and Aston University's Life and Health Sciences Research Ethics Committee.

Anonymizing results to protect confidentiality and the use of the same researcher, who has no prior knowledge of the interviewees (or ability to routinely impact on their care such as changes to their prescribed treatment) should have increased the likelihood of individuals sharing their personal views and experiences [42–44]. The interviews were conducted by a qualified pharmacist with many years of experience of working in mental health and substance misuse services.

### *2.2. Study Design: Participant Selection and Setting*

Potential participants were contacted by their RC (who identified that the person had experience of NPS) and individuals were provided with an information sheet and consent form which provided a full explanation of the study. The person's ability to provide informed consent [45,46] and eligibility to participate was confirmed immediately prior to the interview. The interviews took place at one of the SMSs or established partner agency sites, where the individual usually attends for their treatment reviews. The presence of non-participants such as the person's RC was permitted if requested by the individual.

Inclusion criteria: Previous experience of using NPS and receiving community treatment (pharmacological/psychosocial) for substance use with the charities RISE in Devon or Addaction in Cornwall.

Exclusion criteria: In receipt of in-patient or prison services; known in a clinical capacity by the Researcher; presented with significant risk issues (after assessment by their RC); additional needs could not be met (for example if they required an interpreter because their first language was not English and the SMS was unable to facilitate) or lacked capacity to consent: particular care was taken if the person was thought to have a disability, mental health problem or thought to be under the influence of substances [47,48].

### 2.3. Study Design: Data Collection

Halo is the electronic record system utilized by SMSs in the South-West Peninsula of England. Quantitative data was collated from the Halo system to identify key characteristics including the participants age, sex, employment, housing status and primary substances they use (such as opiates, cannabis, stimulants and alcohol), which the system classifies in accordance with PHE [15] for the NDTMS [16].

The interview guide (Supplementary Information 1 (SI1)) was piloted to ensure it was suitable for use, and open questions were used to avoid leading the person's responses. The piloting process involved local SMS managers and experienced HCPs reviewing the questions. The interviews were digitally recorded and fully transcribed verbatim [41]. The intention was to undertake approximately twenty interviews to achieve a degree of data saturation, where no new or relevant information is elicited; however, research suggests that as few as eleven or twelve may be required [49], and this was found to be the case in this study.

### 2.4. Data Analysis

During the transcription process any potentially identifying information was deleted and only Halo identification codes used to identify participants. Thematic analysis, which has been specifically designed for applied qualitative research that commences deductively from specified aims and objectives, was used to organize and make sense of the data using a framework approach [41–44]. Initially, a framework was developed from existing literature; this was then updated based on the new data obtained from the interviews using a stepwise approach: (a) interviews were audio-recorded and transcribed verbatim; (b) familiarization: initial recurrent themes were identified following immersion in the transcripts; (c) coding: researcher applied line-by-line codes to describe key issues, concepts and themes by which the data was examined and referenced; (d) developing an analytical framework: after coding the initial transcripts, the researcher in consultation with supervisor, developed a set of codes that could be applied to all subsequent transcripts. Codes were then grouped into categories; (e) applying the analytical framework: data was attached to the framework of codes and categories; (f) developing a framework matrix: to manage and summarize the data, it was put on to the framework to which the data related. At this stage all transcripts were actively searched for results, which contradicted the key conclusions; (g) data interpretation: the framework matrix was used to define concepts and discover associations between the themes to provide explanations for the results; and (h) the end result was a matrix of themes from each source.

## 3. Results

Twelve individuals participated in this study between July and September 2015 and their demographic particulars are summarized in Table 1. All participants were in receipt of psychological interventions, with an age range of 26–59 years (SD = 9; mean 37). Three people (all within Addaction Cornwall) were known to the Criminal Justice Team as they were subject to Court Treatment Orders (CTOs) for their substance use.

During the interviews, one participant ($P_9$) was accompanied by his RC following his request. Interviews had a mean duration of 11 min 23 s (with a range of 4 min 45 s to 24 min 57 s). No individuals had additional needs, which required support during the interviews. The data was collated and manually analyzed by the same researcher. When transcripts were independently reviewed for themes, the findings were discussed, and no differences were identified.

**Table 1.** Summary of information obtained from the electronic record system (Halo for all 12 participants.

| Participant | $P_1$ | $P_2$ | $P_3$ | $P_4$ | $P_5$ | $P_6$ | $P_7$ | $P_8$ | $P_9$ | $P_{10}$ | $P_{11}$ | $P_{12}$ |
|---|---|---|---|---|---|---|---|---|---|---|---|---|
| Age (years) | 28 | 33 | 34 | 31 | 40 | 37 | 36 | 59 | 45 | 44 | 26 | 32 |
| Sex | Male | Male | Male | Male | Male | Male | Male | Male | Male | Male | Male | Male |
| Service attended | RISE Devon | RISE Devon | Addaction Cornwall | Addaction Cornwall | RISE Devon | Addaction Cornwall | RISE Devon | RISE Devon | RISE Devon | Addaction Cornwall | Addaction Cornwall | RISE Devon |
| Under Criminal Justice | No | No | Yes | No | No | No | No | No | No | No | Yes | Yes |
| Housing problem | None | None | None | None | None | None | Acute problem | None | None | None | None | None |
| Employed | Yes | No | No | No | Yes | No | No | No | No | No | No | No |
| Substitute prescription | Methadone oral liquid 40 mg/day | None | Buprenorphine sublingual tablet 8 mg/day | Methadone oral liquid 50 mg/day | None | Methadone oral liquid 30 mg/day | None | None | Methadone oral liquid 100 mg/day | None | None | None |
| Primary Drug * | Morphine | Cocaine | Heroin | Heroin | NPS-stimulant | Heroin | Heroin | NPS-Cannabis | Heroin | Alcohol | Heroin | NPS-other |
| Secondary Drug * | Codeine | NPS–stimulant | Cannabis | None | NPS-Cannabis | None | Diazepam | None | None | None | Cannabis | None |
| Tertiary Drug * | None | None | None | None | None | None | NPS-other | None | None | None | None | None |
| Injecting status (number of days injected in last 28 days) | 0 | 0 | 28 | 0 | 0 | 8 | 0 | 0 | 23 | 0 | 12 | 0 |

* In accordance with PHE classification [15] recorded for NDTMS purposes [16] on Halo.

Using thematic analysis [41–44], data from the interview transcripts were assigned to four core categories:

1. Substance use history;
2. Type and pattern of NPS use;
3. Positive experiences associated with NPS use;
4. Negative experiences associated with NPS use.

Thematic analysis [42–44] enabled further explorations of the data and identified sub-themes which are evidenced in Tables 1–4, including participants' quotations. A summary of the frequencies of the sub-themes is presented in supplementary information (SI2).

1. *Substance use history*

Individuals described a wide range of substance use histories and were at different stages in their recovery journeys; some described more complex histories and most used a variety of substances. There were varying perceptions of the severity of their substance use and some described ongoing entrenched behaviors:

*"I'd been in accidents and the doctors had had me on codeine and dihydrocodeine and slow release morphine and stuff . . . I just gradually got used to it over the years and years and years and because I didn't have a regular doctor, I was seeing a different doctor each time who just kept giving me scripts . . . My body got used to it and I just started taking more and more . . . I'd just split up with my wife, and sort of going through a bit of a dodgy patch"* **P1**

*"I'm a recovering alcoholic . . . Anything that would go up my nose was going"* **P2**

*"Fertiliser–from off the farm . . . I inject heroin . . . tried every drug in the alphabet . . . got a crack addiction . . . started having counselling . . . gotta get my life sorted . . . going to rehab . . . Childhood–stepdad beat me up . . . "* **P3**

*"I fell in with the wrong crowd . . . I lost both my parents in a car crash so sort of went downhill and then sort of started using heroin"* **P4**

*"Started taking mind altering substances when I was 16 . . . these 20 years . . . changing my mental state on a daily basis . . . good help from a drug worker . . . got a job . . . more stable . . . My childhood trauma is what they think kind of led to my habitual use of drugs"* **P5**

*"I can't put drugs away . . . just work my way through them to the bitter end"* **P6**

*"I don't really know why I take them anymore. I think it's just a habit"* **P7**

*"I used to do it [speed-balling] quite a lot . . . since I was a kid . . . once a month or so, I might have a drink but nothing to excess . . . never more than a bottle of whiskey"* **P11**

2. *Type and pattern of NPS use*

**Table 2.** Type and pattern of NPS use. A list of all the themes and sub-themes, with respective quotes by participants.

| Participant | Quote | Theme | Sub-Theme |
|---|---|---|---|
| $P_1$ | *Plant food . . . Snorting it . . . Just a couple of times . . . it wasn't really something I got into heavily or used a lot . . . just a couple of times . . . A mate of mine had it at his house* | NPS type | "Other" (not otherwise specified) only |
| | | Source | Friend only |
| | | Frequency | Occasional |
| | | Route of administration | Nasal only |
| $P_2$ | *Sparkle . . . exodus . . . I'm injecting [i/v] . . . back of my hands, my arms . . . I'm now snorting instead . . . I'm surprised they [veins] haven't collapsed yet to be fair . . . I was taught by the best . . . Sat down for an afternoon . . . talked process and cleanliness [injecting technique] . . . About three or four [times a day] it used to be five or six . . . I'm using another to come down on [synthetic cannabinoid] . . . a couple of tokes . . . at the end of the session, however many days that is-3 or 4 . . . I tend to get my money at the beginning of the fortnight and I'll plan out for it. I'm a typical user . . . [from a headshop] It's easier than buying, chasing a dealer* | NPS type | Stimulating and Cannabinoid |
| | | Source | Headshop only |
| | | Frequency | Daily (several times) |
| | | | Binging |
| | | Route of administration | Nasal and Intra-venous injection |
| | | Concomitant use | Cannabinoid NPS to end stimulant NPS use |
| | | Preference | Accessibility |
| | | | Avoid dealers |

**Table 2.** *Cont.*

| Participant | Quote | Theme | Sub-Theme |
|---|---|---|---|
| | | Harm reduction | Changed route of administration |
| | | | Safer injecting training |
| | | Affordability | Budgeting |
| $P_3$ | *Mephedrone ... Cherry Bomb [cannabis type] ... speedy ... Gocaine ... smoke ... snort powder ... banging up ... It was cheap ... shops and online ... you can buy it ... in a kilo and sell it off in ten bags ... made a lot of money ... dealt loads* | NPS type | Stimulating and Cannabinoid |
| | | Source | Headshop and Online |
| | | Route of administration | Nasal, Smoking and Intra-venous Injection |
| | | Affordability | Cheap |
| | | | Dealing |
| $P_4$ | *Pink Panthers and Eisenberg ... represent speed ... uppers ... Black Mamba ... I smoked them but I have been known to inject a Pink Panther ... I dibbled and dabbled ... it wasn't an everyday thing, only you know once every 3 or 4 weeks ... and then when I would come home, I would do a bit of heroin to go to sleep ... [head] shop* | NPS type | Stimulating & Cannabinoid |
| | | Source | Headshop only |
| | | Frequency | Occasional |
| | | Route of administration | Smoking and Intra-venous Injection |
| | | Concomitant use | Opiates to end stimulant NPS use |
| $P_5$ | *[Speedy ones] the names they had for them were things like Gogaine, or Posh ... Stimulants were either taken orally or snorted ... if I was smoking synthetic cannabis, I would be using tobacco with it ... constantly ... either be becoming high on synthetic stimulants or coming down off that and using synthetic cannabis ... if I'd just been paid ... in one hit and then top up throughout the week ... I go in there for one thing, the temptation to buy something else ... My willpower was helped by a change of circumstances and that change of circumstances in that the shop's no longer selling it* | NPS type | Stimulating and Cannabinoid |
| | | Source | Headshop only |
| | | Frequency | Daily (several times) |
| | | Route of administration | Oral, Nasal and Smoking |
| | | Concomitant use | Cannabinoids with tobacco |
| | | | Cannabinoid NPS to end stimulant NPS use |
| | | Preference | Accessibility |
| | | Affordability | Budgeting |
| $P_6$ | *The pot ones ... Spice ... Scorpion ... Clockwork Orange ... Pandora's Box ... Toxic Waste ... Smoking it neat in a pipe ... in a rolled cigarette ... I found that the dosage is important ... I'd do very small amounts ... I was writing it down, how much I was doing, taking tiny puffs ... I was on methadone at the time ... I substituted it [with NPS] ... At the newsagent, you were able to buy them pre-rolled and my friend who smokes pot ... headshop ... online from some dodgy retailer ... Couldn't get any marijuana* | NPS type | Stimulating and Cannabinoid |
| | | Source | Headshop, Friend, Online and Other (newsagent) |
| | | Route of administration | Smoking only |
| | | Concomitant use | Displacement (prescribed opiates) |
| | | | Cannabinoids with tobacco |
| | | Preference | Accessibility |
| | | Harm reduction | Changed dose |
| $P_7$ | *Diamond Dust, Lush, Sparkle [speedy types] ... Crystal ... IV ... In my arms ... Since I've been doing legal highs I haven't touched it [heroin] ... legal high shop* | NPS type | Stimulating only |
| | | Source | Headshop only |
| | | Route of administration | Intra-venous injection only |
| | | Concomitant use | Displacement (illicit opiates) |
| $P_8$ | *Low Rider, Cotton Candy, Strawberry Cough ... cannabis types ... Smoking them, putting them into joints or into a pipe ... just this and tobacco ... Every 20 min ... buy it in bulk of tens ... headshop* | NPS type | Cannabinoid only |
| | | Source | Headshop only |
| | | Frequency | Daily (several times) |
| | | Route of administration | Smoking only |
| | | Concomitant use | Cannabinoids with tobacco |
| | | Affordability | Bulk-buying |
| $P_9$ | *Mephedrone ... Devil's Dust ... an upper, a stimulant ... synthetic cannabinoids ... IV [groin] ... smoking [cannabinoids] ... No more often than once a day [cannabinoids] ... About every quarter of an hour [stimulants] ... obviously there were sleep breaks but it was about a 6-month period ... I didn't withdraw from opiates ... it took me away from heroin ... Group of friends and from a chap* | NPS type | Stimulating and Cannabinoid |
| | | Source | "Street dealer" and Friend |
| | | Frequency | Daily (several times) |
| | | | Binging |
| | | Route of administration | Smoking and Intra-venous Injection |
| | | Concomitant use | Displacement (illicit opiates) |
| $P_{10}$ | *The powders and the puff ... Smoking it. Injecting it ... snorting everything ... Stopped me drinking ... no withdrawals ... Legal high shop ... Dealers as well* | NPS type | Stimulating and Cannabinoid |
| | | Source | "Street dealer" and Headshop |
| | | Route of administration | Nasal, Smoking & Intra-venous Injection |
| | | Concomitant use | Displacement (alcohol) |

**Table 2.** *Cont.*

| Participant | Quote | Theme | Sub-Theme |
|---|---|---|---|
| $P_{11}$ | *Mephedrone . . . Methalone. A couple of hallucinogenic ones. And the pills that they did . . . Hawaiian Woodrose . . . They're a seed basically and they've got an LSA in them which is like a precursor to LSD . . . smoking . . . Usually I would just have a couple of Valium [to help come down from NPS] . . . Internet . . . It was just a sort of weekend thing . . . Not very regularly.* | NPS type | Stimulating, Dissociative and Hallucinogenic |
| | | Source | Online only |
| | | Frequency | Occasional |
| | | Route of administration | Smoking only |
| | | Concomitant use | Benzodiazepines to end NPS use |
| $P_{12}$ | *Crystal, Boom Dust . . . Diamond Dust mephedrone . . . smoke the cannabinoids . . . Lotus . . . The speedy ones . . . Crystal Meth ones–the uppers . . . opiates from Italy . . . I snort them . . . dabble them . . . Put it in your mouth, let it dissolve . . . smoking if they're the cannabinoid ones . . . Putting it in with baccy, it makes it last longer . . . If you mix them together, you hallucinate . . . It's opportunist . . . just down the road...just go to the shop and don't get ripped off by the drug dealers . . . every day.* | NPS type | Stimulating, Cannabinoid and Sedating |
| | | Source | Headshop only |
| | | Frequency | Daily (several times) |
| | | Route of administration | Oral, Nasal and Smoking |
| | | Concomitant use | Potentiating effects |
| | | | Cannabinoids with tobacco |
| | | Preference | Accessibility |
| | | | Avoid dealers |
| | | Affordability | Cannabinoids with tobacco |

### 3. *Positive experiences associated with NPS use*

**Table 3.** Positive experiences associated with NPS use. A list of all the themes and sub-themes, with respective quotes by participants.

| Participant | Quote | Theme | Sub-Theme |
|---|---|---|---|
| $P_1$ | *I wasn't thinking about the ex-wife . . . The buzz . . . like being drunk without the drink . . . fuzzy, happy, chilled out sort of feeling* | Psychological effects | Escapism |
| | | | Relaxation |
| | | | Happiness |
| | | | Euphoria |
| $P_2$ | *It allows me not to be me . . . Without them, I'm a totally different person, I would never talk you right now without it . . . allows me to be confident . . . Part of it was to lose weight . . . I was 17 stone when I started out on it . . . just 10 times better than the drink . . . It's stronger than street* | Psychological effects | Escapism |
| | | | Confidence |
| | | Physical effects | Weight loss |
| | | Preference | Strength |
| | | | Quality |
| $P_3$ | *They keep me awake when I was out clubbing . . . Was I allowed to sell them? I thought I was cos it was legal* | Psychological effects | Alertness/Energy |
| | | Preference | Legal status |
| $P_4$ | *It was about a fiver whereas you go out and buy a gram of coke and its 60 quid* | Preference | Affordability |
| $P_5$ | *Wanting to escape from reality any way, or change that reality . . . [stimulants] a heightened sense . . . very energetic . . . happy . . . [cannabinoids] lethargic, very drowsy . . . most of the time dozing on the sofa in front of the TV-that is what I wanted . . . It's hundreds of times stronger . . . would last for ages . . . I got bored . . . I was drawn to try them . . . It's cheaper [than marijuana] . . . 13.5 stone down to about 9.* | Psychological effects | Escapism |
| | | | Relaxation |
| | | | Happiness |
| | | | Alertness/Energy |
| | | Physical effects | Weight loss |
| | | Preference | Strength |
| | | | Affordability |
| | | | Curiosity |
| | | | Boredom |
| | | | Duration |

**Table 3.** *Cont.*

| Participant | Quote | Theme | Sub-Theme |
|---|---|---|---|
| $P_6$ | *More involved in the music, film . . . my playing sounded great . . . [it] wasn't very great . . . they didn't have any downside at all . . . they didn't relax you or send you to sleep–quite the opposite . . . I went back because of the power it had over me. It scared me and I wanted it to . . . I wanted to tame it . . . I wanted to be able to do it without freaking out . . . it would last for ages because it's so strong* | Psychological effects | Alertness/Energy |
| | | | Improved subjective experiences |
| | | | Overcome and control previous negative experiences |
| | | Preference | Strength |
| | | | Duration |
| $P_7$ | *You just get more for your money worth [than "street" amphetamine]* | Preference | Quality |
| | | | Affordability |
| $P_8$ | *I like the relaxing, calming numb feeling . . . The effect, it's quicker than marijuana. You get higher quicker . . . faster* | Psychological effects | Relaxation |
| | | Preference | Onset of action |
| $P_9$ | *It was quite stimulating . . . had an overriding desire to argue with Christians . . . improved my darts. It deepened my appreciation of Johnny Cash . . . You legalise [it] and I'll be back on it . . .* | Psychological effects | Alertness/Energy |
| | | | Improved subjective experiences |
| | | Preference | Legal status |
| $P_{10}$ | *Make myself happy . . . made me stronger . . . gives me confidence . . . I eat every day [resulting in weight gain when previously underweight]* | Psychological effects | Happiness |
| | | | Confidence |
| | | Physical effects | Weight gain |
| $P_{11}$ | *Totally a good feeling basically, made me feel quite happy and cheerful . . . I tried most of them really to see what they were like I stuck to the illegal ones cos they work better . . . I thought, yeah I'll try that–see what happens* | Psychological effects | Happiness |
| | | Preference | Quality |
| | | | Curiosity |
| $P_{12}$ | *[Stimulant NPS] gives me more energy . . . [cannabinoid NPS] calms me down . . . It enhances–changes your perspective on stuff . . . Helps me listen to music . . . I've lost a lot of weight doing them. I was 18 and a half stone before I started doing them . . . I like to keep the weight off . . . I've got a bad leg and it takes that pain away* | Psychological effects | Relaxation |
| | | | Alertness/Energy |
| | | | Improved subjective experiences |
| | | Physical effects | Weight loss |
| | | | Analgesia |

4. *Negative experiences associated with NPS use*

**Table 4.** Negative experiences associated with NPS use. A list of all the themes and sub-themes, with respective quotes by participants.

| Participant | Quote | Theme | Sub-Theme |
|---|---|---|---|
| $P_1$ | *My lip and my front teeth just went numb . . . it makes your eyes water . . . and your nose burnt sometimes. The nostrils would burn [when snorting NPS]* | Physical effects | Administration site |
| $P_2$ | *A little bit dearer [than "street drugs"] . . . It has turned me into a more devious person as well, although I've never stolen . . . I am the nastiest person on it . . . I don't like the shakes . . . it makes me itch a bit . . . eczema . . . it's a really dangerous sweat, it's pretty embarrassing* | Psychological effects | Personality changes |
| | | Physical effects | Tremor |
| | | | Eczema |
| | | | Sweating |
| | | | Itching |
| | | Preference | Affordability |
| $P_3$ | *I've had thoughts of . . . killing myself . . . not wanting to be here . . . I didn't like the effects . . . it'll kill you . . . the heartbeat on the high ones . . . you feel like, I've just injected here and my heart's going. It feels like I'm dying . . . That's a vein there and it's just left a massive lump . . . It's too powerful* | Psychological effects | Suicidal ideation |
| | | Physical effects | Administration site |
| | | | Cardiac |
| | | Preference | Strength |
| $P_4$ | *I couldn't go out, struggled concentrating . . . They don't make you feel good; all they do is make your heart feel like you're having a heart attack . . . heart fluttering, palpitations . . . Too strong, over-powering* | Psychological effects | Concentration |
| | | | Impaired activity of daily living |
| | | Physical effects | Cardiac |
| | | Preference | Strength |

**Table 4.** *Cont.*

| Participant | Quote | Theme | Sub-Theme |
|---|---|---|---|
| $P_5$ | *I stopped cleaning my flat ... go for about 4 days without eating ... lost interest in my home. I wasn't paying my bills ... washing up not done for months ... got sacked ... all I wanted to do was get money and buy legal highs. That was my whole life ... crawling around my carpet on my hands and knees ... try and get enough for another rollie ... that's how addictive they were ... Eventually the police turned up and I basically got detained under the Mental Health Act for 24 h, until the effect of the drugs wore off ... I started fitting in the street and I just couldn't control my body ... it no longer had that kind of kick to it ... I stopped buying it ... you get a variation ... the illegal high stuff is more consistent in its strength* | Legal | Detained (Mental Health Act) |
| | | Psychological effects | Impaired activity of daily living |
| | | | Self-neglect |
| | | | Loss of control |
| | | | Dependency/Addiction |
| | | Physical effects | Seizures |
| | | Preference | Strength |
| | | | Quality |
| $P_6$ | *Too potent ... I hate the fact that this is controlling me ... I don't have control ... Couldn't remember what I was doing ... completely confused ... Gave me panic attacks ... Wouldn't have been in any fit state to go out ... It seemed to speed my heart up to a frightening degree ... I really thought I was gonna have a heart attack ... my heart was thumping away madly ... Hundreds of times stronger ... it's easy to go over-board ... the intensity of it was just on another level ... I think they're more dangerous because they are just so intense ... It could be a little bit hit and miss ... it wouldn't have the same sort of effect* | Psychological effects | Impaired activity of daily living |
| | | | Confusion |
| | | | Impaired memory |
| | | | Panic attacks |
| | | | Loss of control |
| | | Physical effects | Cardiac |
| | | Preference | Strength |
| | | | Quality |
| $P_7$ | *It was pretty strong and I thought I was gonna collapse and die ... It was the strength of it* | Preference | Strength |
| $P_8$ | *I want to keep to that high all the time ... sleep [to stop] ... It might make you cough ... sweats* | Psychological effects | Dependency/Addiction |
| | | Physical effects | Coughing |
| | | | Sweating |
| $P_9$ | *Abscesses* | Physical effects | Administration site |
| $P_{10}$ | *You get more addicted. You wanna another bag, another bag and another* | Psychological effects | Dependency/Addiction |
| | | | Cravings |
| $P_{11}$ | *I stuck to the illegal ones cos they work better* | Preference | Quality |
| $P_{12}$ | *I need them, cos I've been doing them for 6–7 years ... I don't like having to wake up when I haven't got the money for them. Then I have to try to get the money for them. I don't like that part of it ... they're quite addictive ... done some quite reckless stuff to get them ... trouble with the police ... Makes me shake a lot ... all the time* | Psychological effects | Dependency/Addiction |
| | | Physical effects | Tremor |
| | | Legal | Police involvement |

## 4. Discussion

This study contributes to existing knowledge of how NPS are used by individuals, who engage with specialist adult SMSs. Seven (58%) reported opiates (illicit heroin/morphine) as their primary substance of use; this is in keeping with the finding that five (42%) of participants were in receipt of opiate substitution prescriptions. For a quarter of individuals, NPS was their primary substance of use in accordance with PHE classification [15], suggesting that while not as common as opiates (which SMSs are more familiar with treating [15]), NPS use is prevalent among individuals accessing treatment services, as previously suggested by both national and international findings [7,8,39].

The interviews allowed individuals to describe their experiences with all types and routes of administration of NPS; therefore, adding to the existing evidence base, particularly since previous studies [24,40] have largely focused on stimulant NPS, which were injected. Audio recordings allowed for more complete data and detailed transcriptions than relying on memory or notes alone and piloting should have increased the likelihood of individuals sharing their personal views and experiences [42–44].

Harm reduction measures aim to reduce the harm that someone may experience because of their ongoing substance use [45,46]. These include but are not limited to avoiding poly-pharmacy, administering by routes associated with less risk (such as smoking rather than injecting), not sharing drug paraphernalia and using smaller amounts. This study, as with other research, found that individuals did not usually know exactly which chemical they were taking [19,50]. Amount of experience with NPS and frequency of use varied greatly, from very occasional up to every 20 min. Frequent use was mainly observed with synthetic cannabinoid receptor agonists (SCRAs) and stimulant NPSs. Due the wide chemical diversity of SCRAs, little is known on their pharmacokinetics [51]. However, stimulants such as mephedrone may have a short duration of action warranting repeated dosing [52]. Overall substance use patterns fluctuated over time (with varying self-perceptions), which may be explained by individuals being at different stages in their recovery journeys. Participant ages ranged from 26 to 59 (SD = 9); other studies have found and that most people using NPS are under 30 years old [1]. The difference may be because this study unlike national data reflects the age of those requiring treatment. Our results therefore show that SMSs need to manage individuals with a range of ages presenting with NPS use.

Previous studies and national reports have outlined a complex relationship between NPS and other substances, and the need for further investigation. Factors affecting use include substance availability, effects, safety profile, quality, price, purity and legal status [1,16,21–23,38]. This study equally found that NPS were favored over other substances for their perceived legal status, improved price, availability and higher quality, including quicker onset and duration of action, therefore adding to the existing knowledge base.

The large proportion ($n$ = 9; 75%) of participants who stated they had experience with SCRAs is perhaps to be expected (SI2), given that cannabis, the traditional illicit substance, which these substances are attempting to mimic, has the highest prevalence rate of all illicit substances [53]. Preference for NPS type appeared to be dependent upon the required effect (usually stimulating or sedating). Some wanted to gain confidence, energy and alertness; others wanted to "escape reality", experience euphoria, feel happy, relaxed or were potentially self-medicating for underlying psychological trauma (and in one case ($P_{12}$) for leg pain). This has been found in other studies [30,54], where stimulating effects were particularly popular [21,31,54]. One study found that psychedelic effects were commonly favored [30]; although this could be due to the differing study environments (such as dance venues and festivals). Individuals also reported using NPS to alleviate feelings of boredom and out of curiosity, which has also been found previously [1,21,55] and similarly for traditional illicit substance use [1].

NPS were often mixed with other substances [34,50] and administered by a variety of routes, although snorting/injecting stimulant NPS and smoking SCRAs, the latter in combination with tobacco ($n$ = 4; 33%) predominated (SI2). Stimulant and SCRA NPS were also used sequentially to balance the effects of each other. Excessive binging for long durations on stimulant NPS, followed by substances with sedating and relaxing effects to "come down" supports the results of another study [24]. Poly-pharmacy is associated with an increased risk of drug interactions and side-effects including overdose and death [7,45], so harm reduction advice, which SMSs offer, should include: overdose awareness, how to reduce frequency, avoid "binges", minimize polysubstance use, manage altered tolerance levels as well as the provision of take home naloxone [24,56].

The amount participants spent on their NPS varied widely and was affected by how much money they had access to, the source of NPS supply and pattern of use. To reduce costs NPS were bought in bulk or smoked with tobacco and one person ($P_3$) also described dealing NPS to fund his habit. NPS were described as comparatively cheap to traditional illicit drugs which has been similarly suggested by the Home Office [1]. A Dutch study has found them to be similar in price to the substances they are attempting to mimic [30] and this may be accounted for by differences between England and Holland drug markets.

Strength of NPS was perceived as both a positive and negative. Some found them to be too strong, leading to unwanted effects and overdoses; others preferred them for their strength, considering them to be more cost-effective and of higher quality. Overall, NPS use reduced if strength and quality was variable, and the NPS was viewed as inferior rather than superior to traditional illicit drugs; this may be highly dependent on the local drug markets and has been similarly identified by the Home Office [1].

Our findings support other research, which identified that the rapid proliferation of NPS use may be changing drug taking habits [22]. Several individuals reported NPS alleviating withdrawal symptoms including cravings, from other substances and in some cases completely substituted with NPS. SMSs should therefore provide individuals with advice on how to manage withdrawals (from all substances). Using NPS in addition to traditional illicit drugs or prescribed substitute medication to potentiate effects was also reported, particularly when then the person was presenting as more chaotic as found in similar studies [24]. This is unsurprising since individuals in the early stages of recovery commonly present with more complex and riskier patterns of substance use.

Participants reported obtaining NPS from various sources; the majority had experience of using headshops ($n = 9$; 75%) (SI2) in contrast to a qualitative study that found that NPS were usually obtained from friends or online [30]. Headshops were often preferred for their convenience (particularly if they could avoid "dealers"), with usage reducing when they could no longer be legally sold. However, legal status did not always deter use, supporting Home Office findings, which suggest this may be due to the impact of legal status upon the quality of NPS [1,3]. Previous studies have equally conflicted in their findings on the effect of legal status on the decision to use NPS [24,30]. Purchasing them from high street vendors may add to the perception of this being "normal" behavior and the risk of them being considered as "safe" and "legal" and consequently increase NPS use. For example, one person ($P_3$) felt it was permissible to sell them because they did not consider them to be "drugs" in the same way as traditional illicit substances. Recent studies showed that there is an underlying competition between cryptomarkets and street networking, which may drive high quality of illicit substances as well as NPS [25–28]. However, an international drug testing service that was offered to cryptomarket users suggested that this may not be the case [25].

Participants described a wide range of physical and psychological problems including symptoms of NPS dependency reflecting national and international findings [4,8,57,58]. Similar to the findings of other studies [31,57,58], reported physical health effects included tremor, coughing, itching, seizures, eczema and sweating, and problems associated with specific routes of administration such as venous abscesses. Like other studies, cardiac effects were reported ($n = 3$; 25%) (SI2), usually following stimulant NPS use and sometimes lasting a few days [31,57,58]. While individuals described some of these effects as sometimes being prolonged, the long-term effects remain unknown. Individuals were not specifically asked about their experiences of acute compared to chronic effects or to distinguish between side-effects and withdrawal symptoms. This suggests further study development and provides additional support for the need for longitudinal research [1]. Unpleasant psychological effects, included feelings of loss of control, difficulties concentrating, impaired memory, confusion, personality changes, panic attacks and cravings; sometimes leading to crime, impaired activities of daily living and self-neglect. Suicidal ideation and in one case ($P_5$), being sectioned under the Mental Health Act following prolonged NPS use was reported. Individuals with pre-existing mental health conditions ("dual diagnosis") may be particularly at risk of psychological problems and local integrated pathways should outline how to obtain the required support quickly and effectively, especially in acute situations such as the person disclosing suicidal ideation.

High risk administration practices and side-effects such as vein damage as a direct result of the route of administration were described, although not as significant as identified by a similar Irish study, perhaps because it only included NPS mainly administered by injection [24]. To ameliorate this, individuals actively undertook harm reduction approaches such as switching from injecting to snorting and using less [45]. It is important that SMSs appropriately signpost to additional sources of help and support, for example tissue bioavailability services.

### *4.1. Limitations of the Study*

Repeat interviews and member-checking was not implemented due to difficulties in re-establishing contact with the participants, time constraints and geographical problems. The purposive sampling [42–44] approach enabled suitable participants to be identified. Although small, tentative data saturation was achieved, as has been found to occur in other research [24,42–44,49]. A larger sample size may have enabled more generalizability; however, this smaller sample size allowed for more in-depth analysis.

Interviews require people to discuss their experiences in an artificial environment, which may lead to problems with reliability. However, this approach of using semi-structured interviews to obtain detailed information from individuals regarding their NPS use has been successfully used previously [23,24,30].

Data was collected in a predominantly rural environment and further research should be conducted in more urban areas. The Devon RISE and Addaction Cornwall SMSs were almost equally represented (7:5 respectively). Men dominate SMSs and reflecting this, all our participants were men [1,7]. With a larger sample size, women may have been included, providing the opportunity for comparison.

Data was collected in 2015, when many NPS were sold openly in headshops and NPS markets have since changed. Currently, under the UK NPS Act 2016, headshops can no longer legally sell NPS and a clear shift from the surface to the dark net was observed [59] and motivation for NPS use may have consequently evolved. Implications of the new legislation include intentional poor disclosure of NPS use to HCPs and NPS emerging on the illicit market, often sold as the traditional illicit drug the NPS mimics, to increase profit margins [55]. The delayed reporting of this study is due to the time needed for the necessary approval for publication

*4.2. Implications for HCPs and Policy-Makers*

The way that the participants described NPS, easily made them identifiable in accordance with PHE categories used by NDTMS, therefore providing support for this approach in clinical practice [15]. However, there were significant discrepancies between NPS use recorded on Halo for the purposes of NDTMS [16] and disclosures made by individuals during the interviews. Therefore, all individuals presenting to SMSs should be asked about their use of NPS, the name of the substance, and reassessed regularly, because they may not routinely present or perceive this as an issue, especially if other substances dominate their pattern of substance use or if it changes over time. Additionally, this study highlights that individuals should be asked about NPS regardless of their age. With the increasing emergence of NPS (from approximately 478 in 2015 when this data was collected [14] to 740 in 2016 [11]), increasing chemical diversity, potency, and changing degree of purity [14,25], it is important that HCPs reassess regularly the use of novel or existing NPS and tailor harm reduction approaches to individuals. The importance of offering harm reduction interventions was demonstrated by the positive impact that they had on individuals; however, the reports of managing withdrawal symptoms by diverting prescribed medication or otherwise using polypharmacy must not be underestimated in clinical practice. HCPs must check that prescribed doses are optimized to reduce cravings and "on top" use. Additionally, adherence to medication regimens must be checked and community pharmacy teams must promptly notify prescribing services of missed doses.

Consequently, treatment needs may also fluctuate over time, so SMSs need to be able to accommodate this and regularly review the person's progress. These findings also provide support for using interviews to elicit more accurate data regarding people's NPS use and highlights that reviewing NDTMS data in isolation to assess the extent of NPS use is inadequate. This may be for a variety of reasons, including lack of staff vigilance when completing the required data set and suggests a potential training need.

Because of their overall experiences, some strongly felt that they would never use NPS again, while others continued to use despite their negative consequences. These findings corroborated with previous research on SCRAs, where users reported that these substances completely "hijacked their personalities" [60]. These negative effects may have a significant impact upon the person, including their employment, housing status and criminal record, and the wider community. SMSs are traditionally skilled in providing support with such problems but promoting awareness among staff about how best to identify individuals requiring more intensive support, or those whose needs may need to be prioritized, such as individuals with pre-existing conditions, those who are homeless or subject to CTOs, may enable this to be provided more promptly.

There was evidence that the SMSs were raising awareness of harm reduction by advising on alternative routes of administration, such as switching from injecting to snorting and offered safer injecting technique sessions. Risks may be further reduced if the substance could be tested to confirm its content prior to administration and harm reduction advice [5,61] was provided at the time of purchase. Currently, neither is currently permissible in UK SMSs, therefore adding further weight to reviewing existing legislation.

SMSs need to understand the motivation for using NPS: when individuals disclosed their substance use histories, they were highly variable. In one case, iatrogenic dependency ($P_1$) was described, though reasons for use were frequently associated with traumatic life events, often from childhood. This has been found to occur in other NPS studies [21] and SMSs should therefore be sensitive to the needs of these individuals and tailor psychological interventions accordingly. When more significant disclosures are made, other services such as bereavement counselling and mental health teams should be signposted so that any unresolved issues can be managed effectively.

Some described improved abilities and experiences with NPS, often acknowledging this was perceived because of the mind-altering effects of the substance, such as having energy while on a night out and enjoyment of activities such as playing music. Such information may be of interest to policy-makers, where psychoactivity of newly emerging NPS has not yet been demonstrated. One individual ($P_6$), reported a desire to use NPS to overcome their previous negative experiences with these substances, alongside entrenched addictive behaviors and boredom due to a lack of meaningful daytime activities. This highlights the need for SMSs to promote a variety of psychosocial interventions to help occupy an individual's time in substance-free environments, which are tailored to the person's needs to enable them to progress with their recovery. Supporting people to develop skills which will enable them to find work is important because the number of participants in employment was comparatively low and boredom was cited as a reason for NPS use, which may be compounded by rural locations. Some may require more intensive RC support and there should be adequate provision for this.

The main positive physical health effects reported were upon weight: three (25%) stated that using predominantly stimulant NPS to keep their weight down was one of their main motivators for use. This may be a particular problem once the person stabilizes their NPS use and weight gain is observed, which may result in the occurrence of other eating disorder symptoms. In contrast, one individual ($P_{10}$) reported appetite stimulating effects which they found to be beneficial as they were otherwise losing weight due to self-neglect because of their chaotic drug use. However, it cannot be assumed that the food they were selecting to eat included "healthy options". In these situations, individuals should be offered supportive explanations that if their substance use stabilizes their weight will usually return without the need for stimulants. Malnutrition may be common in people in substance use treatment, which is one of many reasons why SMSs supporting activities such as "breakfast clubs" and the provision of "life-skills" courses which incorporate cooking techniques and general nutritional advice, should be actively encouraged. Everyone involved in the care of people with substance use problems (including GPs and community pharmacists in addition to specialist SMSs) should be vigilant for eating disorder behaviors and provide the required support or signpost as required: there may be training needs.

Three participants were subject to CTOs because of their substance use and would therefore require regular drug testing for SMSs to report on their progress. Since NPS may not always be detectable in routine drug screens and can produce false positives [5,55,61], SMSs could consider more specialist NPS-specific tests. These may be expensive (and not always possible due to the novelty of the substances), but if used sparingly and appropriately, they may be a useful tool. However, this is not without risk, since it may also perpetuate the demand for "new" NPS that are not detectable. Half of the participants were in receipt of a prescription for oral opiate substitution treatment and using NPS as a replacement for such medication was reported. The diversion of prescribed medication is highly likely in such situations. Therefore NPS-specific tests may also be useful for supporting decisions around continued prescribing in circumstances where there is evidence of "on top" use or diversion is suspected. Staff should receive appropriate training so that they are vigilant for "on-top" use, diversion and substitution of the person's prescribed intervention with NPS, particularly if the individual is under a CTO.

NPS treatment systems are complex and require structured partnerships between multidisciplinary teams with a broad range of competencies. This includes: A&E departments, sexual, social care and mental health services, prison, probation staff and Young Offender teams, community adult and young people SMSs, youth services and organizations such as the police [6]. This is required to manage the myriad of health, social and criminal problems associated with NPS use and to address the diverse needs of individuals including young people, MSM, prisoners, and the homeless population. This approach should also involve people who use NPS and their carers. Drug detection is key to support diagnosis and treatment planning, adherence and outcomes [5,6,55,61]. Proactive, engaging and competent SMSs are needed to respond appropriately to meet the needs associated with NPS use. Regular education and training is of paramount importance to inform about types and degrees of harm, new patterns and trends of recreational drug use and changes to the drug scene [6]. NPS use should be considered in clinical assessments and management plans should be devised accordingly [20].

## 5. Conclusions

This study found that NPS are used by individuals across a range of ages, presenting to SMSs in Devon and Cornwall, but is highly variable. NPS may be favored over other substances for their perceived legal status, price, strength, availability and better quality, including quicker onset and duration of action and improved side-effect profile. Consequently, NPS use may be dependent on local drug markets and reduce if perceived to be variable in strength and quality in comparison to traditional illicit drugs. SCRAs and stimulant NPS are most frequently used and preference for NPS type is often dependent upon the required effect. Using poly-pharmacy (including NPS, traditional illicit substances and prescribed medication) to potentiate effects, manage side-effects and withdrawal symptoms occurs, sometimes resulting in displacement of substances. Therefore, SMS must remain vigilant and consider the use of NPS-specific tests, especially when substitute medication is prescribed. NPS are frequently administered by a variety of routes, including high risk injecting practices, though individuals can respond well to harm reduction interventions, which should be routinely provided and include the management of withdrawals. Results showed that a wide range of problematic physical and mental health effects may occur, including symptoms of dependency, which may lead to criminal activity, impaired activities of daily living and self-neglect. People's perception of the severity of their use, frequency and amount used varies widely and may change depending on their recovery journey, consequently fluctuating for individuals over time. People use NPS for a variety of reasons, including stimulant types taken for the intention of losing weight. As malnourishment is often an issue for individuals accessing SMS, the multidisciplinary team must be attentive, frequently revisit the current pattern of substance use and any associated issues, promptly refer to other services accordingly and may require further training. Local integrated pathways for individuals presenting with more complex issues and particular needs such as dual diagnosis and tissue bioavailability should be established to enable prompt access. SMSs should engage individuals with psychosocial interventions and meaningful daily activities, especially in more rural areas. It is important that current approaches to existing treatment strategies are adapted and recovery plans tailored to an individual's needs. Education and training is needed for HCPs working within various services where people who use NPS are encountered. Multidisciplinary and multiagency approaches should be nationally adopted to capture changing trends of NPS use.

**Supplementary Materials:**
Supplementary Information 1 (SI1): Semi-structured Interview Guide; Supplementary Information 2 (SI2): Summary of Themes and Sub-themes

**Acknowledgments:** No funding or grants were provided to conduct this study. Addaction and RISE had no roles in study design, in the collection, analysis, and interpretation of data, in the writing of the report, or in the decision to submit the paper for publication. The views expressed here reflect only the authors' views. The authors would like to acknowledge the help of Julie Bonning-Snook for assisting with transcription processes and the Addaction/RISE staff and clients without whom the data collection would not have been possible. Photo of NPS packaging in the graphical abstract (taken by RG) is reproduced with permission from Addaction, UK.

**Author Contributions:** R.G. conceived the project and undertook the data collection, supervised by I.M. A.G. conceived the paper and led on writing. F.S. advised on paper as a whole; R.G., A.G., F.S. and I.M. reviewed the paper. All authors contributed to the writing of the paper.

## References

1. Stephenson, G.; Richardson, A. *New Psychoactive Substances in England: A Review of the Evidence*; Crime and Policing Analysis Unit, Home Office Science; Home Office: London, UK, 2014.
2. Simonato, P.; Corazza, O.; Santonastaso, P.; Corkery, J.; Deluca, P.; Davey, Z.; Blaszko, U.; Schifano, F. Novel psychoactive substances as a novel challenge for health professionals: Results from an Italian survey. *Hum. Psychopharmacol.* **2013**, *28*, 324–331. [CrossRef] [PubMed]
3. Bright, S.J.; Bishop, B.; Kane, R.; Marsh, A.; Barratt, M.J. Kronic hysteria: Exploring the intersection between Australian synthetic Cannabis legislation, the media, and drug-related harm. *Int. J. Drug Policy* **2013**, *24*, 231–237. [CrossRef] [PubMed]
4. Abdulrahim, D.; Bowden-Jones, O. *Guidance on the Clinical Management of Acute and Chronic Harms of Club Drugs and Novel Psychoactive Substances*; Novel Psychoactive Treatment UK Network (NEPTUNE): London, UK, 2015.
5. Guirguis, A.; Girotto, S.; Berti, B.; Stair, J.L. Identification of new psychoactive substances (NPS) using handheld Raman Spectroscopy employing both 785 and 1064 nm laser sources. *J. Forensic Sci. Int.* **2017**, *273*, 113–123. [CrossRef] [PubMed]
6. Independent Expert Working Group. *Drug Use and Dependence. UK Guidelines on Clinical Management*; Crown: London, UK, 2017.
7. UNODC. World Drug Report. United Nations Office on Drugs and Crime: Vienna, Austria, 2014. Available online: https://www.unodc.org/documents/wdr2014/World_Drug_Report_2014_web.pdf (accessed on 21 March 2018).
8. Royal College of Psychiatrists (RCPsych). *One New Drug a Week. Why Novel Psychoactive Substances and Club Drugs Need a Different Response from UK Treatment Providers (FR/AP/02)*; Faculty Report; Faculty of Addictions Psychiatry, Royal College of Psychiatrists: London, UK, 2014.
9. Psychoactive Substances Act 2016. The Stationery Office Limited, 2016. Available online: http://services.parliament.uk/bills/2015-16/psychoactivesubstances.html (accessed on 21 September 2015).
10. Drug Watch. *A Simple (ish) Guide to the Psychoactive Substances Act (PSA)*, version 1.5; Linnell Communications: Prestwich, UK, 2016.
11. United Nations Office on Drugs and Crime (UNODC). *Global Synthetic Drugs Assessment. Amphetamine-Type Stimulants and New Psychoactive Substances*; United Nations Office on Drugs and Crime: Vienna, Austria, 2018.
12. United Nations Office on Drugs and Crime (UNODC). *The Challenge of New Psychoactive Substances. Global SMART Programme*; United Nations Office on Drugs and Crime: Vienna, Austria, 2013.
13. Adley, M. The Drug Wheel. 2017. Available online: http://www.thedrugswheel.com/downloads/TheDrugsWheel_2_0_2_colour.pdf (accessed on 2 February 2017).
14. Zloh, M.; Samaras, E.G.; Calvo-Castro, J.; Guirguis, A.; Stair, J.L.; Kirton, S.B. Drowning in diversity? A systematic way of clustering and selecting a representative set of new psychoactive substances. *RSC Adv.* **2017**, *7*, 53181–53191. [CrossRef]
15. Public Health England (PHE). *New Psychoactive Substances: A Toolkit for Substance Use Commissioners*; Public Health England: London, UK, 2014.
16. Public Health England (PHE). *Healthcare Professionals and Partners*; National Drug Treatment Monitoring System (NDTMS): Manchester, UK, 2016.

17. Department of Health (England) and Devolved Administrations. *Drug Misuse and Dependence, UK Guidelines on Clinical Management*; Department of Health (England); Scottish Government; Welsh Assembly Government and Northern Ireland Executive: London/Edinburgh, UK, 2007.
18. Guirguis, A.; Corkery, J.M.; Stair, J.L.; Kirton, S.B.; Zloh, M.; Goodair, C.; Schifano, F.; Davidson, C. Survey of knowledge of legal highs (novel psychoactive substances) amongst London pharmacists. *Drugs Alcohol Today* **2015**, *15*, 93–99. [CrossRef]
19. Wood, D.M.; Ceronie, B.; Dargan, P.I. Healthcare professionals are less confident in managing acute toxicity related to the use of new psychoactive substances (NPS) compared with classical recreational drugs. *QJM* **2016**, *109*, 527–529. [CrossRef] [PubMed]
20. Badachha, S. *New Psychoactive Substances: The Response by Probation and Substance Use Services in the Community in England. A Joint Inspection by HM Inspectorate of Probation and the Care Quality Commission*; Crown: London, UK, 2017.
21. Sweet, A.D. Free return trajectories or enmeshment? Some psychodynamic factors and thoughts on the role of social capital in the use of substituted cathinones (M-cats). *Drugs Alcohol Today* **2014**, *14*, 2–9. [CrossRef]
22. Moore, K.; Dargan, P.I.; Wood, D.M.; Measham, F. Do novel psychoactive substances displace established club drugs, supplement them or act as drugs of initiation? The relationship between mephedrone, ecstasy and cocaine. *Eur. Addict. Res.* **2013**, *19*, 276–282. [CrossRef] [PubMed]
23. Van Hout, M.; Brennan, R. 'Heads Held High': An Exploratory Study of Legal Highs in Pre-Legislation Ireland. *J. Ethn. Subst. Abuse* **2011**, *10*, 256–272. [CrossRef] [PubMed]
24. Van Hout, M.C.; Bingham, T. "A Costly Turn On": Patterns of use and perceived consequences of mephedrone based head shop products amongst Irish injectors. *Int. J. Drug Policy* **2012**, *23*, 188–197. [CrossRef] [PubMed]
25. Caudevilla, F.; Ventura, M.; Fornís, I.; Barratt, M.J.; Vidal, C.; Quintana, P.; Calzada, N. Results of an international drug testing service for cryptomarket users. *Int. J. Drug Policy* **2016**, *35*, 38–41. [CrossRef] [PubMed]
26. Van Buskirk, J.; Naicker, S.; Roxburgh, A.; Bruno, R.; Burns, L. Who sells what? Country specific differences in substance availability on the Agora cryptomarket. *Int. J. Drug Policy* **2016**, *35*, 16–23. [CrossRef] [PubMed]
27. Van Hout, M.C.; Hearne, E. New psychoactive substances (NPS) on cryptomarket fora: An exploratory study of characteristics of forum activity between NPS buyers and vendors. *Int. J. Drug Policy* **2017**, *40*, 102–110. [CrossRef] [PubMed]
28. Wadsworth, E.; Drummond, C.; Deluca, P. The Dynamic Environment of Crypto Markets: The Lifespan of New Psychoactive Substances (NPS) and Vendors Selling NPS. *Brain Sci.* **2018**, *8*, 46. [CrossRef] [PubMed]
29. Norman, J.; Grace, S.; Lloyd, C. Legal high groups on the Internet—The creation of new organized deviant groups? *Drugs Edu. Prev. Policy* **2014**, *21*, 14–23. [CrossRef]
30. Van Amsterdam, J.G.C.; Nabben, T.; Keiman, D.; Haanschoten, G.; Korf, D. Exploring the Attractiveness of New Psychoactive Substances (NPS) among Experienced Drug Users. *J. Psychoact. Drugs* **2015**, *47*, 177–181. [CrossRef] [PubMed]
31. Measham, F.; Wood, D.; Dargan, P.I.; Moore, K. The rise in legal highs: Prevalence and patterns in the use of illegal drugs and first- and second-generation "legal highs" in South London gay dance clubs. *J. Subst. Use* **2011**, *16*, 263–272. [CrossRef]
32. Archer, J.; Dargan, P.; Rintoul-Hoad, S.; Hudson, S.; Wood, D. Nightclub urinals—A novel and reliable way of knowing what drugs are being used in nightclubs. *Br. J. Clin. Pharmacol.* **2012**, *73*, 985.
33. Kalyanam, J.; Katsuki, T.; Lanckriet, G.R.G.; Mackey, T.M. Exploring trends of non-medical use of prescription drugs and polydrug abuse in the Twittersphere using unsupervised machine learning. *Addict. Behav.* **2017**, *65*, 289–295. [CrossRef] [PubMed]
34. Shafi, A.; Gallagher, P.; Stewart, N.; Martinotti, G.; Corazza, O. The risk of violence associated with novel psychoactive substance use in patients presenting to acute mental health services. *Hum. Psychopharmacol.* **2017**, *32*, E2606. [CrossRef] [PubMed]
35. Pirona, A.; Bo, A.; Hedrich, D.; Ferri, M.; van Gelder, N.; Giraudon, I.; Montanari, L.; Simon, R.; Mounteney, J. New psychoactive substances: Current health-related practices and challenges in responding to use and harms in Europe. *Int. J. Drug Policy* **2017**, *40*, 84–92. [CrossRef] [PubMed]
36. Abdulrahim, D.; Whiteley, C.; Moncrieff, M.; Bowden-Jones, O. *Club Drug Use among Lesbian, Gay, Bisexual and Trans (LGBT) People*; Novel Psychoactive Treatment UK Network (NEPTUNE): London, UK, 2016.

37. Lovett, C.; Yamamoto, T.; Hunter, L.; White, J.; Dargan, P.I.; Wood, D.M. Problematic recreational drug use: Is there a role for outpatient sexual health clinics in identifying those not already engaged with treatment services? *Sex Health* **2015**, *12*, 501–505. [CrossRef] [PubMed]
38. Stanley, J.L.; Mogford, D.V.; Lawrence, R.J.; Lawrie, S.M. Use of novel psychoactive substances by inpatients on general adult psychiatric wards. *BMJ Open* **2016**, *6*, e009430. [CrossRef] [PubMed]
39. Kapitány-Fövény, M.; Farkas, J.; Pataki, P.A.; Kiss, A.; Horváth, J.; Urbán, R.; Demetrovics, Z. Novel psychoactive substance use among treatment-seeking opiate users: The role of life events and psychiatric symptoms. *Hum. Psychopharmacol.* **2017**, *32*, e2602. [CrossRef] [PubMed]
40. Csak, R.; Demetrovics, Z.; Racz, J. Transition to injecting 3,4-methylene-dioxy-pyrovalerone (MDPV) among needle exchange program participants in Hungary. *J. Psychopharmacol.* **2013**, *27*, 559–563. [CrossRef] [PubMed]
41. Brod, M.; Tesler, L.E.; Christensen, T.L. Qualitative research and content validity: Developing best practices based on science and experience. *Qual. Life Res.* **2009**, *18*, 1263–1278. [CrossRef] [PubMed]
42. Green, J.; Thorogood, N. *Qualitative Methods for Health Research*, 3rd ed.; Seaman, J., Ed.; Sage Publications: London, UK, 2014.
43. Braun, V.; Clarke, V. Using thematic analysis in psychology. *Qual. Res. Psychol.* **2006**, *3*, 77–101. [CrossRef]
44. Gale, N.K.; Heath, G.; Cameron, E.; Rashid, S.; Redwood, S. Using the framework method for the analysis of qualitative data in multi-disciplinary health research. *BMC Med. Res. Methodol.* **2013**, *13*, 117. [CrossRef] [PubMed]
45. United Nations Office on Drugs and Crime (UNODC). Reducing the Harm of Drug Use and Dependence. Available online: https://www.unodc.org/ddt-training/treatment/VOLUME%20D/Topic%204/1.VolD_Topic4_Harm_Reduction.pdf (accessed on 11 May 2016).
46. Guirguis, A.; Corkery, J.M.; Stair, J.L.; Kirton, S.B.; Zloh, M.; Schifano, F. Intended and unintended use of cathinone mixtures. *Hum. Psychopharmacol.* **2017**, *32*. [CrossRef] [PubMed]
47. Department for Constitutional Affairs. *Mental Capacity Act 2005: Code of Practice*; Stationary Office: Norwich, UK, 2007.
48. General Pharmaceutical Council (GPhC). *Guidance on Consent*; GPhC: London, UK, 2012.
49. Guest, G.; Bunce, A.; Johnson, L. How Many Interviews Are Enough? An Experiment with Data Saturation and Variability. *Field Methods* **2006**, *18*, 59–82. [CrossRef]
50. Harris, C.R.; Brown, A. Synthetic cannabinoid intoxication: A case series and review. *J. Emerg. Med.* **2013**, *44*, 360–366. [CrossRef] [PubMed]
51. Schifano, F.; Orsolini, L.; Papanti, D.; Corkery, J. NPS: Medical consequences associated with their intake, in Neuropharmacology of New Psychoactive Substances (NPS): The Science Behind the Headlines. In *Current Topics in Behavioral Neurosciences*; Springer International Publishing: Basel, Switzerland, 2016.
52. Adams, R.D.; Good, A.M.; Thomas, S.H.L.; Thompson, J.P.; Vale, J.A.; Eddleston, M. TOXBASE and its use in collecting data on new and uncommon products of interest. *Clin. Toxicol.* **2015**, *53*, 398.
53. UNODC. World Drug Report. United Nations Office on Drugs and Crime: Vienna, Austria, 2017. Available online: https://www.unodc.org/wdr2017/field/Booklet_1_EXSUM.pdf (accessed on 21 March 2018).
54. Chen, C.; Kostakis, C.; Irvine, R.J.; White, J.M. Increases in use of novel synthetic stimulant are not directly linked to decreased use of 3,4-methylenedioxy-N-methylamphetamine (MDMA). *Forensic Sci. Int.* **2013**, *231*, 278–283. [CrossRef] [PubMed]
55. Ralphs, R.; Williams, L.; Askew, R.; Norton, A. Adding Spice to the Porridge11 'Porridge' is British slang for a prison sentence. e.g., 'Doing his porridge'. The term is most commonly thought to be an allusion to the fact that porridge is, or used to be, a common food in prison. The term is also thought to be a pun on the much older slang word for prison, 'stir': The development of a synthetic cannabinoid market in an English prison. *Int. J. Drug Policy* **2017**, *40*, 57–69. [PubMed]
56. Guirguis, A. New psychoactive substances: A public health issue. *Int. J. Pharm. Pract.* **2017**, *25*, 323–325. [CrossRef] [PubMed]
57. Soussan, C.; Kjellgren, A. "Chasing the high"—Experiences of ethylphenidate as described on international internet forums. *Subst. Abuse* **2015**, *9*, 9–16. [CrossRef] [PubMed]

58. Mounteney, J.; Bo, A.; Griffiths, P. The internet and drug markets: Shining a light on these complex and dynamic systems. In *The Internet and Drug Markets*; Mounteney, J., Bo, A., Oteo, A., Eds.; European Monitoring Centre on Drugs and Drug Addiction: Lisbon, Portugal, 2016; Chapter 1.
59. Tracy, D.K.; Wood, D.M.; Baumeister, D. Novel psychoactive substances: identifying and managing acute and chronic harmful use. *BMJ* **2017**, 365. [CrossRef] [PubMed]
60. Kassai, S.; Pintér, J.N.; Rácz, J.; Böröndi, B.; Tóth-Karikó, T.; Kerekes, K.; Gyarmathy, V.A. Assessing the experience of using synthetic cannabinoids by means of interpretative phenomenological analysis. *Harm Reduct. J.* **2017**, *14*, 9. [CrossRef]
61. Assi, S.; Guirguis, A.; Halsey, S.; Fergus, S.; Stair, J.L. Analysis of 'legal high' substances and common adulterants using handheld spectroscopic techniques. *Anal. Methods* **2015**, *7*, 736–746. [CrossRef]

# 5

# A Study on Photostability of Amphetamines and Ketamine in Hair Irradiated under Artificial Sunlight

**Giorgia Miolo [1,*], Marianna Tucci [2], Luca Menilli [1], Giulia Stocchero [2], Susanna Vogliardi [2], Salvatore Scrivano [3], Massimo Montisci [2] and Donata Favretto [2,*]**

1 Department of Pharmaceutical and Pharmacological Sciences, University of Padova, 35131 Padova, Italy; luca.menilli@phd.unipd.it
2 Legal Medicine and Toxicology, University Hospital of Padova, 35121 Padova, Italy; marianna.tucci@gmail.com (M.T.); giulia.stocchero@aopd.veneto.it (G.S.); susanna.vogliardi@unipd.it (S.V.); massimo.montisci@unipd.it (M.M.)
3 School of Specialization in Legal Medicine, University Hospital of Padova, 35121 Padova, Italy; salvatore.scrivano@studenti.unipd.it
* Correspondence: giorgia.miolo@unipd.it (G.M.); donata.favretto@unipd.it (D.F.);

**Abstract:** Drugs incorporated into hair are exposed to the environment, and cosmetic and chemical treatments, with possible decreases in their content. Knowledge concerning the effect of sunlight on drug content in hair can be helpful to forensic toxicologists, in particular, when investigating drug concentrations above or below pre-determined cut-offs. Twenty authentic positive hair samples were selected which had previously tested positive for amphetamines and/or ketamine. Washed hair were divided into two identical strands, with the former exposed at 765 W/m$^2$ (300–800 nm spectrum of irradiance) for 48 h in a solar simulator, and the latter kept in the dark. Hair samples were extracted and analyzed by liquid chromatography high-resolution mass spectrometry detection. The percentage of photodegradation was calculated for each analyte (i.e., amphetamine, methamphetamine, methylendioxyamphetamine, ketamine, and norketamine). In parallel, photodegradation processes of standard molecules dissolved in aqueous and organic solutions were studied. In 20 hair samples positive for the targeted analytes, exposure to artificial sunlight induced an appreciable decrease in drug concentrations. The concentration ranges in the non-irradiated hair samples were 0.01–24 ng/mg, and 65% of samples exhibited a decrease in post-irradiation samples, with reduction from 3% to 100%. When more drugs were present in the same hair sample (i.e., MDMA and ketamine) the degradation yields were compound dependent. A degradation product induced by irradiation of ketamine in aqueous and methanol solutions was identified; it was also found to be present in a true positive hair sample after irradiation. Ketamine, amphetamines, and their metabolites incorporated in the hair of drug users undergo degradation when irradiated by artificial sunlight. Only for ketamine was a photoproduct identified in irradiated standard solutions and in true positive irradiated hair. When decisional cut-offs are applied to hair analysis, photodegradation must be taken into account since sunlight may produce false negative results. Moreover, new markers could be investigated as evidence of illicit drug use.

**Keywords:** hair; solar light; photodegradation; amphetamines; MDMA; ketamine

---

## 1. Introduction

The main advantage of hair as a testing matrix is the ability to provide information relating to historical drug exposure. Hair analysis has many applications within forensic (e.g., drug-related deaths, drug-facilitated crimes (DFCs), child protection) and clinical toxicology (e.g., drug rehabilitation programs, workplace drug testing) [1–4].

The stability of drugs in hair, however, is affected by exposure to sunlight and weathering, cosmetic chemical treatments (i.e., oxidative dyeing, bleaching, or permanent wave), and physical damage [5–7]. In particular, exposure to sunlight and/or artificial light for many hours per day can induce photodegradation (i.e., photolysis) of licit/illicit drugs through the formation of free radicals (produced by the drug itself or formed by eumelanin and pheomelanin, and their oxidative products oxyeumelanin, and oxypheomelanin) or photosensitization reactions by intermolecular energy transfer. [8]

Previous studies on this matter have been published by Skopp et al. [9] in which cannabinoids detected in hair and affected by solar radiation were shown to reduce in concentration. More recently, Favretto et al. [10] evaluated the effect of light exposure on methadone, cocaine, and heroin metabolites in hair.

In order to better understand the role and underlying mechanisms of solar light exposure on decreasing concentrations of drugs in hair, and following our previous [10] photodegradation studies on UVA- and UVB-induced changes, the aim of the present work was to evaluate the photodegradation of several common stimulant drugs (i.e., amphetamines and ketamine (KET)) in true positive hair samples exposed to the whole spectrum of sunlight in a solar simulator. The use of a solar simulator, including visible light (400–800 nm) and part of UV radiation from 400 nm to 3 μnm (UVA = 400–315 nm, UVB = 315–280 nm), mimics exposure to environmental sunlight.

Amphetamine-based drugs are illegal synthetic stimulants that share a common structural backbone. The four amphetamines considered in the present work are the most used in Europe: amphetamine (AMF), methamphetamine (MA), 3,4-methylenedioxymethamphetamine (MDMA), and 3,4-methylenedioxyamphetamine (MDA).

Amphetamine can be metabolized along two pathways: either by hydroxylation of the aromatic ring to 4-hydroxyamphetamine or by deamination of the side chain to benzyl methyl ketone, which can then be degraded to benzoic acid. Methamphetamine is metabolized by cytochrome P450 (CYP), mainly by the CYP2D and CYP3A subfamilies, leading to the production of 4-hydroxyamphetamine and AMF. The half-life of MA is about 10 h, and 35–45% of a dose is excreted unchanged in the urine over a period of several days. Other metabolites, such as 4-hydroxymethamphetamine, norephedrine, and 4-hydroxynorephedrine, can also be found in urine in substantial quantities [11–13].

In addition, MDMA (i.e., 3,4-methylenedioxymethamphetamine, ecstasy) is a widely abused psychostimulant drug that acts as a powerful releaser and/or reuptake inhibitor of serotonin (5-HT), dopamine (DA), and norepinephrine (NE). Its metabolism depends on the following main metabolic pathways: (1) *O*-demethylenation followed by catechol-*O*-methyltransferase (COMT) methylation and/or glucuronide/sulfate conjugation; and (2) *N*-dealkylation, deamination, and oxidation. MDMA *N*-demethylation gives rise to 3,4-methylenedioxyamphetamine (MDA). The elimination half-life of MDMA is about 8–9 h, lower than those reported for MA (10–12 h) or AMF (12–15 h) [14,15].

Ketamine is a dissociative anesthetic drug that functions as an antagonist of the *N*-methyl-D-aspartate receptor and enhances the antinociceptive effects of conventional opioid analgesia, binding to μ opioid and σ receptors. Ketamine is increasingly misused as a recreational and "club drug" because of its hallucinogenic and stimulant effects, and also as a "date-rape" drug (to facilitate sexual assault). Ketamine is metabolized in the liver by the P450 system, and CYP3A4 is the main enzyme responsible for transforming *N*-demethylation into norketamine (NKET), 4-hydroxy-ketamine, and 6-hydroxy-ketamine. The elimination half-life is about 2 h, and the predominant metabolite of urinary excretion over a 72 h period is dehydronorketamine (DHNK) (16%), along with conjugates of hydroxylated ketamine metabolites [16,17].

The consumption of alcohol and/or drugs is associated with an increased risk of being the victim of a sexual assault. A retrospective case series in London on 1014 cases of claimed drug-facilitated sexual assaults (DFSAs) showed that in 34% of samples (blood and/or urine), an illicit drug (with or without alcohol) was found, of which 10.8% contained cocaine, 4.6% "ecstasy" (MDMA), and 2.3% AMF [18,19]. In DFC cases, alleged victims are often unconscious leading up to the assault due to the amnesiac effects of the drug(s) administered, thus a considerable amount of time may be spent before the victim reports the incident. Consequently, hair analysis is of primary importance compared to blood and urine analysis, particularly when the occasional consumption is sufficiently high; however, exposure to the environment may affect the stability of drugs in the keratin matrix.

For these reasons, reliable interpretation of the analytical results is fundamental for a correct interpretation of a positive or negative result, and general knowledge of the photostability of drug analytes in the biological matrix must be considered. However, no data have been published until now on the effect of light on KET and amphetamines, and their respective metabolites in the keratin matrix; only morphine and 6-monoacetylmorphine (6-MAM) photodegradation have been studied by UVA and UVB irradiation [20].

In the present paper, levels of AMF, MA, MDMA, MDA, KET, and NKET were determined by means of liquid chromatography high-resolution mass spectrometry (HPLC-HRMS) [21,22] in authentic hair samples from drugs users before and after irradiation under the whole spectrum of sunlight in a solar simulator.

Although the photodegradation of a molecule not only depends on the wavelength used, but also on its physical state (solid or liquid) and the environment in which it is irradiated (i.e., solvent, polarity, pH, and the presence of salts, oxygen, and other compounds in the sample), we tested the same analytes in a pure methanol and water solution irradiated under the whole spectrum of sunlight to gather general information on their behavior and to study their kinetics of photodegradation.

## 2. Experiments

### 2.1. Chemicals

Amphetamine, MA, MDMA, MDA, KET, and NKET were purchased from LGC Promochem Cerilliant (Teddington, Middlesex, UK) as pure solutions in methanol at 1.0 mg/mL. The internal standards (IS) MA-D5, AMF-D5, MDMA-D5, MDA-D5, and KET-D3 were methanol solutions also from LGC Promochem at 1.0 mg/mL.

Methanol, dichloromethane, and acetonitrile (Merck, Darmstadt, Germany) were high-performance liquid chromatography (HPLC) grade. Trifluoroacetic acid (TFA) was from Sigma (Sigma-Aldrich, Milan, Italy). High-performance liquid chromatography water was prepared using a Milli-Q Plus (Millipore, Molsheim, France) system. All other reagents were from Sigma-Aldrich (St Louis, MO, USA).

### 2.2. Hair Samples

Authentic positive hairs were selected from samples at the laboratory that had previously tested positive for amphetamines and/or KET. Hair samples were collected with scissors from the posterior vertex and cut as close to the scalp as possible, wrapped in aluminum foil, and kept at room temperature until analysis. As recorded in donor interviews, all samples had not been submitted to previous cosmetic or chemical treatments.

### 2.3. Irradiation Procedure

Irradiation was performed in a Suntest CPS+ (Atlas, Linsengericht, Germany) equipped with a 1.8 kW xenon lamp and a glass filter (cut-off 310 nm) according to Option 1 of ICH Guideline Q1B (European Medicines Agency, London, UK, ICH Topic Q1B–Photostability testing of new active substances and medical products, 1998). The dark samples were maintained at solar box temperature during irradiation.

### 2.4. Photolysis Experiments in Solution (In Vitro Study)

Solutions of the compounds at concentrations ranging from $10^{-5}$ to $10^{-4}$ M in methanol and water were irradiated in the Suntest CPS+ with times increasing from 1 h up to 3 h.

Photolysis was evaluated using Cary 50 UV-Vis spectrophotometer (Varian, Milan, Italy) analyzing the change in the original spectrum upon irradiation, as already described [20], and by high-resolution mass spectrometry (HRMS). At selected UV doses, the solutions were diluted to $10^{-6}$ M in methanol and water, and analyzed by direct injection HRMS to measure the photodegradation of the analytes by recording the decrease of the ion signal of protonated molecules obtained by electrospray ionization (ESI) of solutions kept in the dark. The results are the mean of at least three experiments.

### 2.5. Photolysis Experiments in Hair Samples (In Vivo Study)

Hairs 5–7 cm long were divided into two approximately identical strands: the former was put between two 5 × 5 cm optical glasses and exposed at 765 W/$m^2$ (spectrum of irradiance: 310–800 nm) for 48 h in the solar simulator to an endpoint corresponding to two months exposure under the sunlight, and the latter was kept as a dark control in the same chamber of irradiation covered with an aluminum foil.

### 2.6. Hair Sample Preparation and Extraction

Hair samples were decontaminated with 3 mL of water and 3 mL of methanol. Pulverization was applied by the automatic homogenizer Precellys® Evolution (Bertin Technologies, Genoa, Italy) at a speed of 6000 RPM, cycle 9 × 30 s, pause 30 s. Solid phase extraction (SPE) was performed by Oasis MCX (Waters, Milford, MA, USA) cartridges. Sample preparation consisted of the addition of 2 ng/mg of IS and 3 mL of a methanol/TFA (90:10, *v*/*v*) solution to 25 mg powdered hair samples, ultrasonication for 1 h, and incubation overnight at 45 °C. After centrifugation, the methanolic solutions were dried under a stream of nitrogen at 40 °C. The residues were reconstituted in 3 mL of 0.1 M phosphate buffer pH 6 and subjected to SPE. After, cartridges of the sample conditioned with 3 mL methanol and 3 mL 0.1 M phosphate buffer pH 6 were loaded. Cleanup was accomplished by sequential washes with 3 mL of water, 3 mL of 0.1 N hydrochloric acid, and 3 mL of methanol. Cartridges were dried for 10 min under vacuum before elution with 2 mL of dichloromethane: 2-propanol (80:20, *v*/*v*) 2% ammonium hydroxide. Eluates were evaporated to dryness with nitrogen at 40 °C, reconstituted in 200 µL of water (0.1% formic acid)/acetonitrile 9:1 mixture, and 25 µL were injected into the LC-HRMS system.

### 2.7. High-Resolution Mass Spectrometry (HRMS)

All measurements were performed on an LTQ-Orbitrap (Thermo Fisher Scientific, Bremen, Germany) high-accuracy, high-resolution mass spectrometer operating in positive ESI mode and equipped with a Surveyor MS Pump.

### 2.8. Electrospray Ionization HRMS

For the analysis of pure standard solutions, direct injection analysis was performed with a syringe pump delivering solutions at 10 µL/min directly into the ESI source. The positive ion ESI parameters were as follows: capillary voltage 10 V, sheath gas flow rate 20 (arbitrary units, a.u.), auxiliary gas ($N_2$) flow rate 5 (a.u.), sweep gas flow rate 5 (a.u.), and capillary temperature 275 °C. Profile full-scan mass spectra were acquired in the Orbitrap in the $m/z$ range 120–700 with a target mass resolution of 100,000 (FWHM as defined at 400 $m/z$) and a scan time of 0.65 s.

### 2.9. High-Performance Liquid Chromatography HRMS

For the determination of drug concentrations in hair and in standard solutions, 25 µL of solutions or extracts were injected into an Atlantis T3 (150 × 1.0 mm, 3 µm) column (Waters Corporation, Milford, MA, USA). High-performance liquid chromatography separation was achieved by gradient elution at a constant flow rate of 300 µL/min. High-performance liquid chromatography conditions: A (water, 0.1% formic acid) and B (methanol, 0.1% HCOOH); initial conditions 10% B, linear gradient to 25% B in 4 min, 25% B hold from 4 min to 7 min, then ramped to 40% B in 5 min, to 60% B in 4 min and to 90% B in 2 min; 90% B hold from 18 min to 26 min. The column temperature was 40 °C. Mass spectrometry conditions were: positive ion ESI; capillary voltage 10 V, sheath gas flow rate 50 (arbitrary units, a.u.), auxiliary gas ($N_2$) flow rate 5 (a.u.), sweep gas flow rate 5 (a.u.), and capillary temperature 275 °C. Profile full-scan mass spectra were acquired in the Orbitrap in the $m/z$ range 120–700 with a target mass resolution of 60,000 (FWHM as defined at 400 $m/z$) and a scan time of 0.45 s. Detection of the analytes and the IS was based on retention time, accurate mass measurements of $MH^+$ ions, and correspondence of the observed isotopic pattern to the calculated one. Drug concentrations were determined from peak area ratios of analyte to its IS compared to calibrator curves of peak area ratios to concentrations. The method was fully validated exhibiting a linear range from 0.1 ng/mg to 50 ng/mg (determined from regression with $1/x^2$ weighting utilizing six calibration points), lower limits of quantification of 0.01 ng/mg and limits of detection of 0.005 ng/mg for all the target analytes, intra-day imprecision, inaccuracy always lower than 19% and 20%, and inter-day imprecision and inaccuracy always lower than 21% and 22%, respectively. Extraction efficiency was determined in the range of 85–100% for the different substances.

## 3. Results

### *3.1. Photodegradation in Methanol and Water Solutions Exposed to Suntest CPS+*

Preliminary, stock methanol, and water solutions for all the analytes diluted to $10^{-4}$ M were irradiated inside the photostability test chamber from 1 h to 3 h (each hour corresponding to about 70 J/cm$^2$), and their absorption spectra before and after irradiation were recorded (Supplementary Figures S1A1–S1F2).

Amphetamine dissolved in methanol was characterized by the only band at around 205–210 nm, mainly corresponding to the solvent, thus remaining unmodified in all the irradiated solutions (see Supplementary Figure S1A1). However, a shift to 205 nm and a small increase in spectral intensity were detected by increasing irradiation. When irradiated in water, AMF was characterized by two bands (around 220 nm and 240 nm) decreasing as irradiation dose increased (see Supplementary Figure S1A2).

Methamphetamine, both in methanol and water (Figures S1B1 and B2, respectively), presented curves similar to AMF, with the unique difference being the absorption at 205 nm in water which increased under irradiation.

In addition, MDA in methanol (Figure S1C1) was characterized by three bands at 208 nm, 235 nm, and 285 nm. The irradiated solutions presented similar curves with increasing absorption and a small blue shift at 230 nm and 280 nm. Similar spectra were obtained for MDA in water (Figure S1C2), with two bands at 230 nm and 285 nm increasing in relation to irradiation time.

Furthermore, MDMA in methanol showed two bands centered at 235 nm and at 285 nm, indicating a small absorption increase and a small blue shift (Figure S1D1). A new band of absorption (300–340 nm) appeared which increased upon irradiation. In water, MDMA presented the same absorption band with a higher increase at 235 nm than at 285 nm, and the appearance of a band at 320 nm (Figure S1D2).

Ketamine in methanol was characterized by a single absorption band (205–230 nm). When irradiated, this band slightly increased and a shoulder (230–270 nm) appeared, as evidenced in Supplementary Figure S1E. On the contrary, in water, KET did not change its absorption spectrum upon irradiation (Figure S1E2). Absorption spectrum of NKET in methanol increased upon irradiation at 210–220 nm and in the range of 240–250 nm (Figure S1F1). In water, NKET showed a similar behavior upon irradiation for the band 240–250 nm, with slight changes (Figure S1F2).

### 3.2. Identification of New Photoproducts

All the irradiated solutions in the solar simulator, including the control solutions kept in the dark, were diluted to $10^{-5}$ M either in methanol or water, and analyzed by direct infusion HRMS, with the aim of identifying the compounds eventually formed upon irradiation. Interestingly, for KET and NKET only, some new species were observed in irradiated solutions. In HRMS spectrum of KET irradiated in water solution, its $[M+H]^+$ ion at 238.0993 $m/z$ ($C_{13}H_{17}ClNO$) was accompanied by a new ionic species at 220.0888 $m/z$ ($C_{13}H_{15}ClN$), corresponding to the loss of $H_2O$. In methanol, two species were observed at 220.0888 $m/z$ and at 252.0786 $m/z$ ($C_{13}H_{15}ClNO_2$), with the latter corresponding to the loss of $H_2$ and to the photo-addition of one oxygen atom. The proposed structures of KET photoproducts are shown in Figures 1 and 2. It must be highlighted that the ionic species identified were new protonated molecules present in solution, and they are not fragment ions produced by collisional experiments on precursor ions.

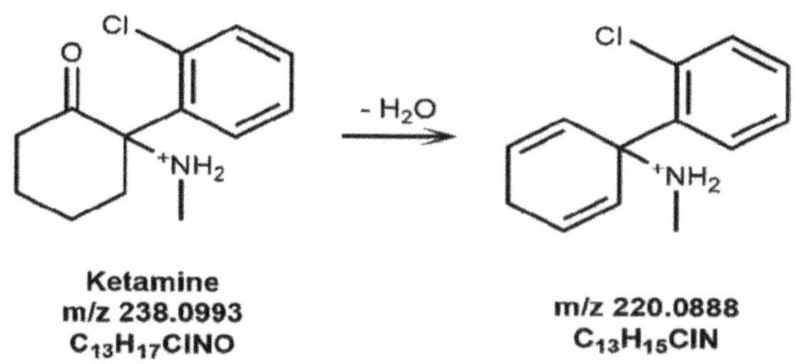


**Figure 1.** Proposed structures of ketamine (KET) photoproducts formed in a water solution upon irradiation for 3 h.

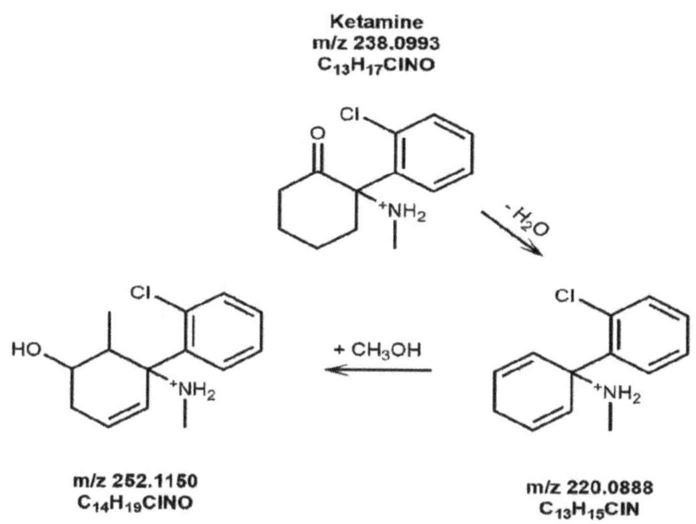


**Figure 2.** Proposed structures of KET photoproducts formed in a methanol solution upon irradiation for 3 h.

In HRMS spectrum of the methanol solution of NKET irradiated in the solar simulator, $[M+H]^+$ ions at 224.0837 $m/z$ ($C_{12}H_{15}ClNO$) were accompanied by a new species at 206.0731 $m/z$ ($C_{12}H_{13}ClN$), corresponding to the loss of $H_2O$. The proposed structure of NKET photoproducts formed in methanol is shown in Figure 3 analogously to KET. However, differently from KET, no photoproduct was detected in HRMS spectrum of NKET irradiated in water solution.

Vice versa, for all the other analytes (i.e., AMF, MA, and MDMA), both in water and methanol solutions, no photoproducts were evidenced by direct HRMS analysis. To avoid ionization suppression phenomena that could occur in a mixture and shield the presence of less abundant species, irradiated solutions were also analyzed by HPLC-HRMS. The ratios of peak areas observed for samples upon irradiation vs those analogous samples kept in the dark were calculated as "percent degradation". In Figure 4, the yields of photodegradation obtained for all the analytes after 1 h, 2 h, and 3 h of irradiation are reported.

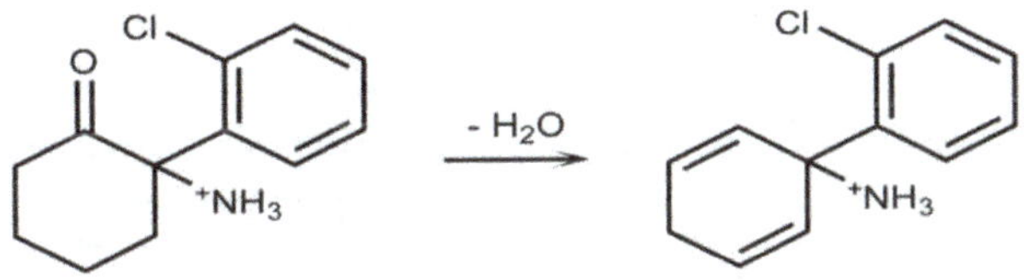


**Norketamine**
**m/z 224.0837**
**$C_{12}H_{15}ClNO$**

**m/z 206.0731**
**$C_{12}H_{13}ClN$**

**Figure 3.** Proposed structures of norketamine (NKET) photoproducts formed in a methanol solution upon irradiation for 3 h.

As may be observed, AMF and MA in water show the highest photostability: the photodegradation was 1% and 4%, respectively, while in methanol it increased up to 15%. In addition, MDMA and MDA in methanol and water both presented similar photodegradation with a linear relationship with irradiation time: MDMA from 23% to 42% and MDA from 13% to 36%. For KET and NKET, the photodegradation yield was significantly higher in methanol (KET 61%; NKET 36%) than in water (KET 16%; NKET 13%) after 3 h.

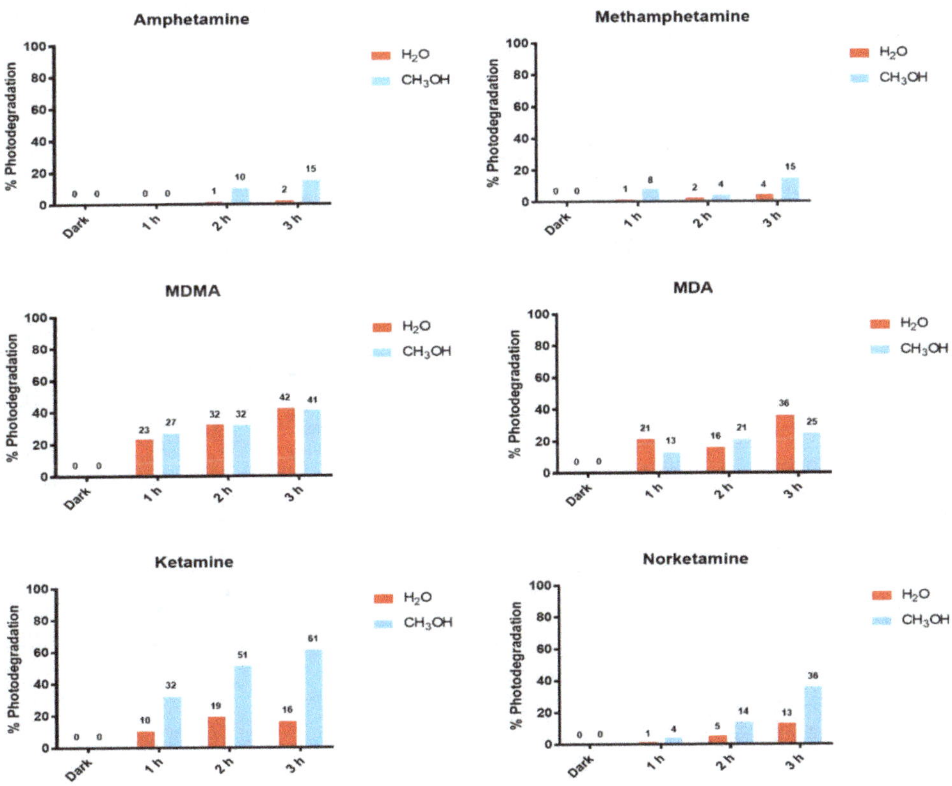


**Figure 4.** Relative degradation of target drugs in methanol and water solutions with increasing time of irradiation in the solar simulator (% photodegradation calculated using the peak area of protonated molecules in solutions kept in the dark as controls for 0% degradation).

### 3.3. Photodegradation in Hair Exposed to Solar Box

The main goal of the study was to observe the photo-induced degradation of drugs in hair. In Figure 5, the concentrations of each drug for all seventeen hair samples irradiated in the solar simulator or kept in the dark (control) are presented.

| Physical characteristics | | | | Dark | | | | | | Irradiated | | | | | |
|---|---|---|---|---|---|---|---|---|---|---|---|---|---|---|---|
| Color | Thickness | Straight | Curly | MET (ng/mg) | AMP (ng/mg) | MDMA (ng/mg) | MDA (ng/mg) | KET (ng/mg) | NKET (ng/mg) | MET (ng/mg) | AMP (ng/mg) | MDMA (ng/mg) | MDA (ng/mg) | KET (ng/mg) | NKET (ng/mg) |
| Brown 1 | Thin | ● | | -* | - | - | - | 0.02 | - | -* | - | - | - | 0.02 | - |
| Brown 2 | Thin | ● | | - | - | - | - | 0.04 | 0.02 | - | - | - | - | 0.03 | 0.01 |
| Brown 3 | Thin | ● | | - | - | 2.34 | 0.34 | 23.8 | 3.17 | - | - | 0.34 | 0.34 | 4.2 | 0.85 |
| Brown 4 | Thick | | ● | - | - | - | - | 0.12 | - | - | - | - | - | 0.05 | - |
| Brown 5 | Thin | ● | | - | 0.06 | - | - | 0.10 | 0.03 | - | 0.04 | - | - | 0.07 | 0.01 |
| Brown 6 | Thick | ● | | - | - | 0.20 | - | - | - | - | - | 0.118 | - | - | - |
| Brown 7 | Thin | ● | | - | - | 0.69 | 0.05 | - | - | - | - | 0.76 | 0.04 | - | - |
| Brown 8 | Thick | ● | | - | - | 0.09 | - | - | - | - | - | 0.07 | - | - | - |
| Brown 9 | Thick | | ● | - | - | - | - | 0.06 | 0.06 | - | - | - | - | 0.04 | 0.04 |
| Brown 10 | Thin | ● | | - | - | - | - | 0.15 | 0.02 | - | - | - | - | 0.09 | 0.01 |
| Brown 11 | Thick | ● | | - | - | - | - | 0.28 | 0.02 | - | - | - | - | 0.22 | 0.03 |
| Brown 12 | Thick | | ● | - | - | - | - | 0.05 | 0.01 | - | - | - | - | 0.02 | 0.01 |
| Dark Brown 1 | Thick | ● | | - | - | - | - | 0.34 | 0.02 | - | - | - | - | 0.09 | 0.02 |
| Black 1 | Thin | ● | | - | 0.99 | 1.40 | 0.07 | 14.3 | 2.43 | - | 0.64 | 1.63 | 0.06 | 8.85 | 1.46 |
| Black 2 | Thin | ● | | 0.97 | - | - | - | - | - | 0.84 | - | - | - | - | - |
| Black 3 | Thin | ● | | 24.1 | 0.93 | - | - | - | - | 12.7 | 0.7 | - | - | - | - |
| Black 4 | Thin | ● | | - | - | 0.45 | - | - | - | - | - | 0.32 | - | - | - |

**Figure 5.** Drug concentrations in hair samples with their physical characteristics calculated by high-performance liquid chromatography high-resolution mass spectrometry (HPLC-HRMS) in both aliquots kept in the dark or irradiated in the solar simulator. -: absent at limit of detection (LOD, 0.005 ng/mg); (—) observed % increase.

In Figure 6, the percentages of photodegradation are reported. Calculations were made using the concentrations of samples kept in the dark as control:

$$\%\ \text{photodegradation} = (\text{drug conc.}_{\text{dark}} - \text{drug conc.}_{\text{irradiatied}})/\text{drug conc.}_{\text{dark}} \times 100.$$

| | % PHOTODEGRADATION | | | | | | | | | | | | | | | | Average % | SD | Range % |
|---|---|---|---|---|---|---|---|---|---|---|---|---|---|---|---|---|---|---|---|
| | BROWN 1 | BROWN 2 | BROWN 3 | BROWN 4 | BROWN 5 | BROWN 6 | BROWN 7 | BROWN 8 | BROWN 9 | BROWN 10 | BROWN 11 | BROWN 12 | DARK BROWN 1 | BLACK 1 | BLACK 2 | BLACK 3 | BLACK 4 | | | |
| MET | | | | | - | | | | | | | | | - | 13 | 47 | | 30 | 24 | 13-47 |
| AMF | | | | | 33 | | | | | | | | | 35 | - | 25 | | 31 | 6 | 25-35 |
| MDMA | | | 85 | | | 41 | (-)10 | 22 | | | | | | (-)16 | | | 29 | 25 | 37 | (-)16-85 |
| MDA | | | - | | | - | 20 | - | | | | | | 14 | | | | 8 | 11 | 0-16 |
| KET | 0 | 25 | 82 | 58 | 30 | | | | 33 | 40 | 21 | 60 | 74 | 38 | | | | 42 | 24 | 0-82 |
| NKET | - | 50 | 73 | - | 63 | | | | 33 | 50 | (-)50 | 0 | 0 | 40 | | | | 29 | 39 | (-)50-73 |

(-): % increase; -: substance not present

**Figure 6.** Percentage of photodegradation, average, standard deviation, and range of drugs in hair samples irradiated at 765 W/m$^2$ in the solar simulator.

When comparing results from three poly-drug abusers, photodegradation of all the analytes was generally obtained, with the highest comparable photodegradation yields observed in sample Brown 3 (see Figure 7).

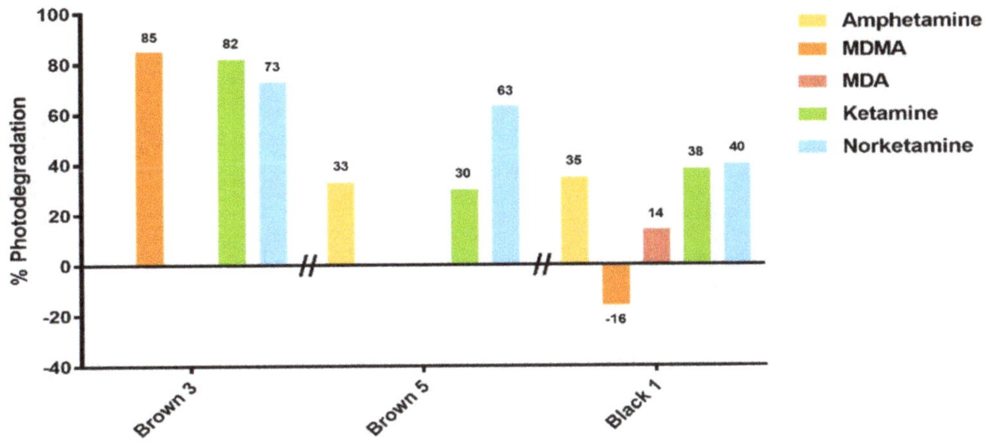


**Figure 7.** Percentage of photodegradation of amphetamine (AMF), KET, and NKET in three different hair samples. In these three samples, photodegradation seems to depend on the hair owner.

## 4. Discussion

From our results, a clearly different behavior of KET and NKET was evidenced when compared to all the other drugs and metabolites under study. Indeed, these drugs seem photo-unstable, both in solution and in hair matrix. In particular, for the experiments in solution, KET and NKET photo-induced products were identified; in hair samples their degradation was higher (average 42% and 29%) than all the other compounds (average 8–30%).

No color effect seems to be present, although no fair hair samples were present in this study, and the number of samples was limited. It is well known that the color of hair depends on the relative amount of pheomelanin (red) and eumelanin (black), the first defense against UV in human hair and skin [23–26]. Generally, a part of the light is absorbed by the hair matrix itself without any photochemical effect. In dark hair, the eumelanin can protect the drugs/metabolites with a higher degree than in fair hair. However, melanin may also react with oxygen under irradiation, producing reactive species, such as superoxide anion, that can induce photolysis of melanin itself [27], thus weakening the photoprotective effect of the pigment. In this context, no clear-cut interpretation of the role of hair color can be made.

Regarding MA and AMF, on the basis of the in vitro experiments, they were expected to photodegrade less readily than KET and NKET. Unexpectedly, the experiments in hair revealed an average degradation of 30% and 31% for MA and AMF, respectively, with a range of 13–47% and 25–35%.

The presence of photoproducts was also investigated in irradiated hair samples. In one sample, the species at 220.08750 $m/z$, corresponding to the photoproduct of KET shown in Figure 1, could be identified by LC-HRMS as evidenced in Figure 8.

The importance of this finding must be highlighted, since no previous study has identified stable photoproducts in hair for KET, nor for any other substance previously investigated (i.e., cannabinoids, cocaine, opiates, methadone [9,10,20,21]).

The "apparent production" of NKET upon irradiation of sample Brown 11 was at first sight surprising, but could be reasonably related to the physical decomposition of the matrix, leaving KET more labile during the irradiation experiment and favoring its transformation to the metabolite. Furthermore, the increase of MDMA in sample Black 1 and Brown 7 upon irradiation can be rationalized (as already demonstrated in previous studies) by a greater lability of the keratin matrix with consequent greater yield during the extraction of the analytes in the liquid acid phase with access to deeper layers of the hair structure.

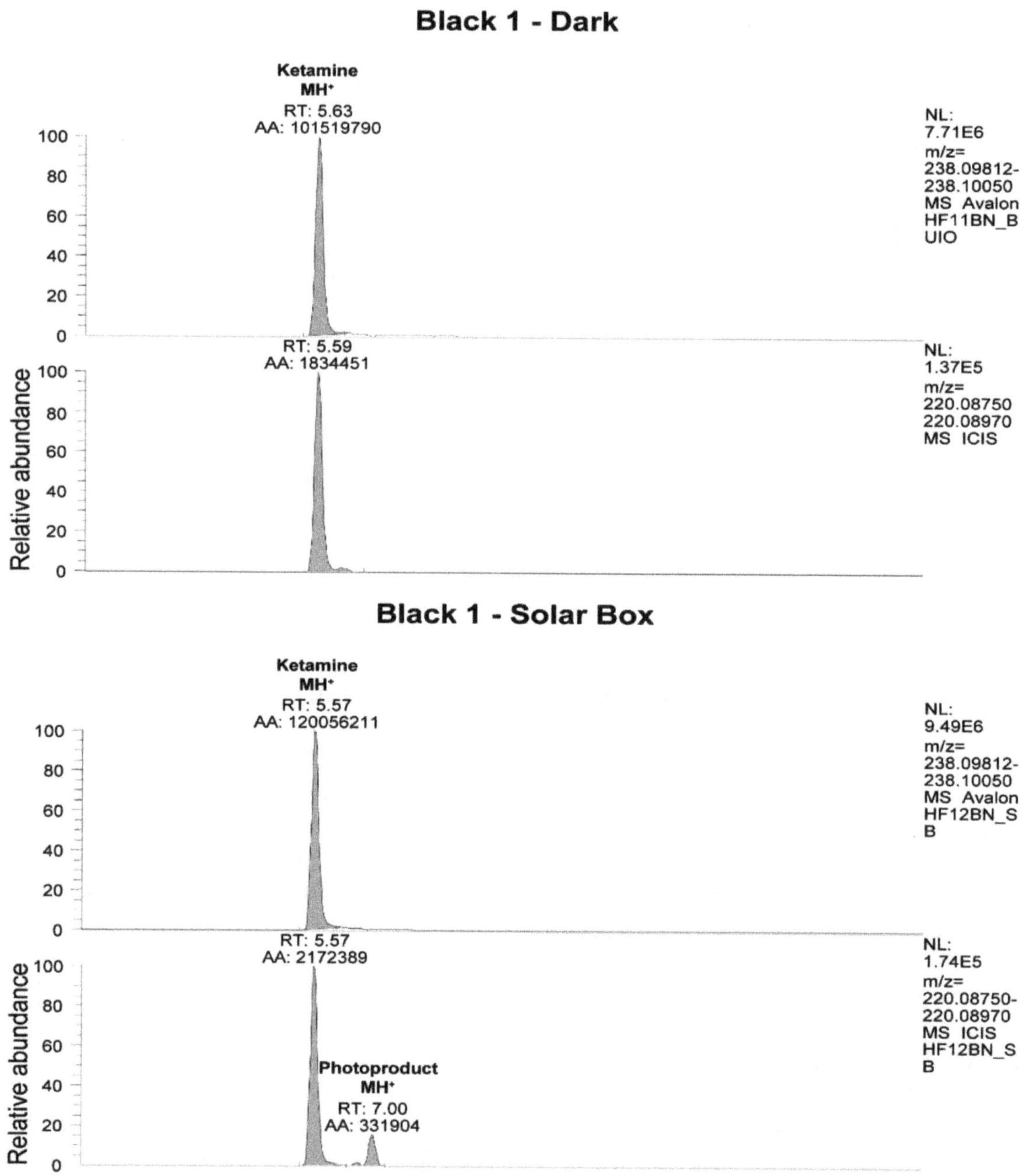


**Figure 8.** LC-HRMS analysis of hair sample Black 1 taken in the dark and after irradiation in the solar simulator. In the irradiated sample, the presence of a KET photoproduct with 220.08750 $m/z$ is evident.

## 5. Conclusions

Amphetamine, MA MDA, MDMA, KET, and NKET incorporated in hair undergo degradation when irradiated by artificial sunlight, suggesting that they can suffer photodegradation under natural sunlight. With this work, for the first time, the presence of a photoproduct of KET was evidenced in one true positive sample.

Since the detection of drugs in hair is often used as evidence of illegal acts with consequences on the freedom of persons, the UV-Vis effects on the integrity of the drugs and their metabolites should be considered when single administration needs to be evidenced. When decisional cut-offs are applied to hair analysis (e.g., for granting a driving license, a job, or a child custody), it must be taken into account that hair exposed to sunlight may produce false negative results and lead to misjudgment. When possible, the detection of photoproducts of a drug under investigation can be a key factor in a case management.

**Supplementary Materials:**
Fig S1A1/A2. UV spectrum of AMF (10-4 M) in methanol/water, by increasing exposure time in solar simulator;
Fig S1B1/B2. UV spectrum of MA (10-4 M) in methanol/water, by increasing exposure time in solar simulator;
Fig S1C1/C2. UV spectrum of MDA (10-4 M) in methanol/water, by increasing exposure time in solar simulator;
Fig S1D1/D2. UV spectrum of MDMA (10-4 M) in methanol/water, by increasing exposure time in solar simulator;
Fig S1E1/E2. UV spectrum of KET (10-4 M) in methanol/water by increasing exposure time in solar simulator;
Fig S1F1/F2. UV spectrum of NKET (10-4 M) in methanol/water, by increasing exposure time in solar simulator.

**Author Contributions:** G.M. and D.F. conceived and designed the experiments; L.M., M.T., G.S., and S.V. performed the experiments; D.F., G.M., L.M., and G.S. analyzed the data; M.M. contributed reagents/materials/analysis tools; D.F., G.M., L.M., M.T., and S.S. wrote the paper.

## References

1. Cooper, G.A.; Kronstrand, R.; Kintz, P. Society of Hair Testing. Society of Hair Testing guidelines for drug testing in hair. *Forensic Sci. Int.* **2012**, *218*, 20–24. [CrossRef] [PubMed]
2. Salomone, A.; Tsanaclis, L.; Agius, R.; Kintz, P.; Baumgartner, M.R. European guidelines for workplace drug and alcohol testing in hair. *Drug Test Anal.* **2016**, *8*, 996–1004. [CrossRef] [PubMed]
3. United Nations Office on Drugs and Crime. *Guidelines for the Forensic Analysis of Drugs Facilitating Sexual Assault and Other Criminal Acts*; United Nations Office on Drugs and Crime: Vienna, Austria, 2011.
4. Cooper, G.A. Hair testing is taking root. *Ann. Clin. Biochem.* **2011**, *48*, 516–530. [CrossRef] [PubMed]
5. Jurado, C.; Kintz, P.; Menedez, M.; Repetto, M. Influence of cosmetic treatment of hair on drug testing. *Int. J. Leg. Med.* **1997**, *110*, 159–163. [CrossRef]
6. Skopp, G.; Potsch, L.; Moeller, M.R. On cosmetically treated hair—Aspects and pitfalls of interpretation. *Forensic Sci. Int.* **1997**, *84*, 43–52. [CrossRef]
7. Rohrich, J.; Zorntlein, S.; Pötsch, L.; Skopp, G.; Becker, J. Effect of the shampoo Ultra Clean on drug concentrations in human hair. *Int. J. Leg. Med.* **2000**, *113*, 102–106. [CrossRef]
8. Janga, K.Y.; King, T.; Ji, N.; Sarabu, S.; Shadambikar, G.; Sawant, S.; Xu, P.; Repka, M.A.; Murthy, S.N. Photostability Issues in Pharmaceutical Dosage Forms and Photostabilization. *AAPS PharmSciTech* **2018**, *19*, 48–59. [CrossRef] [PubMed]
9. Skopp, G.; Pötsch, L.; Mauden, M. Stability of cannabinoids in hair samples exposed to sunlight. *Clin. Chem.* **2000**, *46*, 1846. [PubMed]
10. Favretto, D.; Tucci, M.; Monaldi, A.; Ferrara, S.D.; Miolo, G. A study on photodegradation of methadone, EDDP, and other drugs of abuse in hair exposed to controlled UVB radiation. *Drug Test Anal.* **2014**, *6* (Suppl. 1), 78–84. [CrossRef] [PubMed]
11. Dostalek, M.; Jurica, J.; Pistovcakova, J.; Hanesova, M.; Tomandl, J.; Linhart, I.; Sulcova, A. Effect of methamphetamine on cytochrome P450 activity. *Xenobiotica* **2007**, *37*, 1355–1366. [CrossRef] [PubMed]
12. Harris, D.S.; Boxenbaum, H.; Everhart, E.T.; Sequeira, G.; Mendelson, J.E.; Jones, R.T. The bioavailability of intranasal and smoked methamphetamine. *Clin. Pharmacol. Ther.* **2003**, *74*, 475–486. [CrossRef] [PubMed]
13. Cook, C.E.; Jeffcoat, A.R.; Hill, J.M.; Pugh, D.E.; Patetta, P.K.; Sadler, B.M.; White, W.R.; Perez-Reyes, M. Pharmacokinetics of methamphetamine self-administered to human subjects by smoking S-(+)-methamphetamine hydrochloride. *Drug Metab. Dispos.* **1993**, *21*, 717–723. [PubMed]
14. De la Torre, R.; Farré, M.; Roset, P.N.; Pizarro, N.; Abanades, S.; Segura, M.; Segura, J.; Camí, J. Human pharmacology of MDMA: Pharmacokinetics, metabolism, and disposition. *Ther. Drug Monit.* **2004**, *26*, 137–144. [CrossRef] [PubMed]
15. Green, A.R.; Mechan, A.O.; Elliott, J.M.; O'Shea, E.; Colado, M.I. The pharmacology and clinical pharmacology of 3,4-methylenedioxymethamphetamine (MDMA, "ecstasy"). *Pharmacol. Rev.* **2003**, *55*, 463–508. [CrossRef] [PubMed]

16. Adamowicz, P.; Kala, M. Urinary excretion rates of ketamine and norketamine following therapeutic ketamine administration: Method and detection window considerations. *J. Anal. Toxicol.* **2005**, *29*, 376–382. [CrossRef] [PubMed]
17. Peltoniemi, M.A.; Hagelberg, N.M.; Olkkola, K.T.; Saari, T.I. Ketamine: A Review of Clinical Pharmacokinetics and Pharmacodynamics in Anesthesia and Pain Therapy. *Clin. Pharmacokinet.* **2016**, *55*, 1059–1077. [CrossRef] [PubMed]
18. Scott-Ham, M.; Burton, F.C. Toxicological findings in cases of alleged drug-facilitated sexual assault in the United Kingdom over a 3-year period. *J. Clin. Forensic Med.* **2005**, *12*, 175–186. [CrossRef] [PubMed]
19. Beynon, C.M.; McVeigh, C.; McVeigh, J.; Leavey, C.; Bellis, M.A. The involvement of drugs and alcohol in drug-facilitated sexual assault: A systematic review of the evidence. *Trauma Violence Abuse* **2008**, *9*, 178–188. [CrossRef] [PubMed]
20. Miolo, G.; Tucci, M.; Mazzoli, A.; Ferrara, S.D.; Favretto, D. Photostability of 6-MAM and morphine exposed to controlled UV irradiation in water and methanol solution: HRMS for the characterization of transformation products and comparison with the dry state. *J. Pharm. Biomed. Anal.* **2016**, *126*, 48–59. [CrossRef] [PubMed]
21. Favretto, D.; Vogliardi, S.; Stocchero, G.; Nalesso, A.; Tucci, M.; Ferrara, S.D. High performance liquid chromatography-high resolution mass spectrometry and micropulverized extraction for the quantification of amphetamines, cocaine, opioids, benzodiazepines, antidepressants and hallucinogens in 2.5 mg hair samples. *J. Chromatogr. A* **2011**, *1218*, 6583. [CrossRef] [PubMed]
22. Vogliardi, S.; Favretto, D.; Tucci, M.; Stocchero, G.; Ferrara, S.D. Simultaneous LC-HRMS determination of 28 benzodiazepines and metabolites in hair. *Anal. Bioanal. Chem.* **2011**, *400*, 51. [CrossRef] [PubMed]
23. Miolo, G.; Gallocchio, F.; Levorato, L.; Dalzoppo, D.; van Henegouwen, G.M.J.B.; Caffieri, S. UVB photolysis of betamethasone and its esters: Characterization of photoproducts in solution, in pig skin and in drug formulations. *J. Photochem. Photobiol. B* **2009**, *96*, 75. [CrossRef] [PubMed]
24. Herrling, T.; Jung, K.; Fuchs, J. The role of melanin as protector against free radicals in skin and its role as free radical indicator in hair. *Spectrochim. Acta Mol. Biomol. Spectrosc.* **2007**, *69*, 1429. [CrossRef] [PubMed]
25. Hoting, E.; Zimmermann, M.; Hilterhaus-Bong, S. Photochemical alterations on human hair. Part I: Artificial irradiation and investigations of hair proteins. *J. Soc. Cosmet. Chem.* **1995**, *46*, 85.
26. Hoting, E.; Zimmermann, M.; Hocker, H. Photochemical alterations on human hair. Part II: Analysis ofmelanin. *J. Soc. Cosmet. Chem.* **1995**, *46*, 181.
27. Chedekelt, M.R.; Smitht, S.K.; Postf, P.W.; Pokorat, A.; Vessellt, D.L. Photodestruction of pheomelanin: Role of oxygen. *Proc. Natl. Acad. Sci. USA* **1978**, *75*, 5395. [CrossRef]

# 6

# Synthetic Cannabinoid use in a Case Series of Patients with Psychosis Presenting to Acute Psychiatric Settings: Clinical Presentation and Management Issues

**Stefania Bonaccorso [1,2,*], Antonio Metastasio [1], Angelo Ricciardi [1,3], Neil Stewart [1], Leila Jamal [1], Naasir-Ud-Dinn Rujully [1], Christos Theleritis [4,5], Stefano Ferracuti [6], Giuseppe Ducci [3] and Fabrizio Schifano [7]**

1 Highgate Mental Health Centre, Camden & Islington NHS Foundation Trust, London NW1 0PE, UK; antonio.metastasio@candi.nhs.uk (A.M.); angelo.ricciardi@candi.nhs.uk (A.R.); Neil1.Stewart@candi.nhs.uk (N.S.); leila.jamal@candi.nhs.uk (L.J.); naasir-ud-dinn.rujully@candi.nhs.uk (N.-U.-D.R.)

2 Department of Psychological Medicine, King's College London, London WC2R 2LS, UK

3 Department of Mental Health, ASL Rome 1, 00135 Rome, Italy; angelo.ricciardi@aslroma1.it (A.R.); giuseppe.ducci@aslroma1.it (G.D.)

4 Department of Psychosis Studies, King's College London, London WC2R 2LS, UK; christos.theleritis@kcl.ac.uk

5 National and Kapodistrian University of Athens, Eginition Hospital, 11528 Athens, Greece

6 Department of Human Neurosciences, University of Rome 'La Sapienza', 00185 Rome, Italy; stefano.ferracuti@uniroma1.it

7 Department of Psychopharmacology, University of Hertfordshire, Hertfordshire AL10 9AB, UK; f.schifano@herts.ac.uk

* Correspondence: stefania.bonaccorso@kcl.ac.uk or stefania.bonaccorso@candi.nhs.uk;

**Abstract:** Background: Novel Psychoactive Substances (NPS) are a heterogeneous class of synthetic molecules including synthetic cannabinoid receptor agonists (SCRAs). Psychosis is associated with SCRAs use. There is limited knowledge regarding the structured assessment and psychometric evaluation of clinical presentations, analytical toxicology and clinical management plans of patients presenting with psychosis and SCRAs misuse. Methods: We gathered information regarding the clinical presentations, toxicology and care plans of patients with psychosis and SCRAs misuse admitted to inpatients services. Clinical presentations were assessed using the PANSS scale. Vital signs data were collected using the National Early Warning Signs tool. Analytic chemistry data were collected using urine drug screening tests for traditional psychoactive substances and NPS. Results: We described the clinical presentation and management plan of four patients with psychosis and misuse of SCRAs. Conclusion: The formulation of an informed clinical management plan requires a structured assessment, identification of the index NPS, pharmacological interventions, increases in nursing observations, changes to leave status and monitoring of the vital signs. The objective from using these interventions is to maintain stable physical health whilst rapidly improving the altered mental state.

**Keywords:** synthetic cannabinoids; SCRAs; NPS; novel psychoactive substances; NPS testing; antipsychotics; mental health; physical health; nursing care; psychosis

## 1. Introduction

Recent statistics in England have reported an increased number of hospital admissions with a primary diagnosis of drug-related mental health/behavioural disorders and poisoning by illicit drugs, respectively of 12 and 40% compared to statistics released in 2006/07 [1]. Over the last five years deaths involving Novel Psychoactive Substances (NPS) have sadly increased, with a further 8% increase in 2016 [2]. NPS represent an emerging and concerning global phenomenon [3–5] mainly due to: (1) the difficulties posed in the clinical management, of both mental and physical health; and (2) the absence of a clear and formal/structured description of the clinical presentation of patients using NPS, with obvious repercussions on clinical management.

NPS are a heterogeneous class of typically synthetic molecules including: synthetic cannabinoid receptor agonists (SCRAs), synthetic cathinones, amphetamine-derivatives, psychedelic phenethylamines, ketamine derivatives, novel tryptamines, synthetic opioids and sedatives (GABA-A/B agonists) [3,6,7]. Trends in illicit drug use over the last decade clearly show that adolescents and young adults give preference to NPS instead of traditional psychoactive substances (TPS) (e.g., cannabis, cocaine, heroin, amphetamines, LSD, ecstasy, ketamine, etc), because NPS are cheap and easily available either on the street or from websites [6–8]. They are difficult to identify in blood or urine drug screening (UDS) [9]. Lifetime NPS consumption was reported by 8% of young individuals in 2015 [10] up from 5% in 2011 [6]. Young adults (aged 16 to 24) are around twice as likely to have used an NPS in their lifetime compared to older adults (aged 16 to 59) [11]. It has recently been reported that the three psychiatric diagnoses most frequently associated with NPS use are bipolar disorder (23.1%), personality disorders (11.8%), and schizophrenia and related disorders (11.6%) [12].

In comparison to TPS users, poly NPS users are more likely to be young males [11], with daily use of traditional cannabis, weekly or more use of ecstasy, recent LSD use, higher levels of poly drug use, and a history of overdose on any drug in the past year [13]. Young adults attending nightlife events in pubs and discos are also more prone to poly-substance use, mainly combining NPS with alcohol and cocaine [14]. NPS users also tend to have a forensic history and a history of promiscuous sexual activity (e.g., chem-sex) [13].

Few studies have attempted to provide a psychopathological description of the clinical presentation of NPS users in acute settings. For example, in an observational cohort study enrolling consecutive adult patients presenting to an Emergency Department (ED) in London, the most common clinical features identified were seizures and agitation [15]. In a recent study looking into the impact of NPS misuse on admissions to an acute psychiatric facility in London, increased levels of violence in the group of NPS users were identified ([16]. Data collected in the Accident and Emergency departments (A&Es) of ten European countries have shown that the association between NPS use and the occurrence of psychosis varied considerably, depending on the type of drug used [17]. In particular, psychotic symptoms were noted in 6.3% of a large sample (5529 consecutive cases), with psychosis being more common amongst NPS users that had used tryptamines, methylenedioxypyrovalerone (MDPV), methylphenidate, SCRAs and amphetamine-type compounds [17]. A mounting range of evidence suggests that SCRAs can trigger the onset of acute psychosis in vulnerable individuals and/or exacerbate psychotic episodes in those patients with a previous psychiatric history. The literature reports a wide range of psychopathological issues such as paranoid thoughts, increases in aggressive and combative behavior, together with confusion, agitation and suicidal thoughts [18]. It has been suggested that SCRAs may have a higher psychosis-inducing potential compared to natural cannabis [19] because of the lack of cannabidiol—a substance associated with the medicinal effects of cannabis. For a review on existing studies and models of cannabis induced psychosis see a review from Murray et al [20].

Professionals usually report feeling less confident about managing NPS compared to TPS users, specifically because of the lack of clear guidance regarding the clinical management and the increased risk of toxicity [10–18,21]. For example, with the ingestion of NPS with high serotonergic activity (e.g.: psychedelic phenethylamines), misusers may present with hyperthermia, seizures, and hyponatraemia.

Conversely, NPS with high dopaminergic activity (e.g., methylphenidate-like drugs such as some synthetic cathinones) are highly addictive and associated with prolonged stimulation, insomnia, agitation, and psychosis [22,23]. Furthermore, most SCRAs are at times associated with medical emergencies such as hypertension, myocardial infarction, renal failure [24], elevated heart rate, hyperglycaemia, nausea, vomiting, hypokalaemia, and seizures [18]. Moreover, in view of the increased use of latest generation of sedatives or ultra-high potency fentanyl derivatives, the assessment of vital parameters is of paramount importance when NPS users are presenting to an emergency or acute facility [3–6].

The implementation of an appropriate and safe clinical management plan is commonly based on patients' accounts on which kind of NPS have been used. Acute mental health and emergency services are not routinely equipped with urine drug screening tests (UDS) for NPS in order to identify and provide an appropriate toxicological confirmation [15]. This causes considerable limitations when offering a targeted treatment strategy that can address patients' presentations and potentially life-threatening intoxications [9,13,25].

At present, there is a dearth of detailed information relating to the clinical presentation of NPS users in acute mental health settings, especially in terms of: (1) descriptions of behavioural and psychopathological features using structured assessment and psychometric scales; (2) analytical toxicology and identification of the index NPS used; and (3) appropriate and evidence-based clinical management plans. This results in a range of difficulties in formulating targeted/individually tailored treatment plans.

The aims of this case series are: (1) to offer a standardized description of NPS users' clinical presentations to provide clinicians with objective and measurable clinical pictures aimed at shaping protocols and standard operating procedures when NPS use is suspected and/or detected; (2) to provide best practice advice in the management of mental state alterations and medical complications, with the goal of reducing the number of serious adverse outcomes associated with NPS use.

## 2. Materials and Methods

### 2.1. Study Design and Recruitment

Data on presentation and clinical management of 4 cases, selected amongst patients consecutively admitted to two acute psychiatric wards from June 2017 to June 2018 at Highgate Mental Health Centre—Camden & Islington NHS Foundation Trust—were retrospectively collected using a database. Patients were aged 18 and 65 years and admitted because of presenting with psychotic illnesses and with a history of NPS use before or during admission. Data were collected using a standardized database to capture a range of information at baseline i.e., the time of the admission, and then during and after NPS intake. The information collected revolved around: (1) the clinical presentation, with a formal description of the psychotic symptoms; (2) the type of recreational drug(s) used; (3) the physical health outcomes; (4) the levels of psychiatric inpatient observation and leave status.

The clinical presentation was identified with the help of clinical notes and corroborated by the retrospective scoring of the Positive and Negative Syndrome Scale (PANSS), a multi-item questionnaire widely used to quantify disease severity in schizophrenia and psychosis [26]. Monitoring data of vital signs were collected using the National Early Warning Signs tool (NEWS) [27]. Data on the type of substance used were collected using routine drug screening tests for traditional psychoactive substances whilst a more thorough analysis (urine and/or oral fluids tests; Alere Laboratories technologies) was carried out to identify the index drug(s) used by both NPS and TPS patients. All subjects identified received medications included in the British National Formulary (BNF), such as benzodiazepines (BZO) and antipsychotics (first and second generation), with the choice guided by the clinical presentation and the drug testing results. Levels of nursing care, such as close or general observations, were also recorded together with the possibility of leave in the hospital grounds , either accompanied by staff (escorted) or alone (unescorted).

### 2.2. Participants

#### 2.2.1. Inclusion Criteria

Cases were selected amongst patients with recent or current histories of NPS use, aged 18–65 years, presenting to acute services with a psychotic illness classified by the International Classification of Diseases, Mental and Behavioral Disorders [28] as schizophrenia, schizotypal, delusional, and other non-mood psychotic disorders (ICD-10 codes: F20-29), mood (affective) disorders (ICD-10 codes: F30-39), and mental and behavioral disorders due to psychoactive substances (ICD-10 codes: F10-19).

#### 2.2.2. Exclusion Criteria

Patients were excluded from the study if: (1) the psychotic symptoms were precipitated by an organic cause; (2) they had moderate or severe learning disability; (3) they suffered from a medical or neurological illness or (4) had an insufficient command of the English language.

### 2.3. Measures

#### 2.3.1. Psychometric Measures

The Positive and Negative Symptoms Scale (PANSS) is a multi-item questionnaire widely used to quantify disease severity in schizophrenia and to assess the severity of positive (or productive) and negative (or deficit) symptoms of psychosis [26]. PANSS is easy to administer and is based on the clinician's interview with the patient; data are gathered looking at the patient's mental state over the previous week, with the patient's family and/or his/her acquaintances being able to provide further information. PANSS consists of 30 items and takes 45–50 min to be completed by the clinician.

The National Early Warning Score (NEWS; Royal College of Physicians, London, UK) [27] is a standardized system for the assessment of acute illness in adults. It is based on six vital signs such as respiratory rate, oxygen saturation, temperature, blood pressure, pulse/heart rate, and alertness. Each parameter yields a score of between 0 and 3 so that when the scores for all the parameters are summed a total NEWS score of between 0 and 18 is achieved. A score of 7 or greater indicates that a patient is likely to be critically medically unwell.

#### 2.3.2. Laboratory Measures

Standard urine drug screening tests were used to detect TPS such as heroin, cocaine, amphetamine, THC, and methadone. For NPS, the Alere drug screening urine and oral fluids tests were used. The urine tests provided a rapid screening of 30 synthetic cannabinoids at once whilst the oral screening test was able to detect mephedrone.

## 3. Clinical Vignettes

### 3.1. Case 1—Mr A

28 years old Caucasian male, single and unemployed, living alone, with a positive forensic history and a diagnosis of Paranoid Schizophrenia. The patient had a 4 years' history of psychosis with frequent relapses (5 admissions in 4 years). He was transferred to an acute treatment ward from a psychiatric intensive care unit (PICU). At the time of the transfer the patient was stable and on treatment with Risperdal Consta 37.5 mg fortnightly + Olanzapine 10 mg daily + Pregabalin 100 mg daily. The PANSS score was 73/210 and his psychopathology was mainly characterized by positive symptoms: delusional mood, persecutory and grandiose delusions and second and third person auditory hallucinations. The UDS was initially negative but, one week after the transfer, Mr A's mental state deteriorated suddenly and he became very agitated and verbally and physically aggressive. He presented with a bizarre and repetitive behaviour consisting of stopping and remaining immobile for a few minutes and then running fast along the ward corridor. He also had second and third person

auditory hallucinations, persecutory delusions and thought disorganization. He started to fear the hospital ward's electronic fire alarms. He believed that the fire alarms were cameras that were spying on him and he was very preoccupied with specific members of the staff whom he believed were there to kill him. The hallucinations also became very severe and he was responding to internal stimuli constantly throughout the day. The total PANSS score was 109/210 and the UDS was positive for SCRAs. We decided to increase Olanzapine to 20 mg, daily and to add Clonazepam 8 mg, daily to manage the agitated behaviour and the psychotic symptoms. We also increased the level of monitoring of his vital measures by completing the NEWS scores twice a day. NEWS scored 2 with increased heart rate and fluctuating blood pressure. We considered a transfer to PICU but since the patient was starting to respond well to the new treatment plan and the reason for the relapse was evident (NPS intake), we decided to continue to treat the patient on the acute ward. Mr. A responded well to the change/increase of medications, his symptoms improved in 24 h and within 7 days from the acute intoxication the PANSS scores reduced to 74/210.

### 3.2. *Case 2—Ms T*

32 years old Caucasian woman, single and unemployed, living alone, with no forensic history and a diagnosis of Schizoaffective Disorder and poly-substance misuse (mainly crack cocaine and heroin). Ms T was stabilized on a combination of Aripiprazole 30 mg, daily + Lithium carbonate 800 mg, at night. The PANSS score was 95/210 and the UDS was negative for all illicit substances. Four weeks later, the patient's mental state deteriorated suddenly. She became physically and verbally very aggressive with severe features of sexual disinhibition. The patient presented with delusional mood and with complex grandiose and persecutory delusions such that she believed she was part of a secret army and she had powers to kill people with her thoughts. She also believed she was being chased by the Albanian mafia and had to fight for her life. The patient also became very aggressive with members of staff and on four occasions it was necessary to call the emergency team to provide extra sedation. The PANSS score was consistent with the deterioration of her mental state, scoring 115/210 and the UDS tested positive for both SCRAs and THC. The clinical team felt that the patient needed a more robust pharmacological treatment plan and therefore Haloperidol 10 mg daily + Clonazepam 8 mg daily were added. The patient remained acutely unwell for more than 72 h. Ten days after the intoxication Ms T remained still irritable and agitated. The PANSS score was 115/210, 10 points higher than the baseline, and the UDS continued to test positive for SCRAs. NEWS were increased to twice a day but the score was always within range (0 or 1) with tachycardia being the only altered parameter. Meanwhile, other patients on the ward tested positive for SCRAs and it was suspected that Ms T was bringing SCRAs to the ward. At that stage, leave was suspended and a stricter search policy was enforced on the ward. The patient's mental state improved further and ten days later her urine tests were negative for SCRAs.

### 3.3. *Case 3—Mr Y*

20 years old Black-Caribbean male, single and unemployed, living with friends and with no forensic history, was quickly re-admitted to a treatment ward following the sudden onset of bizarre behaviour after an earlier discharge from another ward. The diagnosis was First Psychotic Episode in the context of poly-substance misuse. On admission, Mr Y was on Haloperidol Decanoate 50 mg, monthly + Haloperidol 10 mg, at night (on reducing regime). He appeared severely thought-disordered, sexually disinhibited and aroused, approaching other patients for sex or suddenly becoming physically aggressive by spitting on others. The PANSS score was 116/210 with prominent positive symptoms (positive symptoms subscale 40/49). He presented as being severely disruptive, chaotic, and intrusive into other patients' care, attacking staff and other patients, urinating on the floor and spitting at other people's faces. Mr Y was therefore treated with Aripiprazole 9.75 mg three times a day + Clonazepam 6 mg daily in divided doses. Observation levels were increased to 2:1 arms' length to reduce risks of retaliation from others due to sexually inappropriate and aggressive behaviour. NEWS monitoring

was increased to hourly to monitor any possible deterioration in physical health. UDS were positive for benzodiazepines and SCRAs. The patient remained unwell. Observation levels were maintained at 2:1 arms' length and NEWS monitoring decreased to TDS once physical outcomes remained stable for 12 h. After 72 h the clinical condition improved with a reduction of PANSS score to 98/210. Eventually, because of the continued high risk of retaliation from others Mr. Y was transferred to a Psychiatric Intensive Care Unit (PICU).

### 3.4. Case 4—Mr G

39 year old Asian British man, married and unemployed, living with his family and with a long forensic history. Mr G had a long-standing history of Bipolar Disorder since the age of 28. He had a history of numerous admissions, was non-compliant with his medications, and engaged poorly with his community team. He presented with a long-term history of poly-substance misuse (e.g., alcohol, cocaine, MDMA, cannabis, "legal highs"). He had previously been treated with a mood stabilizer (Sodium Valproate); Zuclopenthixol and Risperidone Depot (both stopped due to sexual dysfunction); Olanzapine and Quetiapine (both stopped due to poor response). At the time of his admission to Highgate Mental Health Centre, he was administered Abilify Depot 400 mg, monthly with no or little efficacy. He was transferred from another ward on Section 3 due to a manic relapse, with no leave and a diagnosis of Bipolar Affective Disorder (BPAD, current episode manic). Mr. G had a long history of violence towards staff and patients (he broke a nurse's nose and stabbed another patient with a pen). At the time of the admission, he was very agitated, aggressive and intimidating, banging his fist on the table and threatening staff with a glass bottle. He also showed bizarre behavior, e.g., wearing sunglasses whilst indoors, holding pieces of paper with some incomprehensible notes on Hitler, quantum physics and aliens. He was thought disordered with grandiose delusional beliefs regarding him being the King of Egypt and able to cause a nuclear war. It proved very difficult to verbally de-escalate him and he did not agree to change his medication regime as he believed that he should be treated "only with love". The PANSS score was 108/210. Abilify was withdrawn and Zuclopenthixol started whilst he continued the rest of his medications. On admission, UDS was negative for both NPS and TPS. A week later, UDS was positive for both benzodiazepines and SCRAs, and NEWS was increased to TDS. Two weeks later, UDS continued to be positive to SCRAs, no changes to his leave status were made, with garden leave being maintained. Three weeks after admission, UDS was positive for benzodiazepines and THC and four weeks later the admission UDS was positive for THC and SCRAs. After admission, his mental state remained unsettled with refractory manic positive symptoms and a poor response to medication. The PANSS score was 123/210. Hence, his leave was stopped and, a week later, his UDS became negative for all substances, SCRAs included. His positive symptoms started to improve with a reduction of PANSS to 66/210. Over the following four weeks Mr. G appeared well kempt and settled on the ward, with no grandiose delusions and no further episodes of aggression. He showed a satisfactory response to Zuclopenthixol 300 mg, weekly + Sodium Valproate 1200 mg. UDS was negative for all substances and, therefore, Mr. G was safely discharged to the community team.

## 4. Discussion

NPS misuse is a recent phenomenon and knowledge of its effects, either in the short or the long term, on the population is relatively poor [3]. There is an increasing amount of knowledge regarding the effect that NPS have on individuals with severe mental illness [12]. However, well documented evidence of the negative impact are limited and most cases have not been corroborated by analytic chemistry evidence of the NPS used [15]. Furthermore, there is a paucity of data to guide the monitoring and management of patients with severe mental illness who take NPS, and then suffer from acute psychopathology and physical ill-health [3].

To the best of our knowledge, our case series is the first and only attempt made at describing, with the use of a specific psychometric scale (PANSS), the effects of acute intoxication with NPS (mainly

SCRAs) identified through UDS in an acute hospital setting in patients suffering from severe psychotic disorders. All four cases show how clinically significant the impact of SCRAs use was on their mental states. The cases showed marked and sudden clinical deteriorations, with intense exacerbations of positive symptoms, psychomotor agitation, sexual disinhibition, verbal/physical aggression, and poor responses to medications. The latter phenomenon makes the clinical and risk management of these patients more difficult, and it is therefore necessary to develop appropriate management plans to minimize such risks.

In order to set up an appropriate and safe Informed Clinical Management Plan (ICMP) (Table 1), the first step advised here is to establish, whenever possible, which NPS is responsible for the intoxication due to their wide range of effects. We advocate, therefore, the use and further development of reliable drug tests to identify the specific NPS types associated with particular clinical presentations. Accurate testing for NPS would assist in establishing clear diagnoses, formulating ICMPs and identifying the most effective treatments for intoxications with particular NPS.

**Table 1.** Description of the Camden & Islington—Informed Clinical Management Plan (ICMP).

| **Camden & Islington—Informed Clinical Management Plan (ICMP)** | |
|---|---|
| MENTAL STATE assessment | |
| Using a psychometric scale (PANSS) | Monitoring mental state |
| NPS detection | |
| Using specific analytic toxicology to detect NPS (UDS and/or oral swabs) | Monitoring access to substances and leaves (reduced/suspended—escorted/unescorted) |
| MEDICATION & PHYSICAL HEALTH monitoring | |
| Using benzodiazepines (BDZ) and/or second generation antipsychotics (SGA) when possible | Monitoring physical health (NEWS) Levels of nursing observations |

The cases described here were all characterized by acute SCRA intoxications. The clinical presentations were characterized by an acute onset of agitation and aggressive behavior; the symptoms decreased in intensity and frequency in no less than 72 h. The management of acute intoxications was by identifying the substances responsible for the sudden deteriorations, and by treating the symptoms with benzodiazepines and antipsychotic medications. In addition vital parameters were monitored, nursing observations were increased, and leave statuses were changed. These measures led to rapid and successful resolutions of symptoms and reduced the need for transfer to more intensive care settings. Furthermore, they promoted more rapid step-down and recovery in the community.

In general terms, pharmacological treatment remains the mainstay of treatment. However, the novelty of the use of medications according to our protocol is that pharmacological interventions are guided by NEWS and toxicology results. For example, haloperidol should be avoided in patients that have used cathinones for the toxic effect on cardiac rhythm; and benzodiazepines should be avoided in patient with a NEWS score of 3 because of low oxygen saturations levels.

In terms of pharmacological treatment, the use of BDZ has been recommended with or without a second-generation antipsychotic (SGA) to reduce the risk of cardiac side effects [22,23]. Benzodiazepines remain the first line treatment, although their use needs to be weighed against the risk of respiratory depression when given to subjects who have ingested alcohol and/or unknown substances [6–18]. Amongst the SGAs, whilst aripiprazole is probably the safest antipsychotic to be used in such scenarios because of its negligible effect on QTc, olanzapine has proven to be effective in treating psychotic symptoms caused by NPS [29].

## 5. Limitations

We are aware that four cases are not representative of the multi-faceted spectrum of presentations with NPS use/intoxication and observation of a wider sample size is necessary. However, we believe that this study is important in generating hypotheses that may lead to more comprehensive projects such as case control studies.

Furthermore, although the four cases presented were objectively described by using the PANSS to provide an objective measurement of the clinical observation, this was made retrospectively. We are also aware that the patients described were intoxicated with SCRAs. No other NPS such as cathinones or mephedrone were detected in our sample population. Therefore, our clinical description-albeit exhaustive and comprehensive-is limited to a subgroup of NPS users using only SCRAs. Moreover unfortunately, the UDS screening tests that were available were not able to identify with higher specificity the type of SCRAs used.

It is worth noting how in terms of diagnostic categories our patients sample was not homogenous as one of the four patients was presenting with bipolar disorder. This may be an additional confounding factor; and, in a large enough sample, patients should be divided according to diagnoses.

Finally, a randomized controlled trial (RCT) to establish which ICMP is necessary to establish which treatment plan is most effective in the management of individuals with a severe mental illness intoxicated with NPS would be helpful.

**Author Contributions:** Conceptualization, S.B., A.M., A.R. and F.S.; Methodology, N.-U.-D.R. and L.J.; Writing, S.B., A.M. and A.R.; Review & Editing, F.S., N.S., C.T., S.F. and G.D.; Visualization, C.T., N.S., S.F. and G.D.; Supervision- S.B. and F.S.

**Acknowledgments:** We would like to acknowledge the nursing teams of Topaz, Jade and Coral ward at Highgate Mental Health Centre for their hard work and contribution to the manuscript.

## References

1. Statistics on Drug Misuse: England. 2018. Available online: https://digital.nhs.uk/data-and-information/publications/statistical/statistics-on-drug-misuse/2018 (accessed on 16 June 2018).
2. Statistical Bulletin: Deaths Related to Drug Poisoning in England and Wales: 2016 registrations. Available online: https://www.ons.gov.uk/peoplepopulationandcommunity/birthsdeathsandmarriages/deaths/bulletins/deathsrelatedtodrugpoisoninginenglandandwales/2016registrations#deaths-involving-new-psychoactive-substances-continue-to-increase (accessed on 16 June 2018).
3. Abdulrahim, D.; Bowden-Jones, O.; On Behalf of the NEPTUNE Expert Group. Guidance on the Management of Acute and Chronic Harms of Club Drugs and Novel Psychoactive Substances. Novel Psychoactive Treatment UK Network (NEPTUNE) London. 2015. Available online: http://neptune-clinical-guidance.co.uk/wp-content/uploads/2015/03/NEPTUNE-Guidance-March-2015.pdf (accessed on 16 June 2018).
4. Barrio, P.; Reynolds, J.; García-Altés, A.; Gual, A.; Anderson, P. Social costs of illegal drugs, alcohol and tobacco in the European Union: A systematic review. *Drug Alcohol. Rev.* **2017**, *36*, 578–588. [CrossRef] [PubMed]
5. EU Drug Report. 2017. Available online: http://www.emcdda.europa.eu/system/files/publications/4541/TDAT17001ENN.pdf (accessed on 16 June 2018).
6. Schifano, F.; Orsolini, L.; Papanti, G.D.; Corkery, J.M. Novel psychoactive substances of interest for psychiatry. *World Psychiatry* **2015**, *14*, 15–26. [CrossRef] [PubMed]
7. Miliano, C.; Serpelloni, G.; Rimondo, C.; Mereu, M.; Marti, M.; De Luca, M.A. Neuropharmacology of New Psychoactive Substances (NPS): Focus on the Rewarding and Reinforcing Properties of Cannabimimetics and Amphetamine-Like Stimulants. *Front Neurosci.* **2016**, *10*, 153. [CrossRef] [PubMed]
8. Martinotti, G.; Lupi, M.; Carlucci, L.; Cinosi, E.; Santacroce, R.; Acciavatti, T.; Chillemi, E.; Bonifaci, L.; Janiri, L.; Di Giannantonio, M. Novel psychoactive substances: use and knowledge among adolescents and young adults in urban and rural areas. *Hum. Psychopharmacol.* **2015**, *30*, 295–301. [CrossRef] [PubMed]

9. Vallersnes, O.M.; Persett, P.S.; Øiestad, E.L.; Karinen, R.; Heyerdahl, F.; Hovda, K.E. Underestimated impact of novel psychoactive substances: laboratory confirmation of recreational drug toxicity in Oslo, Norway. *Clin. Toxicol.* **2017**, *55*, 636–644. [CrossRef] [PubMed]
10. Tracy, D.K.; Wood, D.M.; Baumeister, D. Novel psychoactive substances: types, mechanisms of action, and effects. *BMJ* **2017**, *356*. [CrossRef] [PubMed]
11. Home Office. Drug Misuse: Findings from the 2016/17 Crime Survey for England and Wales, Statistical Bulletin 11/17, Edited by Broadfield, D. July 2017. Available online: https://assets.publishing.service.gov.uk/government/uploads/system/uploads/attachment_data/file/642738/drug-misuse-2017-hosb1117.pdf (accessed on 16 June 2018).
12. Acciavatti, T.; Lupi, M.; Santacroce, R.; Aguglia, A.; Attademo, L.; Bandini, L.; Ciambrone, P.; Lisi, G.; Migliarese, G.; Pinna, F.; et al. Novel psychoactive substance consumption is more represented in bipolar disorder than in psychotic disorders: A multicenter-observational study. *Hum. Psychopharmacol.* **2017**, *32*, 3. [CrossRef] [PubMed]
13. Sutherland, R.; Peacock, A.; Whittaker, E.; Roxburgh, A.; Lenton, S.; Matthews, A.; Butler, K.; Nelson, M.; Burns, L.; Bruno, R. New psychoactive substance use among regular psychostimulant users in Australia, 2010–2015. *Drug Alcohol. Depend.* **2016**, *161*, 110–118. [CrossRef] [PubMed]
14. Vento, A.E.; Martinotti, G.; Cinosi, E.; Lupi, M.; Acciavatti, T.; Carrus, D.; Santacroce, R.; Chillemi, E.; Bonifaci, L.; Di Giannantonio, M.; et al. Substance Use in the Club Scene of Rome: A Pilot Study. *Biomed. Res. Int.* **2014**, *2014*. [CrossRef] [PubMed]
15. Abouchedid, R.; Hudson, S.; Thurtle, N.; Yamamoto, T.; Ho, J.H.; Bailey, G.; Wood, M.; Sadones, N.; Stove, C.P.; Dines, A.; et al. Analytical confirmation of synthetic cannabinoids in a cohort of 179 presentations with acute recreational drug toxicity to an Emergency Department in London, UK in the first half of 2015. *Clin. Toxicol.* **2017**, *55*, 338–345. [CrossRef] [PubMed]
16. Shafi, A.; Gallagher, P.; Stewart, N.; Martinotti, G.; Corazza, O. The risk of violence associated with novel psychoactive substance misuse in patients presenting to acute mental health services. *Hum. Psychopharmacol.* **2017**, *32*, 3. [CrossRef] [PubMed]
17. Vallersnes, O.M.; Dines, A.M.; Wood, D.M.; Yates, C.; Heyerdahl, F.; Hovda, K.E.; Giraudon, I.; Euro-DEN Research Group; Dargan, P.I. Psychosis associated with acute recreational drug toxicity: A European case series. *BMC Psychiatry* **2016**, *16*, 293. [CrossRef] [PubMed]
18. Papanti, D.; Schifano, F.; Botteon, G.; Bertossi, F.; Mannix, J.; Vidoni, D.; Impagniatiello, M.; Pascolo-Fabrici, E.; Bonavigo, T. "Spiceophrenia": A systematic overview of "Spice"-related psychopathological issues and a case report. *Hum. Psychopharmacol.* **2013**, *28*, 379–389. [CrossRef] [PubMed]
19. Van Amsterdam, J.; Brunt, T.; van den Brink, W. The adverse health effects of synthetic cannabinoids with emphasis on psychosis-like effects. *J. Psychopharmacol.* **2015**, *29*, 254–263. [CrossRef] [PubMed]
20. Murray, R.M.; Englund, A.; Abi-Dargham, A.; Lewis, D.A.; Di Forti, M.; Davies, C.; Sherif, M.; McGuire, P.; D'Souza, D.C. Cannabis-associated psychosis: Neural substrate and clinical impact. *Neuropharmacology* **2017**, *124*, 89–104. [CrossRef] [PubMed]
21. Palamar, J.J.; Martins, S.S.; Su, M.K.; Ompad, D.C. Self-reported use of novel psychoactive substances in a US nationally representative survey: Prevalence, correlates, and a call for new survey methods to prevent underreporting. *Drug Alcohol. Depend.* **2015**, *156*, 112–119. [CrossRef] [PubMed]
22. Schifano, F.; Orsolini, L.; Papanti, D.; Corkery, J. NPS: Medical Consequences Associated with Their Intake. In *Current Topics in Behavioral Neurosciences Neuropharmacology of New Psychoactive Substances (NPS)*; Baumann, M., Glennon, R., Wiley, J., Eds.; Springer: Cham, Switzerland, 2016; Volume 32, pp. 351–380, ISBN 978-3-319-52442-9.
23. Schifano, F.; Papanti, G.D.; Orsolini, L.; Corkery, J.M. Novel psychoactive substances: the pharmacology of stimulants and hallucinogens. *Expert Rev. Clin. Pharmacol.* **2016**, *9*, 943–954. [CrossRef] [PubMed]
24. Liechti, M.E. Novel psychoactive substances (designer drugs): overview and pharmacology of modulators of monoamine signalling. *Swiss Med Wkly.* **2015**, *145*. [CrossRef] [PubMed]
25. Helander, A.; Bäckberg, M.; Hultén, P.; Al-Saffar, Y.; Beck, O. Detection of new psychoactive substance use among emergency room patients: Results from the Swedish STRIDA project. *Forensic. Sci. Int.* **2014**, *243*, 23–29. [CrossRef] [PubMed]
26. Kay, S.R.; Opler, L.A.; Lindenmayer, J.P. Reliability and validity of the positive and negative syndrome scale for schizophrenics. *Psychiatry Res.* **1988**, *23*, 99–110. [CrossRef]

27. Royal College of Physicians. National Early Warning Score (NEWS) 2. Available online: https://www.rcplondon.ac.uk/projects/outputs/national-early-warning-score-news-2 (accessed on 16 June 2018).
28. World Health Organization. *International Statistical Classification of Diseases and Related Health Problems 10th revision (ICD-10)*, 5th ed.; World Health Organization: Geneva, Switzerland, 2016; ISBN 9789241549165.
29. Valeriani, G.; Corazza, O.; Bersani, F.S.; Melcore, C.; Metastasio, A.; Bersani, G.; Schifano, F. Olanzapine as the ideal "trip terminator"? Analysis of online reports relating to antipsychotics' use and misuse following occurrence of novel psychoactive substance-related psychotic symptoms. *Hum. Psychopharmacol.* **2015**, *30*, 249–254. [CrossRef] [PubMed]

# 7

# Octodrine: New Questions and Challenges in Sport Supplements

**Valeria Catalani [1,2], Mariya Prilutskaya [3], Ahmed Al-Imam [4], Shanna Marrinan [5], Yasmine Elgharably [6], Mire Zloh [2], Giovanni Martinotti [7], Robert Chilcott [1,2] and Ornella Corazza [2,*]**

1 Research Centre for Topical Drug Delivery and Toxicology, University of Hertfordshire, Herts SP9 11FA, UK; v.catalani@herts.ac.uk (V.C.); R.chilcott@herts.ac.uk (R.C.)
2 Department of Pharmacy, Pharmacology and Clinical Science, University of Hertfordshire, Herts AL10 9AB, UK; m.zloh@herts.ac.uk
3 Semey State Medical University, Republican Scientific and Practical Center of Mental Health, Pavlodar 140002, Kazakhstan; mariyapril2407@gmail.com
4 Faculty of Medicine, University of Baghdad, Baghdad 10071, Iraq; tesla1452@gmail.com
5 Parliamentary Office of Science and Technology, Houses of Parliament, London SW1A 0AA, UK; marrinans@parliament.uk
6 Navy General Hospital, Cardiovascular department, Alexandria 21513, Egypt; yasmine_elgharably@ymail.com
7 Department of Neuroscience, Imaging and Clinical Sciences, "G.d'Annunzio" University, 66100 Chieti, Italy; Giovanni.Martinotti@gmail.com
* Correspondence: o.corazza@herts.ac.uk

**Abstract: Background:** Octodrine is the trade name for Dimethylhexylamine (DMHA), a central nervous stimulant that increases the uptake of dopamine and noradrenaline. Originally developed as a nasal decongestant in the 1950's, it has recently been re-introduced on the market as a pre-workout and 'fat-burner' product but its use remains unregulated. Our work provides the first observational cross-sectional analytic study on Octodrine as a new drug trend and its associated harms after a gap spanning seven decades. **Methods:** A comprehensive multilingual assessment of literature, websites, drug fora and other online resources was carried out with no time restriction in English, German, Russian and Arabic. Keywords included Octodrine's synonyms and chemical isomers. **Results:** Only five relevant publications emerged from the literature search, with most of the available data on body building websites and fora. Since 2015, Octodrine has been advertised online as "the next big thing" and "the god of stimulants," with captivating marketing strategies directed at athletes and a wider cohort of users. Reported side-effects include hypertension, dyspnoea and hyperthermia. **Conclusions:** The uncontrolled use of Octodrine, its physiological and psychoactive effects raise serious health implications with possible impact on athletes and doping practices. This new phenomenon needs to be thoroughly studied and monitored.

**Keywords:** octodrine; dimethylhexylamine; DMHA; ambredin; fitness; novel psychoactive substance; performance and image-enhancing drugs; anti-obesity agents; weight loss

---

## 1. Introduction

The evolution of trends within drug use has recently been marked by a rapid expansion in the number of commercially-available psychoactive substances [1], with an increased number of young users [2] and relevant psychiatric consequences [3]. This includes both a proliferation of new drugs ('research chemicals' or 'RC's) with a distinct pharmacology and very little associated research evidence on their physiological or side effects, as well as an increase in the abuse of diverted prescription medications [4,5] Octodrine sits somewhere between these two trends, being a traditionally-developed pharmaceutical but with no current, legitimate medical application.

The so-called "Performance and Image-Enhancing Drugs" (PIEDs) taken to enhance human abilities in a myriad of spheres, are one important emerging facet within this. These include substances with a perceived ability to enhance physical performance, psychological status, appearance, cognitive abilities and social relations and as such are sometimes referred to as 'lifestyle drugs' [6–10]. The concept of PIEDs is now well established and is acknowledged particularly in relation to the world of athletics [11,12]. The most well-known PIEDs are the anabolic steroids, peptides and hormones but their use is increasingly giving way to other types of substance to achieve specific goals. These can be physical in nature (e.g., tanning, weight loss, muscle gain, speed, strength, performance) or cognitive, such as the use of nootropics for professional or academic performance [13,14], or for social gain, where various categories of substance as a 'social lubricant' for social anxiety support). Over the past decade, more than 800 NPS were identified in over 102 countries by the EMCDDA and the UNODC Early Warning Systems [15,16] as well as our ongoing monitoring activities [1] and their number is constantly growing. Some of these compounds may represent a serious issue for public health and are changing the face of debates around doping by playing unfairly on the narrow line between legal and illegal [12]. The globalization of the online drugs market has made this a widespread phenomenon, reaching a new cohort of users, which includes not only the body builders and time-pressured professionals, who were initially associated with this trend but also students and others of all demographics [12,17,18].

In November 2016, Octodrine was found in an athlete engaged in a bodybuilding competition, later disqualified as he also tested positive for anabolic and stimulant drugs, included in the World Anti-doping Agency's (WADA) List of Prohibited Substances (Section S6 and S1) [19,20]. Octodrine is a psychoactive central nervous system stimulant. It is an amphipathic primary amine (Figure 1) [21] known under many names, including dimethyl hexylamine (DMHA) and 2-amino-6-methylheptane, 2-metil-5-amino-eptano. Its structure presents some similarities with that of other illegal stimulants like, AMP Citrate (DMBA), Ephedrine and 1.3-DMMA itself. With DMAA and AMP Citrate already phasing or phased out of current supplements, this drug was brought back on market as an alternative in pre-workout and 'fat-burner' products in 2016. Octrodrine was originally developed in the United States as an aerosolized treatment for bronchitis, laryngitis and other conditions [22–24]. Its pharmacology was studied in the early 1950s, was investigated as an antitumor drug and used to be available as a nasal decongestant under the tradenames Vaporpac and Tickle Tackel Inhaler [25]. Sympathomimetic effects of DMHA were explained as alpha adrenergic agonist-mediated via G-protein-coupled receptors (GPCRs) [26]. Limited human data is available just from preliminary studies, while studies on activity and acute toxicity had been conducted on animals (cats, rabbits, dogs and pigs) [27–32]. Octodrine was found to increase the pain threshold, cardiac rate (positive chronotropic effect) and myocardial contractility (positive inotropic effect) [33–35]. The safety of Octodrine as an individual drug remains unknown due to the lack of any placebo-controlled trial but animal experiments suggest a potential for adverse cardiovascular effects. Structurally, there are two forms of DMHA: the naturally occurring 2-amino-5methylpetane and the synthetically derived 2-amino-6-methylheptane. The natural version can be found in extracts of Juglans Regia (Walnut Bark), Aconitum Kusnezoffii's and Kigelia Africana and it is often used for hunting purposes [36–43]. The synthetic version is the most widely used because less expensive and toxic to produce. It is therefore assumed that the DMHA used in supplements is synthetic. As of right now, this molecule is not on the 2016 WADA banned substances list but it fits perfectly in the category of the well-known Performance and Image Enhancing Drugs (PIEDs). Coveted by elite track and field athletes, DMHA is marketed to a broader demographic including beginners and non-professionals.

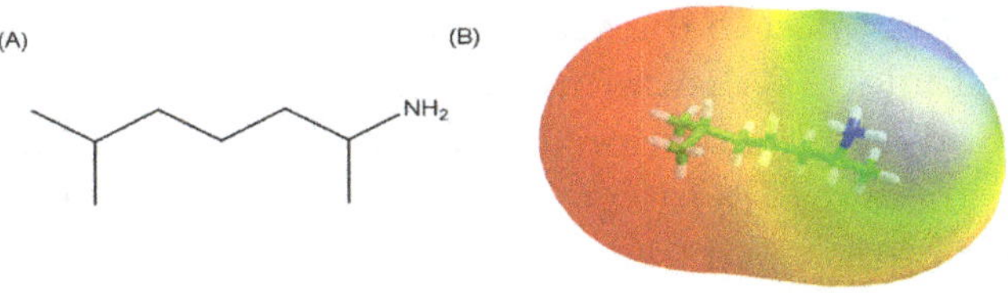


**Figure 1.** Chemical structure (**A**) and molecular lipophilicity potential (MLP) surface (**B**) of octodrine molecule (hydrophobic surfaces are depicted in red and polar surfaces are in blue) [21].

Considering the existing knowledge gap spanning seven decades and the re-emergence of Octodrine as a new drug trend, it was felt the need to further investigate the phenomenon in different communities, while exploring issues related to its e-commerce, consumption, motivations of use and potential negative impacts to health, among other features.

## 2. Materials and Methods

A literature review on Octodrine was carried out in the following databases: Scopus, Medline, EBSCO and Google Scholar (Figure 2). A list of keywords was compiled in accordance with a preliminary pilot study of literature and databases on the surface web and online e-commerce websites. Terms included: "Octodrine," "Ambredin & Vaporpac," "2-aminoisoheptane," "Dimethylhexylamine," "DMHA," "2-amino-6-methylheptane," "6-methyl-2-heptylamine," "2-metil-5-amino-eptano," "5-methyl-2-heptylamine,""Dimethylhexylamine," "Aconitum kusnezoffii, "Aconite extract," among others. The keywords also included synonyms of Octodrine in other languages and names of chemical isomers. Searches were carried out in English, Italian, German, Arabic and Russian.

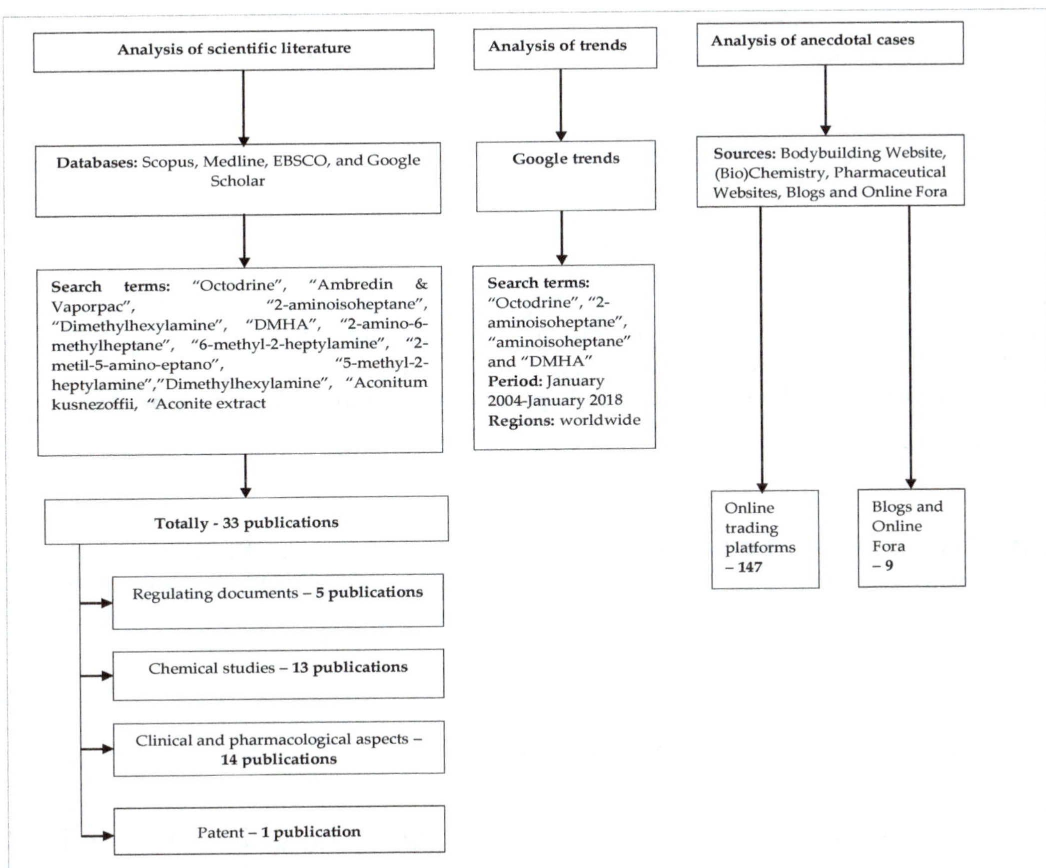


**Figure 2.** Algorithm of the analysis.

No time restrictions were applied to the searches. Inclusion and exclusion criteria for literature data selection are defined in Table 1. Considering the lack of scientific investigations in the field and the absence of experimental and/or interventional studies in humans, additional qualitative systematic searches were carried out in the world-wide web to investigate the extent of diffusion of Octodrine, trading strategies for its distribution and the nature of the self-reported (subjective) experiences by users in English, German, Arabic and Russian. These included bodybuilding websites, chemistry and chemists' websites, pharmaceutical companies, online e-commerce stores as well as a range of fora posts/threads. The web snapshot was carried out on a regular basis (between November 2016 - January 2018) using a Google search. Only publicity available information was considered for the study and no posts/other contributions to fora discussions were made by the researchers. Additional data were also obtained by consulting Google Trends [44].

**Table 1.** Inclusion and exclusion criteria for selection of articles and the web analysed in this study.

| **Inclusion Criteria** |
|---|
| 1. Studies and publication related to Octodrine |
| 2. Studies and publication of octodrine-related compounds and chemicals, in which Octodrine is an ingredient |
| 3. Studies and publication in which octodrine is marginally included |
| 4. English, German and Russian languages |
| 5. All years of publication (no date restriction) |
| 6. Surface web |
| 7. Grey (unpublished) literature, including master's and doctorate theses |
| 8. Fitness and body building websites |
| 9. (Bio)chemistry, pharmacy and pharmaceutical websites |
| 10. Online drug fora |
| 11. Human and animal studies |
| 12. Observational and experimental studies |
| **Exclusion Criteria** |
| 1. Duplicate Articles |
| 2. Initial screening for relevance (reading the title and abstract) |
| 3. Articles found to be irrelevant by analysing the full article |
| 4. Low scoring for an article on CASP critical appraisal tool (poor quality of appraised manuscript) |

Ethical approval for this the study was granted by the School of Pharmacy Ethics Committee, University of Hertfordshire, Hatfield, United Kingdom (November 2013; PHAEC/10-42).

## 3. Results

### *3.1. Medical and Paramedical Database, Grey Literature*

Various articles emerged from our literature searching but only eight of them [23,24,27–31,33] referred to Octodrine, Octodrine derivatives and Octodrine-related compounds in the entire scholarly-published literature (Table 2).

**Table 2.** Pharmacological and clinical properties of Octodrine (analysis of articles).

| Reference | Author | Year of Publication | Name of Studied Substance or Medicament | Key Findings |
|---|---|---|---|---|
| Respiratory system | | | | |
| [28] | Charlier, R.; Philippot, E. | 1950 | theophylline-diethylenediamine ethanoate | The aerosol with Octodrine demonstrated the property to increase respiratory volume |
| [29] | Charlier, R. | 1951 | 2-amino-6-methyl-heptane | Animal experiment (dog) revealed bronchodilation, increased nasal and lung volume caused by 2-amino-6-methyl-heptane |
| [23] | Gode, J. | 1958 | Ambredin | Identification of bronchospasmolitic properties of Ambredin medicament consisting of Aceverine Hydrochloride, Octodrine Phosphate and Theophylline |
| [24] | Tschudin, M.L. | 1960 | Ambredin | |
| Cardiovascular system | | | | |
| [30] | Fellows, E.J. | 1947 | 2-amino-6-methylheptane | 2-amino-6-methylheptane hydrochloride caused an increase in cardiac rate and amplitude of contraction in animal experiment (dog) |
| [27] | Marsh, D.F.; Herring, D.A. | 1951 | Methyl-2-heptylamine | Compared to others sympathomimetic amines, 6-Methyl-2-heptylamine focused the myocardial stimulant activity and increased force of myocardial contraction along with heart rate |
| [29] | Charlier, R. | 1951 | 2-amino-6-methyl-heptane | Animal experiment (with dog) revealed growth in arterial blood pressure after the exposure of 2-amino-6-methyl-heptane |
| [34] | Oelkers, H.A. | 1967 | 2-amino-6-methylheptane (+)-camphor-10-sulfonate | Inotropic properties of 2-amino-6-methylheptane (+)-camphor-10-sulfonate were identified |
| [31] | Trieb, G.; Nusser, E. | 1974 | Ordinal®retard | The medicament Ordinal® retard combining Octodrine, 3-octopamine and adenosine demonstrated pressure effects in treatment of patients with hypotension |
| Nervous system | | | | |
| [30] | Fellows, E.J. | 1947 | 2-amino-6-methylheptane | 2-amino-6-methylheptane demonstrated local anaesthesia and elevation of local pain threshold in experiments with animals (rabbits, cats, dogs) |
| *Antimicrobial activity* | | | | |
| [45] | Kim, K.; Zilbermintz, L.; Martchenko, M. | 2015 | Octodrine | Octodrine demonstrated antifungal activity in experiments with serum-grown *C. albicans* |
| [46] | Niu, H.; Cui, P. | 2015 | Octodrine | Octodrine demonstrated experimental activity against stationary phase *E. coli* |

Reference to its multiple medicinal properties was found in five of these papers, which highlighted its sympathomimetic and broncho-spasmolytic effects, with possible further actions as a stimulant, anti-obesity and appetite suppressant agent. The molecule is cited also as an antimicrobial with specific antifungal activity [45], as a nasal decongestant [47] and as an ingredient of dietary supplements [48]. Other scholarly papers (a total of seven) made passing or limited reference to Octodrine, covering the chemical properties and analyses of several compounds including this one, or providing data on its antimicrobial effects only [45,46]. These are other scattered examples of relevant documentation, including an invention patent from 2012 [49]. However, the lack of experimental randomized controlled trials (RCTs) and other interventional studies on humans has led to a complete absence of systematic reviews and meta-analytic studies related to use of Octodrine as a medicinal agent or food supplement. Two of the three papers found on PubMed were published in the *Journal of Pharmacology and Experimental Therapeutics* in 1947 and 1951 respectively [27,30], while the third paper [29] was published at the *Archives internationales de pharmacodynamie et de thérapie*. Since the 1950s, there have been no other scholarly-published data specific for Octodrine in any peer-reviewed journal, neither observational nor experimental could be found on the entire web, including medical and paramedical databases, or unpublished literature. The substance remerged on the literature in 2017, when Cohen et al. published a study conducted on six different supplements: Game Day, Infrared, 2-Aminoisoheptane, Simply Skinny Pollen, Cannibal Ferox AMPed and Triple X. All these products disclosed on their label the words Octodrine, 2-amino-6-methylheptane and 6-methyl-2-heptanamine or listed the stimulant as if it were an extract of Aconitum kusnezoffii plant. Results showed that only one of them, Game Day, contained Octodrine, while the others contained different or banned stimulants [50].

#### 3.1.1. Limited Data-Reporting in Scholarly Peer-Reviewed Papers and Invention Patents

There is limited mention of Octodrine in invention patents from 2012 in relation to a novel stable anaesthetic for reducing skin reactions [49].Two papers, pertinent to the disciplines of toxicology and chemical chromatography, examined Octodrine in terms of its physiochemical properties including relative retention time (RTT) and its identification in hair samples [51,52]. Furthermore, Niu et al. and Kim et al. [45,47] discussed the broad-spectrum antimicrobial effect, antifungal effect, anti-persister activity and application for the treatment of Candida albicans and uropathogenic strains of Escherichia coli. These two papers also discussed Octodrine microbial resistance. Additionally, Kuo et al. (2004) [26] and Schlessinger et al. (2011) [53], documented the sympathomimetic properties of Octodrine and effects related to norepinephrine transporter (NET) and G-protein-coupled receptors (GPCRs), which was in concordance with the results from 1947 and 1951 animal studies [27,30].

#### 3.1.2. Google Trends

Google Trends provided valuable data in relation to the interest in Octodrine on the Web. Four keywords provided good insight on the trend as far back as the year 2004. These keywords are "Octodrine," "2-aminoisoheptane," "aminoisoheptane" and "DMHA." There was an obvious incremental increase of interest in Octodrine starting in the year 2012. This interest plateaued between 2013 and 2014 and was followed by a steep rise in 2014–2015, followed by a further escalation starting in 2015 before peaking by the January of 2018 [54]. Comparing to other three keywords, DMHA has demonstrated the greatest interest among Google users ranging between 9 searches in July 2008 and 100 searches in September 2017. The leading countries in terms of internet searches of Octodrine (DMHA) were the USA, Canada and Australia. On the Russian-language Internet, users showed no search activity for Octodrine, while intensively searching for DMAA. In June 2017, the quantity of DMAA searches in Russian-language zone was 100. Since 2004 the trend has demonstrated stable growth in this local online area [55]

#### 3.1.3. Bodybuilding Website, (Bio)Chemistry, Pharmaceutical Websites, Blogs and Online Fora

Body building websites provided a major source of data, especially in relation to the analysis of online trading platforms and fora discussing Octodrine and its effects. A multilingual approach used in this part of the study facilitated the characterisation of regional and national features of sport-stimulant markets.

No specific inclusion criteria were imposed upon the body-building websites, beyond demonstrating a mention of DMHA or synonym. All such instances were included in the evaluation.

The English-language domain was investigated with relevant results. No results were produced from searches in Arabic. Thousands of websites can be located using the Google search terms "Octodrine" and its synonyms [56–59]. Popular brand names include: Olympus Labs CONQU3R Unleashed, Total War, Simply Skinny Pollen, AdrenaCLENV2, Game Day, Cannibal Ferox Amped, Giant Sports Giant Rush [57–66]. By January 2018, 68 English- and 6 German-language online shops selling Octodrine were identified. The product is often advertised as the "next big thing" in bodybuilding environments and described as the "new MDAA" whose effects are "just right" for dietary supplement users and/or stimulant-enthusiasts as it can allegedly enhance focus, experience and performance. Many of these sites also provide detailed information around usage and dosage, alongside with warnings on risks and severe side effects of this emerging molecule [56–59]. Professional scientific or pharmaceutical sites regarding the chemistry characterization of this compound can be found on the web, as well as "amateur" websites, displaying more generic scientific information on this potentially dangerous substance [67,68]. Online stores are predominantly American or Australian domains that ship their products all over the world. Octodrine is presented as a DMAA-like stimulant and predominantly sold as a fat-burner product or pre-workout formula. Some websites also recommended it for intensive study sessions, positioning this molecule among the Nootropics;

pharmaceuticals used to improve cognitive and executive function, memory and creativity in healthy individuals. Claims such as "It boosts dopamine and noradrenaline uptake, while slowing down reuptake just long enough for a solid workout or study session" are quite common [58].

Usually Octodrine is sold in powder (e.g., Cannibal Ferox AMPed, Olympus Labs CONQU3R Unleashed, Game Day, Total War) as pre-workout or in capsules (Infrared, Simply Skinny Pollen) as fat burner, with prices ranging from 1.75 to 3.75 dollars per serving.

German online trading platforms focus customers' attention on Octodrine with detailed feedback from the reviewers (estimation of taste, effects, "price-quality") [68] or vague offers of "fitness hardcore pre-workout booster for pumps and focus" [69]. The trader for amazon.de mentions Octodrine as additives "Oct" in "Arginine AKG, Beta-Alanine, Citrullin Malate complex" and omits a description of its side-effects. Standard marketing technologies widely used by German traders are also employed, such as discounts, world-wide express-delivery and even "halal" certification.

In terms of the Russian-language results, the majority consisted of bodybuilding resources linked to 73 online shops delivering Octodrine to the Russian Federation, the Ukraine and 4 Central Asian countries. In contrast, fora did not indicate significant popularity among local athletes and were predominantly arranged within Russian social nets [70,71]. All identified Russian-language websites run their activity legally on the surface web, a fact explained by the absence of any law enforcement restrictions referring to DMHA and DMAA in Russia and Ukraine. The relative lesser popularity of these particular stimulants is no doubt influenced by the availability of much cheaper locally produced analogues. An imported stimulant complex with DMHA and DMAA (from the USA) costs 1.27 ± 0.19 USD per unit compared to a local analogue for 0.49 ± 0.23 USD per unit. The local online platforms offer more than 20 brands of Octodrine. The immense variety of trading names of this substances is attributable to continuous rebranding as attempts to overcome counterfeit production [72]. By offering athletic stimulant complexes, Russian online shops strive to advertise DMHA and DMAA as the active components for the desirable results; less attention is paid to other substances such as vitamins, tyrosine, taurine and DMAE [73,74]. Trading and producing companies announced anti-inflammatory, anaesthetic, spasmolytic and anticonvulsant properties of Octodrine offering the "ideal" substance for "hard-core" training [72]. The use of Octodrine as a weight loss product is rarely advertised (e.g., only 9 Russian-language online shops were identified). Fat burners containing Octodrine are typically sold at a higher price point: 1.3 USD per unit in contrast to the 0.5 USD for the pre-training complex. Taking into account the legality of DMHA and DMAA in Russian-language territories and the absence of relevant trading regulations, local online shops did not notify their customers to possible side and toxic effects of the stimulants. Some shops explicitly claim that Octodrine has no side effects and that is potential is the same as caffeine [75]. For example, berserktakticalfarma.blogspot.com underlined the safety and high effectiveness of DMHA, emphasising that its potency is equal to 90% of DMAA [76]. Only one of 73 identified online websites warned that Octodrine and DMAA can be detected and could possibly mislead sport competition testing and thus advised users to cease Octodrine beforehand [74]. An additional online shop mentioned contraindications generally for stimulant complexes without specification on Octodrine [77].

Discussions on fora include suggested dosages, combinations, duration of action, among others. According to such anecdotal evidence, a "safe dose" is considered to be around 1mg/kg of bodyweight up to 160 mg per day, while others recommend 100 mg of the synthetic DMHA isomer and 75 mg of the natural one to reach the "sweet spot." In the Russian-language internet zone, the recommended dose of DMHA substantially differed between online shops (30 to 400 mg), as did the dosing schedule. For instance, the online retailer hulkfood.ru advised to take Octodrine for 45 days without stopping to gain significant desired stimulating effects before sporting competition [78].

Users suggest an intake approximately 15–30 or 30–60 min prior to working out [79,80]. Alternatively, if used for its appetite suppressant properties, DMHA consumption was advised between meals and never in the evening as it might affect sleeping. According to users, 25 mg twice a day are enough to "keep one's mind off food" [81]. Experienced users shared their insights: "If used predominantly for its appetite suppressant properties, DMHA can be used during the day between meals. However, we recommend taking caution if using this ingredient late in the afternoon or early evening, as it has the potential to hinder your ability to sleep."

DMHA effects will occur ~15 to 60 min after consumption. The substance demonstrates potency to heighten level of mental focus, increase energy and reduce appetite, as well as raise feelings of wellbeing. Bloggers described a three-phase effect for pre-work-out complexes containing DMHA: (1) stimulation, (2) post-stimulation side effect symptoms and (3) sleep disturbances. Octodrine is frequently advised as a substance intensifying the first two phases with no impact on sleep [82]. Because of its stimulants effects, Octodrine has also been used outside fitness settings, including working environments as non-prescribed medication [83,84]. To boost athletic performance, it is sometimes ingested in combination with huperzine A, DMAE, n-acetyl tyrosine, alpha-gpc, noopept, phenotropil and picamilon to gain maximal focusing on training. Phenibut and ladasten strengthen the euphoric effects of Octodrine [82].

Side effects such as mood swings, tremor, concentration deficiency, over-stimulation, energy crashes, anxiety, high blood pressure, dyspnoea, rapid heartbeat and heartburn have been reported 6–8 h after the initial onset of effects [85,86]. Some users also reported eyes twitching (blepharospasm), pulsing sinus area (carotid sinus), mood fluctuation, absent-mindedness; a rise in blood pressure, piloroerection and hyperthermia following ingestion of Octodrine (e.g., Anabolicminds.com, 2016; Project Bodybuilding, 2016; kandeleria.ru). There were only a limited number of indications for professional athletes: some websites suggest avoiding consumption for ethical considerations, or because it could be considered a violation of the WADA restrictions [72,86,87].

Some fora provide information on abuse potential and possibility of dependency on Octodrine. Namely, users warned about withdrawal symptoms and growth of tolerance resulting from the short- and long-term use of the stimulant [71,82]. Experienced athletes recommend alternating 3–4 stimulant complexes each training day to overcome undesirable adaptation [77].

## 4. Discussion and Conclusions

To the best of the authors' knowledge, this study is the first to implement a systematic review of the literature or undertake cross-sectional analysis of the content of the web in relation to the diffusion and e-commerce of Octodrine. The authors also bring to the spotlight the noteworthiness of subsequent studies on Octodrine, specifically chemical analysis and receptor-ligand binding assays, with the aim is of reaching a full understanding of this widely used substance. The restrictions on amphetamine-type stimulants (e.g., DMAA, DMAE) exacerbate demands on new formulas tailored to the ambitions of bodybuilders and athletes. The sympathomimetic properties of Octodrine, inheriting the potential of DMAA, meet the expectations of "new-generation boosting" and stimulate the growth of global trading. Meanwhile discrepancies between practical experience and theoretical knowledge were observed in our study. Very little is known about its pharmacodynamics and pharmacokinetics profiles, or the chemical profile of the commercially-available Octodrine-related products.

On the Internet, Octodrine is misleadingly advertised as a "safe and legal" analogue of banned stimulants (e.g., DMAA and phenethylamine), making it potentially more attractive to new and experienced users. Intensive marketing campaigns with unlimited worldwide delivery, discounting programs and displays of "good" feedback from reviewers, have contributed to the re-emergence and current spread of Octodrine in the drug market. According to anecdotal for a, reports and trading information, motives of use go beyond athletics gyms: more often the drug is recommended as a day-life stimulator.

The psychoactive effects of Octodrine were neither previously described in literature nor studied despite its structural similarity to other drugs of abuse (DMAA, DMAE). Its metabolic pathway and adverse reactions have not been studied in humans, making its use in fitness settings extremely hazardous. A limited number of open claims were found on the potential risk, side effects and complications of Octodrine use, while its properties as "hard-core" for advanced users are often emphasized. Sites exploited fragmented and sporadic "scientific news" describing only favourable effects of Octodrine, with research evidence being completely omitted. Only some English and German sites warned about ceasing Octodrine use before sport competitions. Meanwhile, on Russian-language trading platforms, DMHA was actively offered in combination with DMAA - attributable to the legal status of both in this geographical zone (Russia, Belarus, Kazakhstan, Kyrgyzstan). Amphetamine-type stimulants (such as DMAA) have showed more popularity, especially for the last two years.

The reported side effects of Octodrine suggest the strong need for further research. The desirable, stimulatory effects of Octodrine are accompanied with a range of mental and somatic symptoms, with frequent use of Octodrine being associated with tolerance, withdrawal symptoms and risks of dependence syndrome. We reiterate here the importance of focusing and asking direct questions on the pharmacological and toxicological properties of Octodrine. The addictive potential should be promptly identified and assessed. Hence, attention should be paid to further investigation in the field and consider the incorporation of Octodrine within WADA and FDA prohibited substances lists.

There are some limitations to our study. Only five peer-reviewed papers were directly pertinent to Octodrine and these were mainly published 6–7 decades ago. Other scholarly-published studies addressed Octodrine in a marginal way. The paucity of the available literature, absence of review articles, systematic reviews and meta-analytical studies clearly limit the extent of this present review. Taking into consideration lack of publications on the chemical analysis of Octodrine, a comprehensive chemical analysis is necessary for future research, with the aim of establishing the detection and identification of Octodrine, along with potential contaminants, excipients and other active ingredients in the currently promoted powder-products under the name Octodrine or DMHA. The sympathomimetic effect of Octodrine is well-understood. However, the central effects including the psychostimulant and anti-obesity effects are not adequately explored and/or reported, with no formally documented experimental studies nor case reports. Future studies should focus on the central effect of Octodrine and its correlation with patterns of cerebral dominance and the lateralization of brain function. Moreover, there is an inadequate body of data in relation to the geographic usage of Octodrine, particularly for contrasting the developing world (including the Middle East, North Africa and post-soviet regions) versus the developed world. In terms of multilingual analysis of websites and drug fora, only publicity available information was considered for the study to uphold observational status. Fora requesting registration were not included in the study. Self-reported experiences are only partially reliable and it may be inappropriate to trust such anecdotal evidence without independent verification.

**Author Contributions:** V.C. carried out most of the scientific review and wrote the first version of the paper. M.P., A.A.-I. and Y.E. contributed to the online searches in German, Russian and Arabic. S.M. revised the manuscript at various stages and contributed to the assessment of the literature searches. R.C., G.M. and M.Z. provided inputs on the research work at different stages and reviewed the manuscript before the submission. O.C. oversaw the overall project. O.C. provided guidance and inputs at each stage of the work and reviewed the work before the final submission.

## References

1. Corazza, O.; Assi, S. Promoting Innovation and excellence to face the rapid diffusion of Novel Psychoactive Substances in the EU: The outcomes of the ReDNet project. *Hum. Psychopharmacol. Clin. Exp.* **2013**, *28*, 317–323. [CrossRef] [PubMed]
2. Martinotti, G.; Lupi, M. Novel psychoactive substances: Use and knowledge among adolescents and young adults in urban and rural areas. *Hum. Psychopharmacol.* **2015**, *30*, 295–301. [CrossRef] [PubMed]
3. Martinotti, G.; Lupi, M. Novel psychoactive substances in young adults with and without psychiatric comorbidities. *Biomed. Res. Int.* **2014**, *2014*, 815424. [CrossRef] [PubMed]

4. Van Hout, M.C. Kitchen chemistry: A scoping review of the diversionary use of pharmaceuticals for non-medicinal use and home production of drug solutions. *Drug Test Anal.* **2014**, *6*, 778–787. [CrossRef] [PubMed]
5. Di Nicola, A.; Martini, E. FAKECARE: Developing expertise against the online trade of fake medicines by producing and disseminating knowledge, counterstrategies and tools across the EU. In *eCrime Research Report*; StampaLith Snc: Trento, Italy, 2015; Volume 2.
6. Corazza, O.; Roman-Urrestarazu, A. *Novel Psychoactive Substances: Policy, Economics and Drug Regulations*; Springer: Berlin, Germany, 2017.
7. Rahman, S.Z.; Gupta, V. Lifestyle Drugs: Concept and Impact on Society. *Indian J. Pharm. Sci.* **2010**, *72*, 409–413. [CrossRef] [PubMed]
8. Mooney, R.; Simonato, P. The use of supplements and performance and image enhancing drugs in fitness settings: A exploratory cross-sectional investigation in the United Kingdom. *Hum. Psychopharmacol.* **2017**, *32*. [CrossRef] [PubMed]
9. Corazza, O.; Parrott, A.C. Novel psychoactive substances: Shedding new lights on the ever-changing drug scenario and the associated health risks. *Hum. Psychopharmacol.* **2017**, *32*. [CrossRef] [PubMed]
10. Lanni, C.; Lenzken, S.C. Cognition enhancers between treating and doping the mind. *Pharmacol. Res.* **2008**, *57*, 196–213. [CrossRef] [PubMed]
11. Franques, P.; Auriacombe, M. Sports, use of performance enhancing drugs and addiction. A conceptual and epidemiological review. *Ann. Med. Interne t (Paris)* **2001**, *152*, 37–49.
12. Mazzoni, I.; Barroso, O. Anti-doping Challenges with Novel Psychoactive Substances in Sport. In *Novel Psychoactive Substances: Policy, Economics and Drug Regulations*; Corazza, O., Urrestarazu, A., Eds.; Springer: Berlin, Germany, 2017; pp. 43–56.
13. Van Hout, M.C. SMART: An Internet study of users experiences of synthetic tanning. *Perform. Enhanc. Health* **2014**, *3*, 3–14. [CrossRef]
14. Schifano, F.; D'Offizi, S.; Piccione, M.; Corazza, O.; Deluca, P.; Davey, Z.; Di Melchiorre, G.; Di Furia, L.; Farré, M.; Flesland, L.; et al. Is there a recreational misuse potential for pregabalin? Analysis of anecdotal online reports in comparison with related gabapentin and clonazepam data. *Psychother. Psychosom.* **2011**, *80*, 118–122. [CrossRef] [PubMed]
15. European Drug Report 2017. Available online: http://www.emcdda.europa.eu/publications/edr/trends-developments/2017 (accessed on 20 September 2017).
16. World Drug Report. Available online: http://www.unodc.org/wdr2017/ (accessed on 21 September 2017).
17. Corazza, O.; Bersani, F.S. The diffusion of performance and image-enhancing drugs (PIEDs) on the internet: The abuse of the cognitive enhancer piracetam. *Subst. Use Misuse* **2014**, *49*, 1849–1856. [CrossRef] [PubMed]
18. Vandrey, R.; Johnson, M.W. Novel Drugs of Abuse: A Snapshot of an Evolving Marketplace. *Adolesc. Psychiatry (Hilversum)* **2013**, *3*, 123–134. [CrossRef] [PubMed]
19. The World Antidoping Code. International Standar. Available online: https://www.wada-ama.org/sites/default/files/resources/files/2016-09-29_-_wada_prohibited_list_2017_eng_final.pdf (accessed on 20 September 2017).
20. Australian Sports Anti-Doping Autority. Available online: https://www.asada.gov.au/sanctions/nathan-tait (accessed on 21 September 2017).
21. NIST Chemestry WebBook, SRD 69. Available online: http://webbook.nist.gov/cgi/inchi?ID=C543828&Mask=200 (accessed on 25 September 2017).
22. Eskay's, O. *Physicians Desk Reference 1949*, 3rd ed.; Medical Economics Inc.: Rutherford, NJ, USA, 1949; p. 476.
23. Gode, J. The bronchospasmolytic effect of ambredin. *Therapie der Gegenwart* **1958**, *97*, 106. [PubMed]
24. Tschudin, M.L. Experiences with ambredin in the treatment of asthmoid states. *Praxis* **1960**, *49*, 920. [PubMed]
25. US Food and Drug Administration. Drugs approved 1938-present (including supplements) (Listed by approval date). 1990; p. 1439.
26. Kuo, C.L.; Wang, R.B. G-protein coupled receptors: SAR analyses of neurotransmitters and antagonists. *J. Clin. Pharm. Ther.* **2004**, *29*, 279–298. [CrossRef] [PubMed]
27. Marsh, D.F.; Herring, D.A. The comparative pharmacology of the hydroxy and methyl derivatives of 6-methyl-2-heptylamine. *J. Pharm. Exp. Ther.* **1951**, *103*, 178–186.
28. Charlier, R.; Philippot, E. Action of three aliphatic amines on the respiratory volume. *Arch. Int. Pharmacodyn. Ther.* **1950**, *82*, 243–246. [PubMed]

29. Charlier, R. Pharmacology of 2-amino-6-methyl-heptane. *Arch. Int. Pharmacodyn. Ther.* **1951**, *85*, 144–151. [PubMed]
30. Fellows, E.J. The pharmacology of 2-amino-6-methylheptane. *J. Pharmacol. Exp. Ther.* **1947**, *90*, 351–358. [PubMed]
31. Trieb, G.; Nusser, E. Untersuchungen zur Kreislaufwirkung von Ordinal® retard bei Patienten mit hypotoner (statisch labiler) Blutdruckregulationsstörung. *Herz/Kreislauf* **1974**, *6*, 681–688.
32. Petry, R.; Kolb, K.H. Studies on the intestinal absorption of sympathomimetic substances in man. *Arzneim-Forsch* **1973**, *23*, 1535–1538.
33. Ota, Y. Pharmacological studies on alklaminoheptane deriavatives. IV. Blood pressor, antispasmodic and capillary permeability inhibiting action of *N*-alkyl-1,5-dimethylhexylamine derivatives. *Yakugaku Zasshi* **1961**, *81*, 403–407. [CrossRef]
34. Oelkers, H.A. Pharmacology of 2-amino-6-methylheptane (+)-camphor-10-sulfonate. *Arzneim-Forsch* **1967**, *17*, 25–28.
35. Becker, K.H.; Doerner, J. Circulation studies with 2-amino-6-methylheptane (+)-camphor-10-sulfonate in dogs. *Arzneim-Forsch* **1967**, *17*, 28–32.
36. Ademiluyi, A.O.; Ogunsuyi, O.B. Alkaloid extracts from Jimson weed (DaturastramoniumL.) modulate purinergicenzymes in rat brain. *Neuro Toxicol.* **2016**, *56*, 107–117.
37. Wei, X.Y.; Xu, H.X. Analysis of essential oil of Forsythia suspense (Thunb.) Vahl. By GC-MS and its antioxidant activities. *Shaanxi Shifan Daxue Xuebao* **2010**, *38*, 70–74.
38. Zhao, Y.Y.; Dai, Y. Chemical constituents of Aconitum kusnezoffii volatile oil. *Zhongchengyao* **2007**, *29*, 588–591.
39. Al-Wathnani, H.; Ara, I. Bioactivity of natural compounds isolated from cyanobacteria and green algae against human pathogenic bacteria and yeast. *J. Med. Plants Res.* **2012**, *6*, 3425–3433. [CrossRef]
40. Sadasivan, S.L.; Nair, B.R. GC-MS analysis in two species of Biophytum DC. (Oxalidaceae). *J. Pharm. Res.* **2014**, *8*, 466–473.
41. Xu, Y.; Liu, Y. Determination of volatile compounds in turbot (Psetta maxima) during refrigerated storage by head-space solid-phase microextraction and gas chromatography-mass spectrometry. *J. Sci. Food Agric.* **2014**, *94*, 2464–2471. [CrossRef] [PubMed]
42. Arkhipov, A.; Sirdaarta, J. Metabolomic profiling of Kigelia Africana Extracts with anti-cancer activity by high resolution tandem mass spectroscopy. *Pharmacog. Comm.* **2014**, *4*, 10–32.
43. Xu, Y.X.; Liu, Y. Analysis of volatile compounds in turbot by SPME with different extraction fibers. *Shipin Gongy Keji* **2013**, *34*, 90–97.
44. Google Trends. Available online: https://www.google.com/trends/ (accessed on 10 September 2016).
45. Kim, K.; Zilbermintz, L.; Martchenko, M. Repurposing FDA approved drugs against the human fungal pathogen, Candida albicans. *Ann. Clin. Microbiol. Antimicrob.* **2015**, *14*, 32. [CrossRef] [PubMed]
46. Niu, H.; Cui, P. Identification of anti-persister activity against uropathogenic Escherichia coli from a clinical drug library. *Antibiotics Basel* **2015**, *4*, 179–187. [CrossRef] [PubMed]
47. Lilly, E. NEW and nonofficial remedies: Methylhexamine; forthane. *J. Am. Med. Assoc.* **1950**, *143*, 1156.
48. Yang, C. The New DMAA (DMHA/2-Aminoisoheptane/Octodrine). Available online: https://www.linkedin.com/pulse/new-dmaa-dmha-2-aminoisoheptane-octodrine-cain-yang (accessed 10 September 2017).
49. Portal, T. New Stable Anaesthetic Composition for Reducing Skin Reactions. U.S. Patent Application US 14/693,361, 2015. Galderma Research & Development. Opio, FR.
50. Cohen, A.; Travis, J.C. Four experimental stimulants found in sports and weight loss supplements: 2-amino-6-methylheptane (octodrine), 1,4-dimethylamylamine (1,4-DMAA), 1,3-dimethylamylamine (1,3-DMAA) and 1,3-dimethylbutylamine (1,3-DMBA). *Clin. Toxicol.* **2017**, 1–7. [CrossRef] [PubMed]
51. Dugal, R.; Massé, R. An integrated methodological approach to the computer-assisted gas chromatographic screening of basic drugs in biological fluids using nitrogen selective detection. *J. Anal. Toxicol.* **1980**, *4*, 1–12. [CrossRef] [PubMed]
52. Broecker, S.; Herre, S. General unknown screening in hair by liquid chromatography-hybrid quadrupole time-of-flight mass spectrometry (LC-QTOF-MS). *Forensic Sci. Int.* **2012**, *218*, 68–81. [CrossRef] [PubMed]
53. Schlessinger, A.; Geier, E. Structure-based discovery of prescription drugs that interact with the norepinephrine transporter, NET. *Proc. Natl. Acad. Sci. USA* **2011**, *108*, 15810–15815. [CrossRef] [PubMed]

54. Google Trends. Available online: https://trends.google.com/trends/explore?date=all&q=octodrine,2-aminoisoheptane,aminoisoheptane,DMHA (accessed on 10 January 2018).
55. Google Trends. Available online: https://trends.google.com/trends/explore?date=all&geo=RU&q=DMAA (accessed on 10 January 2018).
56. DMHA (Octodrine). Available online: https://massivejoes.com/articles/supplements-simplified/dmha (accessed on 28 August 2017).
57. Octodrine (DMHA). Available online: http://www.suppreviewers.com/ingredients/octodrine/ (accessed on 28 August 2017).
58. DMHA/2-Aminoisoheptane/Octodrine: 2016's Stimulant. Available online: https://blog.priceplow.com/ (accessed on 28 August 2017).
59. DMHA is Here. Available online: https://www.pinterest.com/pin/300544975113533041/ (accessed on 29 August 2017).
60. Cannibal Carnage Killer Bombsicle. Available online: https://www.chaosandpain.com/cannibal-carnage-killer-bombsicle/ (accessed on 16 January 2018).
61. CONQU3R UNLEASHED. Available online: https://olympus-labs.com/conqu3r-unleashed/ (accessed on 29 August 2017).
62. REDCON1-TOTAL WAR. Available online: https://www.thesuppstop.com.au/shop/pre-workouts/redcon1-total-war/ (accessed on 25 August 2017).
63. Simply Skinny Pollen. Available online: https://www.downtoearth-solutions.com/simply-skinny-pollen.html (accessed on 16 January 2018).
64. Stealth Sports–AdrenaClen. Available online: https://www.vfsupplements.com.au/stealth-sports-adrenaclen.html (accessed on 27 August 2017).
65. Game Day from MAN Sports: Review. Available online: http://muscles.zone/pre-workout/game-day-man-sports-review (accessed on 12 January 2018).
66. Giant Sports Giant Rush. Available online: https://www.powermyself.com/giant-sports-giant-rush-60-servings.html (accessed on 25 August 2017).
67. WEBMD. Available online: http://www.webmd.com/vitamins-supplements/ingredientmono-1538-octodrine.aspx?activeingredientid=1538&activeingredientname=octodrine (accessed on 10 January 2018).
68. GANNIKUS.COM. Available online: https://www.gannikus.com/review-uebersicht/goldstar-triple-x-im-test/ (accessed on 19 January 2018).
69. Amazon.de. Available online: Amazon.de/Pre-Workout-Preworkout-Supplement-Beta-Alanine-Citrullin (accessed on 20 January 2018).
70. PVSport.ru. Available online: https://vk.com/pvsport (accessed on 29 January 2018).
71. Weekend Rambler. Available online: https://weekend.rambler.ru/items/36735347-zdes-vse-chto-nado-znat-o-zhiroszhigatelyah-i-predtrenirovochnyh-kompleksah/ (accessed on 29 January 2018).
72. Fit Magazine. Available online: http://fitmagazine.kandeleria.ru/?s=DMHA&post_type=product (accessed on 29 January 2018).
73. Smart Nutrition. Available online: https://smartnutrition.kz/index.php?route=product/search&filter_name=DMAA (accessed on 29 January 2018).
74. Big Blog. Available online: http://bigblog.com.ua/ (accessed on 29 January 2018).
75. BCAA.RU. Available online: http://ekb.bcaa.ru/category/predtreniki-i-energetiki/ (accessed on 29 January 2018).
76. Berserk. Available online: http://berserktakticalfarma.blogspot.com/search?q=DMHA (accessed on 29 January 2018).
77. DOM AMBALA. Available online: http://domambala.ru/search/?q=dmha (accessed on 29 January 2018).
78. HULKFOOD.RU. Available online: https://hulkfood.ru/energy/pre_workout/ (accessed on 29 January 2018).
79. MRSUPPLEMENT. Available online: https://www.mrsupplement.com.au/dmha-octodrine (accessed on 29 January 2018).
80. GORILLAZMARKET.RU. Available online: http://gorillazmarket.ru/search/?search=dmha (accessed on 29 January 2018).
81. PROHORMONEFORUM.COM. Available online: http://prohormoneforum.com (accessed on 20 September 2017).
82. DO4A.COM. Available online: https://do4a.com/search/30585319/?q=dmha&o=date (accessed on 29 January 2018).

83. Geekzone. Available online: https://www.geekzone.co.nz/forums.asp?forumid=161&topicid=217945 (accessed on 29 January 2018).
84. PHPBB. Available online: http://www.chemport.ru/forum/viewtopic.php?f=16&t=121426 (accessed on 29 January 2018).
85. LeanBulking.com. Available online: https://leanbulking.com/dmha-2-aminoisoheptane-review (accessed on 29 January 2018).
86. SpotrBaza. Available online: http://sportbaza52.ru/shop/valhalla-labs/berserk.html (accessed on 29 January 2018).
87. AnabolicMinds.com. Available online: http://anabolicminds.com (accessed on 29 January 2018).

# 8

# Hallucinogen Persisting Perception Disorder: Etiology, Clinical Features and Therapeutic Perspectives

Giovanni Martinotti [1,2], Rita Santacroce [1,2,*], Mauro Pettorruso [3], Chiara Montemitro [1], Maria Chiara Spano [1], Marco Lorusso [1], Massimo di Giannantonio [1] and Arturo G. Lerner [4,5]

1 Department of Neuroscience, Imaging and Clinical Sciences, University "G. d'Annunzio", 66100 Chieti, Italy; giovanni.martinotti@gmail.com (G.M.); chiara.montemitro@gmail.com (C.M.); m.chiara.spano@gmail.com (M.C.S.); doloma2012@gmail.com (M.L.); digiannantonio@unich.it (M.d.G.)
2 Department of Pharmacy, Pharmacology, Postgraduate Medicine, University of Hertfordshire, Herts AL10 9AB, UK
3 Institute of Psychiatry and Psychology, Catholic University of Sacred Heart, 00168 Rome, Italy; mauro.pettorruso@hotmail.it
4 Lev Hasharon Mental Health Medical Center, Pardessya 42100, Israel; alerner@lev-hasharon.co.il
5 Sackler School of Medicine, Tel Aviv University, Ramat Aviv 69121, Israel
* Correspondence: rita.santacroce82@gmail.com

**Abstract:** Hallucinogen Persisting Perception Disorder (HPPD) is a rare, and therefore, poorly understood condition linked to hallucinogenic drugs consumption. The prevalence of this disorder is low; the condition is more often diagnosed in individuals with a history of previous psychological issues or substance misuse, but it can arise in anyone, even after a single exposure to triggering drugs. The aims of the present study are to review all the original studies about HPPD in order to evaluate the following: (1) the possible suggested etiologies; (2) the possible hallucinogens involved in HPPD induction; (3) the clinical features of both HPPD I and II; (4) the possible psychiatric comorbidities; and (5) the available and potential therapeutic strategies. We searched PubMed to identify original studies about psychedelics and Hallucinogen Persisting Perception Disorder (HPPD). Our research yielded a total of 45 papers, which have been analyzed and tabled to provide readers with the most updated and comprehensive literature review about the clinical features and treatment options for HPPD.

**Keywords:** Hallucinogen Persisting Perception Disorder; flashbacks; hallucinogenic substances; LSD; psychedelics; visual disturbances; perceptual disturbances

---

## 1. Introduction

Hallucinogens represent an enormous group of natural and synthetic agents [1,2]. The core features of hallucinogens include their being empathogenic and being able to induce alterations of consciousness, cognition, emotions, and perception. Their main characteristic is to profoundly affect a person's inner processes and the perception of the surrounding world. The perceptual distortions are mainly visual, as in the vast majority of induced psychoses [3–5]. The hallucinogenic properties of many natural products were known for thousands of years: popular healers, "brujos", and shamans used these substances in ancient times for medical, religious, spiritual, ritual, divination, and magical purposes. Nevertheless, the attention of western culture was drawn to psychedelics only at the beginning of the 20th century, but the turning point is considered to be 1938, the year in which the lysergic acid diethylamide, better known as LSD, was synthesized by Albert Hofmann. In the 1950s and 1960s, LSD was considered to have a therapeutic potential in the psychiatric field, allowing patients to access unconscious material in therapeutic settings. This has been recently re-evaluated with uncertain results. After a mass diffusion of hallucinogens in the 1960s and 1970s, current prevalence data [6] from the United States highlight that more than 180,000 Americans report a recent use of LSD, and 32,000 a recent use of phencyclidine. Nowadays, the intake of hallucinogens is associated with shamanic ceremonies, workshops of underground therapy and self-experiences. In these frameworks, hallucinogenic substances are most commonly used alone, while in rave parties and social events they are often part of a heavy polyvalent use that frequently includes Novel Psychoactive Substances. These compounds, easily available on the Internet without any cultural barrier and sometimes without any advice from the group of peers, have profoundly changed the drug scenario [7–10]. Their use is becoming widespread, also due to their low cost and appealing market strategies [11,12]. However, significant medical and psychiatric problems have been reported for subjects using these drugs [13], regardless of previous psychiatric antecedents [14].

This paper will focus on a rare, and therefore, poorly understood aspect of hallucinogen consumption: the total or partial recurrence of perceptual disturbances that appeared during previous hallucinogenic "trips" or intoxications and re-emerged without recent use [4,5]. These returning syndromes are defined "benign flashbacks", or pervasive Hallucinogen Persisting Perception Disorder (HPPD). LSD is the model and prototype of the classical synthetic hallucinogen, and it is certainly the most explored and investigated substance associated with the etiology of this unique and captivating state [15]. HPPDs do not have a notable prevalence [16], and, therefore, they are frequently unrecognized [17,18].

Classifications used to delineate and outline persisting perceptual disorders are now clearer than in the past [18]. Two major subtypes of hallucinogenic substance-use related recurring perceptual disturbances have been identified and reported [18]: (1) HPPD I, also described and named as benign Flashback and Flashback Type; and (2) HPPD II, also named HPPD Type II [17,18]. HPPD I has a short-term, reversible and benign course. Although visual images may provoke unpleasant feelings, re-experiencing the first hallucinogen intoxication may not lead to significant concern, distress, and impairment in individual, familial, social, occupational, or other important areas of functioning [17,18]. The impairment is mild and the prognosis is usually good. Some of the patients do not report being annoyed by these phenomena: they may indeed consider them as "free trips" resembling psychedelic experiences without consuming a psychoactive substance. Contrarily and conversely, HPPD II has a long-term, irreversible or slowly reversible and pervasive course [17,19]. The impairment of HPPD II is severe and the prognosis is worse. Some of the patients fail to adapt and live with these long-lasting recurrent "trips", and a consistent fraction needs to be constantly treated [19,20]. It has to be considered that the distinction between HPPD type I and HPPD type II has not yet been made in the Diagnostic and Statistical Manual of Mental Disorder, fifth edition (DSM-5) and it is still debated. HPPD type I is consistent with the diagnostic definition expressed by the International Classification of Disease, 10th (ICD-10), while HPPD type II better matches the DMS-5 criteria.

A vast list of psychoactive substances has been identified and linked with the development of this condition, including Magic Mushrooms (psilocybin) [21] and muscimol (*Amanita muscaria* (L.) Lam.) [22]; San Pedro cactus and Peyote (mescaline) [16,23]; ketamine [24]; dextromethorphan [25]; MDMA and MDA [26]; and cannabis and synthetic cannabinoids [27–33]. This condition has also been associated with the consumption of Ayahuasca, *Datura stramonium* L., *Salvia divinorum* Epling & Játiva, and *Tabernanthe iboga* (L.) Nutt., which contains ibogaine [17,18]. It is, therefore, clear that HPPD is not strictly associated with psychedelic consumption, but a number of hallucinogen-inducing substances may be correlated with its arising.

The aim of the present study is to review all the original studies about HPPD in order to evaluate (1) the possible suggested etiologies; (2) the possible hallucinogens involved in HPPD induction; (3) the clinical features of both HPPD I and II; (4) the possible psychiatric comorbidities; and (5) the available and potential therapeutic strategies.

## 2. Materials and Methods

We searched PubMed to identify original studies about psychedelics and Hallucinogen Persisting Perception Disorder (HPPD). The following search terms were used: "Hallucinogen Persisting Perception Disorder" OR "Hallucinogen Persisting Perceptual Disorder". The search was conducted on 15 September 2017 and yielded 46 records. We included all original articles (open-label or double-blind trials, prospective or retrospective observational studies, and case reports) written in English. We included all studies describing perceptual distortions in patients with a previous history of substance consumption. Reviews, commentaries, letters to the editor, and studies enrolling adolescents were excluded. All the authors agreed on the inclusion and exclusion criteria. We excluded 17 records by reading the titles and abstracts. By reading the full texts of the 29 remaining articles, we found 25 papers meeting our inclusion/exclusion criteria, and we, therefore, included them in the qualitative synthesis (Figure 1).

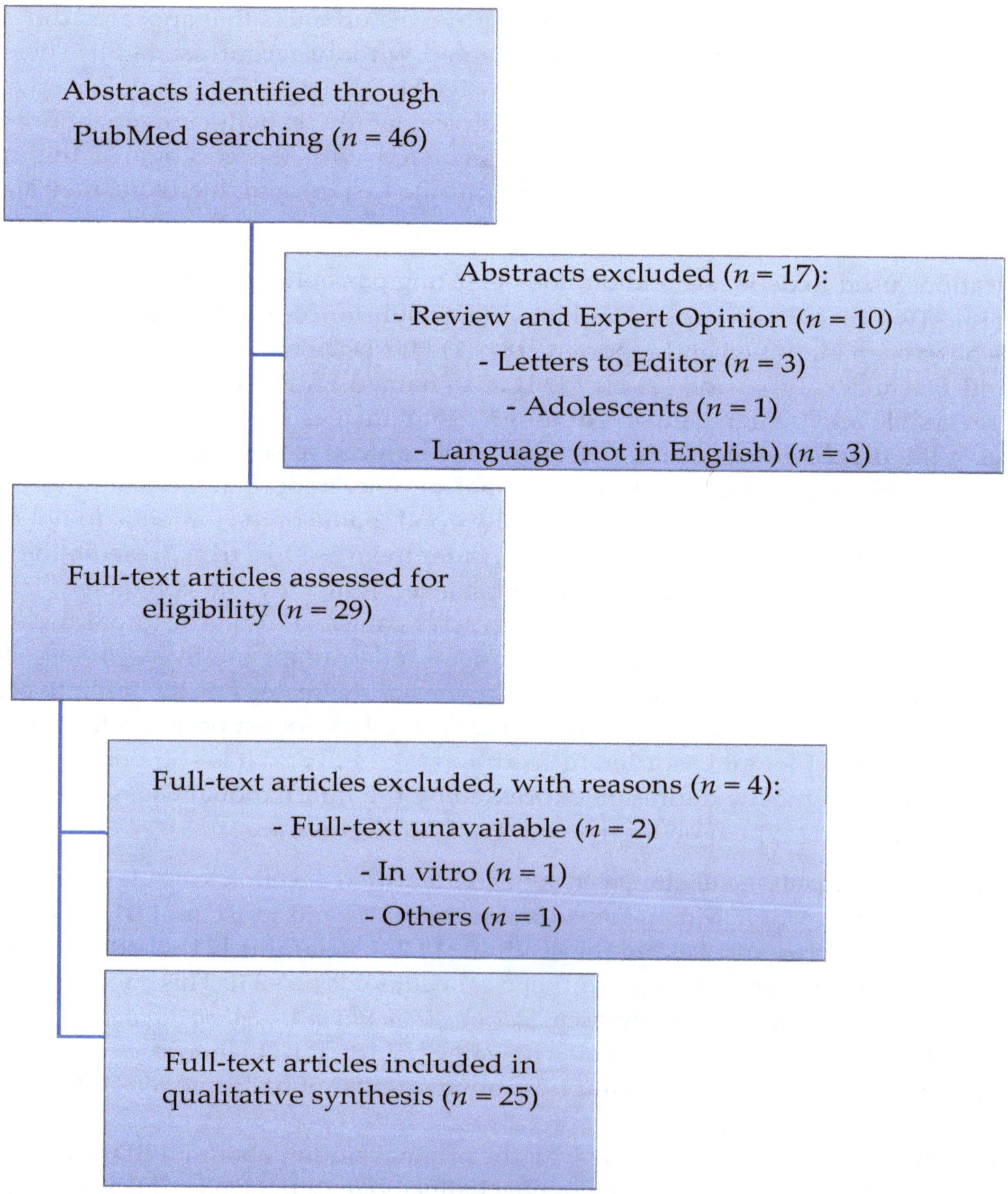


**Figure 1.** Flow-chart describing the data collection process.

## 3. Results

### 3.1. Suggested Etiologies

HPPDs are poorly understood due to the enormous range and variability of recurrent sensory disturbances, and the multiple distinct subtypes [17,18].

The main neurobiological hypothesis is that LSD consumers might develop chronic disinhibition of visual processors and dysfunction in the function of the central nervous system (CNS) [4,34–36]. This disinhibition may be linked to an LSD-generated intense current [37] that may determine the destruction or dysfunction [18] of cortical serotonergic inhibitory interneurons with *gamma*-Aminobutyric acid (GABAergic) outputs, implicated in sensory filtering mechanisms of unnecessary stimuli [34–36,38]. The efficacy of some treatment options in a subject with HPPD, such as pre-synaptic $\alpha_2$ adrenergic agonists, selective serotonin reuptake inhibitor (SSRIs), benzodiazepines, and mood stabilizers would confirm this neurobiological hypothesis (see Section 3.2). Reverse tolerance or sensitization that emerges after LSD exposure may explain recurrent occurrences after the stimulus has been withdrawn [39]. Nonetheless, HPPD-like experiences, such as flashbacks, moments of derealization, and hyper-intense perceptions are reported in healthy populations and non-LSD exposed subjects [40]. Moving from biochemical receptor interactions towards macroscopic areas, a temporary or permanent impairment in the Lateral Geniculate Nucleus (LGN) has been hypothesized [4,41–43]. The LGN, which is located in the thalamus, is associated with visual perception pathways [41–43]. Recent research highlighted a brain dysfunction in patients with visual snow, located mainly in the right lingual gyrus [44], perhaps implying LSD involvement. Halpern et al. [40] suggested that HPPD can be due to a subtle over-activation of predominantly neural visual pathways that worsens anxiety in predisposed subjects after ingestion of arousal-altering drugs, including non-hallucinogenic substances. According to Holland and Passie, environmental triggering by specific situations or stimuli or other elements related to the original experience may be involved in flashback experiences [45].

### 3.2. Substances That Induce HPPD

Different substances have been associated with visual and perceptual disturbances (Table 1).

**Table 1.** Substances that induce Hallucinogen Persisting Perception Disorder (HPPD).

| Authors | Cases (*n*) | Substances Inducing Perceptual Disturbances | Trigger Cues |
|---|---|---|---|
| Zobor, 2015 [29] | 1 | Cannabis | |
| Gaillard, 2003 [46] | 2 | Cannabis | |
| Lerner, 2014 [47] | 2 | Cannabis (Synthetic) | |
| Anderson, 2017 [48] | 1 | Cannabis and MDMA | Stress |
| Brodrick, 2016 [49] | 1 | Cannabis and LSD | |
| Coppola, 2017 [50] | 1 | Cannabis (Synthetic, JWH-122) | Cannabis consumption |
| Lerner, 2003 [51] | 16 | LSD | |
| Lerner, 2002 [20] | 1 | LSD | |
| Lerner, 2000 [52] | 8 | LSD | |
| Gaillard, 2003 [46] | 1 | LSD | Alcohol intake |
| Lev-Ran, 2017 [53] | 40 | LSD | Sexual intercourse or Intentional |
| Hermle, 2012 [54] | 1 | LSD | Stress |
| Lerner, 2014 [19] | 2 | LSD | |
| Abraham, 2001 [35] | 38 | LSD | Dark environment |
| Litjens, 2014 [26] | 31 | LSD | |
| Lerner, 2015 [55] | 1 | LSD | |
| Baggott, 2011 [56] | 104 | LSD | |
| Lev-Ran, 2015 [57] | 37 | LSD | |
| Lev-Ran, 2014 [58] | 12 | LSD | Situation and mental states |
| Lerner, 1997 [59] | 2 | LSD | |
| Abraham, 1996 [34] | 3 | LSD | |
| Espiard, 2005 [21] | 1 | PCP | Cannabis consumption |
| Lauterbach, 2000 [60] | 1 | Risperidone | |

MDMA: 3,4-methylenedioxy-*N*-methylamphetamine; LSD: lysergic acid diethylamide; JWH-122: 4-methyl-1-(naphthalenyl)(1-pentyl-1H-indol-3-yl)-methanone.

According to the literature, we found that the majority of HPPD cases have been induced by LSD or phencyclidine (PCP) (14 studies, 294 patients) [17,19,21,26,35,46,51–53,55–59].

The use of cannabis has been associated with the development of perceptual distortions in seven patients [29,46,48,49,61]. In one case, it was associated with 3,4-Methylenedioxymethamphetamine (MDMA) and in another case with PCP [48,49]. In two patients, visual distortion followed the consumption of synthetic cannabinoids [61].

Lauterbach et al. reported the unique case of HPPD induced by the atypical antipsychotic Risperidone [60].

### 3.3. Clinical Features

According to DSM-5, Hallucinogen Persisting Perception Disorder is the recurrence of perceptive disturbances that firstly develop during intoxication. The contents of the perception and visual imagery range extensively [17,19]. DSM-5 and previous DSM editions report a list of the most common symptoms experienced by HPPD patients, but only a few symptoms have been described in the professional literature. The main group of symptoms reported by Criterion A of the DSM-5 are visual disturbances. In fact, as in the vast majority of induced psychoses, visual hallucinations are notably more common than auditory [3]. Regardless, every perceptual symptom that was experienced during intoxication may re-occur following hallucinogen withdrawal. We report a list of the main literature-reported visual disturbances in Table 2.

A latent period may antecede the onset of returning visual occurrences. This latent period may last from minutes, hours, or days up to years, and re-emerge as either HPPD I or II with or without any recognized or perceived precipitator [17,19]. Episodes of HPPD I and II may appear spontaneously or they may be triggered by identified and non-identified precipitators [18]. Episodes may be continuous, intermittent, or sudden. With regards to this point, neither HPPD I nor HPPD II can really be considered as persisting in a narrow sense of the word. Additionally, their differential diagnosis can only be proposed in terms of prognosis rather than clinical presentation.

However, HPPD I usually onsets with warning "auras", minor feelings of self-detachment, mild bewilderment, and mild depersonalization and derealization [17,18]. Conversely, the onset of HPPD II might be unexpected and abruptly detonate with bursting "auras", deep feelings of self-detachment, acute depersonalization-derealization [19].

The frequency of recurrence of perceptual distortions is lower for HPPD I than HPPD II [18]. Prior substance users can voluntarily elicit or produce visual disturbances with or without known triggers [4,17,18]. After HPPD II onset, hallucinogenic events tend to occur more frequently, and their duration and intensity increase. Subjects might perceive a partial or total loss of control.

**Table 2.** A representative, but not exhaustive, list of reported visual disturbances.

| Symptom | Description |
|---|---|
| **Symptom Reported by Diagnostic and Statistical Manual of Mental Disorder, fifth edition (DSM-5)** | |
| Visual hallucinations | Perceptions in the absence of the objects. False perceived objects are often geometric figures. |
| Altered motion perception | False perceptions of movement in the peripheral visual fields |
| Flashes of color | |
| Color enhancement | Perception of intensified colors |
| Trails or tracers | Lines, stripes or bands that could be observed after animate and inanimate objects have already moved from their previous location. According to DSM-5, images left suspended in the path of a moving object as seen in stroboscopic photography |
| Palinopsia | Positive afterimages that continue to appear in one's vision after the exposure to the original image has ceased. |
| Halos | Colored light around a light source or an object |

**Table 2.** *Cont.*

| Symptom | Description |
|---|---|
| Micropsia | Misperception of images as too small |
| Macropsia | Misperception of images as too large |
| | **Common Symptoms Not Reported by DSM-5** |
| Floaters | Spots that seem to drift in front of the eye |
| Visualizations | Dots, points, particles, mottles or specks emerging in an obscure room |
| Fractals | Self-similarity perception or small parts that are seen having an equal and identical shape or form as the whole |
| Repetitions | Recurrence of inanimate or moving patterns or motives |
| Keenness | Undimmed color contrasts |
| Pareidolia | An image within an image like the imagery of objects or faces in a foggy arrangement |
| Superimpositions | Superimposed or overlapped geometric patterns |
| Distorted Perception of Distance | Objects were seen slightly closer or distant |
| Monochromatic Vision | The visual perception of distinct colors as one unique color with different tinges and tonalities |
| Intense fragmentation | The sense of disintegration of still or moving objects |
| Recurrent Synesthesia | Stimulation of one sensory pathway leads to automatic, involuntary reactions or experiences in a second sensory pathway |
| Geometric Phosphenes | Seeing light without light penetrating the eye. |
| Imagistic Phosphenes | Casual and unplanned formed images like non-humans (zoopsia) and human faces without geometric patterns or figures provoked by closing an eye and pressing it with a finger |
| Acquired Dyslexia | Difficulty with reading notwithstanding normal intelligence |
| Aeropsia or Visual Snow | Virtually seeing particles of air |

### *3.4. Mental Illnesses Comorbid with HPPD*

Recent observations reported a co-occurrence with depressive [20] and anxiety traits [51] and severe mental illnesses such as Major Depressive Disorder [23], Bipolar Disorder [23,62], and Schizophrenia Spectrum Disorders [17,58]. However, HPPD I and HPPD II onsets are not necessarily accompanied by any prominent additional psychiatric disorder, thus representing an independent condition [17,18]. In particular, the onset of HPPD II is often linked to a clear negative mood and affect. Anxiety and depressive features might aggravate new episodes. Anxiety might also evolve into a panic attack. Anticipatory anxiety may antecede future visual aberration events, and avoidant behavior may limit and restrict regular normal functioning [17,18]. Recently, in a study carried out by Halpern, a comprehensive survey of 20 subjects reporting Type-2 HPPD-like symptoms was presented and evaluated. The dissociative symptoms were consistently associated with HPPD, suggesting that HPPD is in most cases due to a subtle over-activation of predominantly neural visual pathways that worsens anxiety in predisposed subjects after the ingestion of arousal-altering drugs, including non-hallucinogenic substances. The authors report that many perceptual symptoms reported were not first experienced while intoxicated, and are partially associated with pre-existing psychiatric comorbidity, tempering the direct role of hallucinogens in the etiopathology of the disorder [40].

Only two observational studies and one case report evaluated psychotic patients with comorbid HPPD [57,58,60] (Table 3). Two observational, cross-sectional studies compared schizophrenic patients with prior use of LSD who developed HPPD (SCZ+HPPD, 49 patients) with those who did not (SCZ, 57 patients), for a total of 106 patients [57,58]. No differences between the two groups have been found with respect to demographic characteristics, age of psychotic onset, age of drug use onset, and type of substances abused [57,58]. As expected, SCZ+HPPD patients reported more distressing and horrific LSD experience ("bad trips") ($p < 0.05$) [57]. Interestingly, the positive subscale of the Positive and Negative Syndrome Scale (PANSS) did not differ between the two groups. On the contrary, SCZ+HPPD patients showed lower scores in the PANSS negative subscale, the PANSS General Psychopathology Subscale, and the PANSS total scores ($p < 0.05$) [57]. Moreover, 67% of the schizophrenic patients comorbid with HPPD were able to distinguish between perceptual distortion and psychotic hallucinations [58], and 9 out of 12 patients could identify precursory cues for perceptual distortion (substance-induced cues, situational cues, and mental cues) [58]. Lauterbach et al. [60] reported a case of HPPD comorbid with psychosis, in which visual distortions were induced by antipsychotic treatment. Interestingly, the patient did not report any history of previous substance abuse [60]. The patient was treated with Risperidone, Clonazepam and Trazodone, and she reported visual disturbances resembling HPPD, in particular, illusions, after three subsequent Risperidone dosage increases [60].

**Table 3.** Observational studies and case reports comparing schizophrenic patients with HPPD (SCZ+HPPD) and schizophrenic patients without HPPD (SCZ) (* $p > 0.05$, ** $p < 0.05$).

| Authors | Study | Number of Patients | Substances | Symptoms Description | Onset Perceptual Disorders | Recurrence of Perceptual Disorders | Treatment |
|---|---|---|---|---|---|---|---|
| Lev-Ran, 2015 [57] | Observational, cross-sectional, control study | 80 hospitalized SCZ patient with past use of LSD<br>43 SCZ (DSM-IV-TR)<br>37 SCZ+HPPD (DSM-IV-TR)<br>Onset of illness: 22.9 SCZ, 23.4 SCZ+HPPD * | Cannabis: 100% SCZ, 92% SCZ+HPPD *<br>MDMA: 60% SCZ, 46% SCZ+HPPD *<br>Opioids: 26% SCZ, 30% SCZ+HPPD 30% *<br>Cocaine: 16% SCZ, 14% SCZ+HPPD *<br>LSD initiation use: SCZ 17.9y, SCZ+HPPD 19.3y * | Adversive LSD experience (bad trip): 28% SCZ, 89% SCZ+HPPD **<br>PANSS: Positive symptoms: SCZ = SCZ+HPPD **<br>Negative symptoms: SCZ > SCZ+HPPD **<br>General psychopathology: SCZ > SCZ+HPPD **<br>Total score: SCZ > SCZ+HPPD ** | | Treatment ineffective in SCZ+HPPD | Antipsychotic medication |
| Lev-Ran, 2014 [58] | Observational | 26 patients<br>14 SCZ (DSM-IV-TR)12 SCZ+HPPD (DSM-IV-TR)<br>Demographic characteristic did not differ between the two groups | Past use of :LSD (100%)<br>cannabis (100%)<br>MDMA (7%)<br>No differences between the two groups in age at onset of drug use and in number of incidences of hallucinogen use | 67% SCZ+HPPD could distinguish HPPD symptoms from hallucination related to a psychotic state | 9 SCZ+HPPD patients recognized precursory cues for perceptual distortion (7 substance-induced, 5 situational, and 2 mental cues) | 12 patients experienced perceptual distortion (SCZ+HPPD) | Antipsychotic treatment.<br>No significant differences in response to APS and adverse effects between the two groups |
| Lauterbach, 2000 [60] | Case report | 1 psychotic patient | No reported substance abuse and hallucinogen exposure<br>Risperidone<br>Clonazepam<br>Trazodone | HPPD-like symptoms: palinopsia, illusions, and visual disturbances | After risperidone treatment | Weekly recurrence. Remission in 48 h each time | |

*3.5. First-Line Medications*

Pre-synaptic $\alpha_2$ adrenergic agonists are a treatment with a low side-effect profile for patients with a previous history of substance-related disorders. Symptoms alleviation has been reported in some patients treated with these drugs [17,18,52,63]. The effectiveness may be based on the evidence that clonidine may elevate plasma GABA levels in humans, having a benzodiazepine-like effect. Clonidine may also decrease locus coeruleus activity, leading to a reduction of adrenergic activity [64], which can be effective in the management of PTSD [65]. Therefore, as in PTSD-related recurring flashbacks, some visual disturbances could be associated with excessive sympathetic nervous activity. Thus, these visual distortions could be ameliorated by Clonidine [52,63].

A dosage of 0.75 mg/die of Clonidine has been evaluated as a treatment option for nine HPPD patients [51,59] (Table 4). The total remission has been reported in a single patient with flashbacks and anxiety treated with 0.25 mg of Clonidine three times a day for two months [59]. In the 2 months open study on eight HPPD patients, the Clinical Global Impression (CGI) and Patient's Severity Perception significantly decreased between entry and endpoint scores [51], although two patients dropped out at week 3 and week 5, respectively [52]. Lofexidine (0.2–0.8 mg/day) is a sympatholytic centrally acting $\alpha_2$ presynaptic adrenergic agonist that showed similar efficacy in some cases [23,65,66].

Benzodiazepines may be useful and effective in eliminating benign HPPD I and ameliorating, but not completely eradicating, pervasive HPPD II symptoms [18,67]. The effectiveness of Benzodiazepines may be related to their activity on the cortical serotonergic-inhibitory inter-neurons with GABAergic outputs [2,4]. Alprazolam (0.25–0.75 mg/day) has been prescribed with some success and Clonazepam (0.5–1.5 mg/day) appears to be the most reliable and effective benzodiazepine even at low doses [17,18,51,67]. Higher doses (4 mg/day) have also been used with good outcomes [68]. Clonazepam may act on serotonergic systems, improving, enhancing, and augmenting transmission [17,18,51,67], thus promoting alleviation and a marked improvement [51,67]. Clonazepam has been evaluated in three case reports and one open-label trial by Lerner [19,50,51]. In the clinical trial, 16 HPPD patients were treated with a Clonazepam dosage of 2 mg/day [51]. Their symptoms improved significantly after treatment initiation and the improvement persisted during a 6-month follow-up after treatment discontinuation [51]. The same author reported two cases of cannabis-induced visual disturbances and correlated anxiety features. In both cases, Clonazepam (2 mg/day) was effective in improving symptoms, but focal visual disturbances without anxiety (trailing phenomena in one case, and black moving spots in the second case) persisted during and after therapy [19]. More recently, Clonazepam (6 mg/day) has been proved to be effective in improving cannabis-induced HPPD symptoms [50]. On the other hand, the intrinsic abuse potential of benzodiazepines might be inconvenient in certain individuals with a past history of substance use [17,18]. Given the benign nature of HPPD I, the use of benzodiazepines should be proposed only for severe cases, in the acute phase, and for the short term.

HPPD patients appear to be sensitive to first-generation antipsychotics at low doses, requiring monitoring of extrapyramidal side effects. Haloperidol [69] and Trifluoperazine [70] were reported to be helpful. Perphenazine (4–8 mg/day) [17,23], Sulpiride (50–100 mg/day) [23], and Zuclopenthixol (2–10 mg/day) [17,23], at very low doses, are well tolerated and may be an effective treatment. Some of the long-acting first-generation antipsychotics may still be useful in co-occurring Psychotic Spectrum Disorders and HPPD II [58]. In one study, haloperidol was noted to reduce hallucinations, but an exacerbation of flashbacks in the early phases of treatment was highlighted as well [1,69].

The use of second-generation antipsychotics in HPPD patients without comorbid psychotic disorders is debated. Anderson recently reported the case of a young woman presenting prolonged and distressing multimodal pseudo-hallucinations, depressive symptoms, and anxiety, who was treated with Risperidone for three months without any significant improvement [48]. At the same time, conflicting evidence exists on the antipsychotics effects in psychotic HPPD patients. One study did not report differences in antipsychotic treatment response between SCZ and SCZ+HPPD patients [58]. On the other hand, a more recent study has shown the ineffectiveness of antipsychotic medications in an SCZ+HPPD population [57].

**Table 4.** Observational studies and case reports evaluating clinical presentation.

| Authors | Study | Number of Patients | Substances | Symptoms Description | Onset Perceptual Disorders | Recurrence of Perceptual Disorders | Treatment |
|---|---|---|---|---|---|---|---|
| Lev-Ran, 2017 [53] | Observational cross-sectional study | 40 (27 males); HPPD (DSM-IV-TR) | Previous use of LSD; Lifetime use of Cannabis | HPPD I: mean age 25.5 (3.7), times of LSD consumption: 7.1 (4.3), use of alcohol; perceptual disorders triggered by sexual intercourse, dark environment, and looking at still or moving objects<br>HPPD II: mean age 22.1 (2.8), times of LSD consumption 24.6 (1.4), use of SCS, stimulants and inhalants; intentionally triggering perceptual disturbances | | | None of the subjects included in the study received medications particularly targeted at treating HPPD |
| Zobor, 2015 [29] | Observational, cross-sectional, control study | Male, 23-year-old | Cannabis, previous 4-year history of heavy consumption (16–20 years) | Visual distortion: visual snow, sperm-like whizzing dot, jittering lights, floaters, photophobia, visual discomfort, positive and negative afterimages, impaired night vision, halos, starburst around lights;<br>Ophthalmological examination: reduction of phosphene threshold, alteration in the EOG | During cannabis use period | Persistence despite cannabis withdrawal | No |
| | | 4 healthy subjects, mean age 25.5 years | Cannabis: Heavy consumption | Not reported | | Not reported | No |
| Lerner, 2014 [19] | Case report | Male, 24-year-old | Cannabis: Three-year past history of social consumption;<br>MDMA, LSD and cocaine (sporadically);<br>Social Alcohol drinking | Visual disturbances (halos, color intensification, flashes of colors, distorted perception of distance) | During LSD intoxication | Recurrence one week after completely stopping all substance use: daily visual distortion<br>Disappearance after one year | Not accepted by the patients |
| | | Female, 25-year-old | Cannabis: Three-year past history of social consumption;<br>MDMA, LSD (sporadically);<br>Social Alcohol drinking | Visual disturbances (positive afterimages, color intensification, flashes of colors, trailing phenomena) | During LSD intoxication | Recurrence four days after completely stopping all substance use: daily visual distortion<br>Improvement after one year;<br>Trailing phenomena continued to appear intermittently | Not accepted by the patients |
| Gaillard, 2003 [46] | Case reports | Female, 18-year-old | Cannabis: Three-year past history of regular consumption | White dots when looking at a white wall or blue sky, "seeing shadows" on the left side, palinopsia, visual vibration upon awakening | During comatose episode following excessive use of cannabis | Recurrence after stopping all substance use: daily visual distortion | |
| | | Male, 25-year-old | Cannabis: Two-year past history of regular and heavy consumption | Visual illusion and dyskinetopsia, difficult in depth perception | After two years of consumption | Symptoms persistence and increase after cannabis withdrawal + memory loss, and concentration deficits | |

**Table 4.** *Cont.*

| Authors | Study | Number of Patients | Substances | Symptoms Description | Onset Perceptual Disorders | Recurrence of Perceptual Disorders | Treatment |
|---|---|---|---|---|---|---|---|
| Abraham, 2001 [35] | Observational | 38 HPPD cases | LSD: first mean use 18.1 (6.0) years; lifetime use 16 times (median) | 7.11 (2.2) different types of visual hallucinations per subject | 21 months after first use | Duration of visual hallucinations: 9.67 (7.68) years | |
| | | | | The majority of subjects reported an intensification of visual hallucinations on emerging into a dark environment | 13.5% subjects experienced symptoms within the first month of use, three subjects after a single use | | |
| Litjens, 2014 [26] | Case series | 31 HPPD cases; Web-questionnaire | MDMA | At least 2 different visual phenomena (visual snow, afterimages, flashes, illusory movement, and increased observation of floaters) with a minimum of one episode of disturbed perception every week (100%); | After a single drug exposure | | |
| | | | Cannabis | | | | |
| | | | LSD | Anxiety or panic in the weeks before or following the use of drugs (71%) | | | |
| | | | | Depersonalization (32%) | | | |
| | | assessment | 80% serotonergic drugs | Derealization (39%) | After a period of extensive drug use | | |
| Lerner, 2015 [55] | Case report | Male, 26-year-old | Cannabis: a Five-year history of occasional consumption; | No distressing macropsia, micropsia, pelopsia and teleopsia, looking at still or moving objects and humans; | LSD intoxication | Recurrence two days after completely stopping all substance use: daily visual distortion | Not accepted by the patients |
| | | | Alcohol: Social Consumption; | | | | |
| | | | LSD: Recreational use | Longer and distressing visual distortion experience with anxiety | | Disappearance after one year | |
| Baggott, 2011 [56] | Observational Web-based questionnaire | 2679 subjects | Median of 5 different drugs used by a single subject | 224 subjects reported having at least one diagnosis associated with unusual visual experiences; | After exposure to LSD | The probability of experiencing constant or near-constant symptoms was predicted by greater past exposure to drugs and exposure to LSD | 104 individuals considered symptoms impairing enough to seek treatment |
| | | 89.5% male, aged 21.6 (3.7) years | | 1487 individuals reported at least one abnormal visual experience; | | | |
| | | | | 587 endorsed at least one experience on a constant or near-constant basis | | | |

Risperidone was usually prescribed due to its proven efficiency in the treatment of perceptual disturbances in Psychotic Spectrum Disorders, mainly in Schizophrenic Disorders. LSD seems to work as a partial agonist of postsynaptic serotonin receptors. Therefore, Risperidone, which is a strong antagonist of both postsynaptic 5-$HT_2$ and $D_2$ receptors, was expected to be convenient. In contrast with this supposition, Risperidone at recommended [71] and lower doses [72] worsens visual disturbances and accompanying anxiety, or does not show any effect [54]. This was presumably due to Risperidone's $\alpha_2$ presynaptic antagonism and noradrenaline release [34]. In addition, Risperidone was associated to the re-experiencing of visual disturbances in some patients suffering from schizophrenia with a past history of LSD use [73]. One psychotic patient treated with Risperidone, Clonazepam, and Trazodone reported visual disturbances resembling HPPD after three subsequent Risperidone dosage increases [60]. At the same time, Risperidone has been shown to be effective in improving PCP-induced HPPD with anxiety in one patient, while in the same patient Olanzapine produced symptoms exacerbation [21].

Evidence not included in our systematic review suggested that low dosages of atypical antipsychotics may be useful, specifically Aripiprazole (5–10 mg/day) [23], also because of its efficacy in substance and alcohol use disorders [74].

Visual oddities and disturbances with sudden paroxysmal onset have been interpreted as visual seizures and prompted the use of antiepileptic drugs in HPPD. This consideration helped to explicate the efficacy of benzodiazepines and led to the prescription of Phenytoin [75,76]. Today, Phenytoin is not used for HPPD treatment due to its troubled side effect profile. Medications such as Valproic Acid (200–600 mg/day), Carbamazepine (200–600 mg/day), Oxcarbamazepine (300 mg/day), Gabapentin (300–900 mg/day), Topiramate (25–100 mg/day), and Lamotrigine (50–100) may be useful [23], also because of their efficacy in substance and alcohol use disorders [77–79]. In a single case of HPPD symptoms and electroencephalographic (EEG) abnormalities, compatible with toxic encephalopathy, the visual hallucinations that recurred at any alcohol ingestion improved, but did not disappear with the use of Valproic Acid (1500 mg/day) [46]. Levetiracetam has shown to reduce some visual symptoms as well as HPPD related-depersonalization and derealization [80]. Lamotrigine has shown to be efficacious in a recent severe case of HPPD with some EEG abnormalities (Anderson et al., 2018). These medications may also be helpful when visual disturbances are accompanied by co-occurring mood swings and mood disorders.

Antidepressant medications could help in the management of co-occurring HPPD II with anxiety and depressive disorders [17,18,20,51,67]. HPPD II alone does not appear to be an appropriate target. There are questionable and controversial results regarding Sertraline, which has been reported to worsen [81] as well as to improve visual disturbances. Amelioration following long-term administration of SSRIs was attributed to the down-regulation of 5-$HT_2$ receptors, providing more evidence to corroborate the serotonergic mechanisms underlying this condition. Other prescribed SSRIs did not show any benefits. Norepinephrine reuptake inhibitors (NRIs) such as Reboxetine have been tried with some success in LSD-induced HPPD symptoms comorbid with Major Depressive Disorder [20]. Agomelatine, given its peculiar function on neurotrophic factors [74], could have some benefits on the syndrome, although no data are available until now.

### 3.6. *Second Line Medications*

Naltrexone has been usually used, alone or with other medications, in chronic patients with continuous visual imagery that previously did not respond to other medications [17,18].

Calcium Channel Blockers and Beta Blockers may be helpful in patients with co-occurring HPPD II and anxiety disorders [18]. Propanolol at low (20–60 mg/day) and high doses (240 mg/day), as well as Atenolol 25–50 mg/day, have been used to diminish accompanying anxiety of visual imagery [18,23]. Investigations of HPPD patients with EEG mapping showed that HPPD is represented by disinhibition [35] in the cerebral cortex [34]. The rationale behind this interesting and novel approach is that improving sensory gating by dopaminergic enhancers may cause an inhibition of catechol-*O*-methyl transferase (COMT), that may improve HPPD symptomatology.

### 3.7. Brain Stimulation Treatments

Currently, brain stimulation treatments have been proposed as a possible therapeutic option to enhance the recovery of refractory symptoms in several disorders [82,83]. Repetitive Transcranial Magnetic Stimulation (rTMS) is a non-invasive brain stimulation approach that acts by modulating specific brain circuits. While high-frequency (>5 Hz) stimulation determines a depolarization of nerve cells, with long-term potentiation (LTP) effects, low-frequency stimulation protocols (1 Hz) determine the long-term depression (LTD) of the targeted area, with the possibility to induce the localized inhibition of specific disordered networks. According to the cortical hyperexcitability hypothesis about its pathogenesis, several case reports propose that rTMS could be a promising therapeutic method for refractory visual hallucinations in schizophrenia [84,85].

To date, no studies have investigated the potential use of rTMS in HPPD. Interestingly, Kilpatrick and Ermentrout (2012) [86] studied the spatiotemporal dynamics of neuronal networks in HPPD, with spike frequency adaptation. This study reported that altering parameters controlling the strength of synaptic connections in the network can lead to spatially structured activity suggestive of symptoms of HPPD. Future research is necessary to test the possible effectiveness of the rTMS neuromodulatory effect on HPPD. Putative targets of stimulation could be hypothesized to be located in the visual cortical areas, as well as in the occipitotemporal sulcus [87]. Functional neuroimaging may be beneficial in localizing a specific target for stimulation and may prevent wasting time and money on targets which are not as likely to be involved in the pathogenesis.

## 4. Discussion

It has to be highlighted that a limitation of the study might be represented by the search method: in fact, we decided to limit the literature search to the DSM terminology in order to exclude simple "flashback phenomena" that are commonly reported in psychopathology, and that may not follow the use of hallucinogens. This could have narrowed the results, preventing the inclusion of other studies using the ICD terminology, which is less "technical" about the issue.

The main consideration that has to be done with respect to HPPD is its rare and unpredictable nature [16]: current prevalence estimates are unknown, but DSM-5 suggests 4.2% [88]. The condition is more often diagnosed in individuals with a history of previous psychological issues or substance misuse [56], but it can arise in anyone, even after a single exposure (mostly to LSD, but it has also been reported after use of other psychedelics) [89]. In many cases, HPPD may also be explained in terms of a heightened awareness of and concern about ordinary visual phenomena, which is supported by the high rates of anxiety, obsessive-compulsive disorder, hypochondria, and paranoia seen in many patients [90].

The crucial movement towards a comprehensive clinical understanding of Hallucinogen Persisting Perception Spectrum Disorders (HPPSD) [23] is the establishment of an accepted operative nomenclature. This wide spectrum of disorders encompasses different subtypes, ranging from HPPD I to HPPD II, according to our hypothetical distinction. Among the innumerable triggers able to precipitate HPPD, prospectively, the use of natural and synthetic cannabinoids appears to be the most frequent. This is consistent with the rapid and vast diffusion of these novel psychoactive compounds, nowadays easily available without specific cultural filters and references [91,92]. Distinct substances, with completely different mechanisms of action, might lead or precipitate the genesis of HPPD, therefore suggesting a multifaceted etiology. Thus, it is accordingly conceivable that different medications could be useful and helpful in the treatment of different subtypes of HPPD. Tracers and trailing phenomena appear to be the most resistant symptoms. Concomitant coexisting psychiatric disorders can represent a further clinical challenge, with the clinical construct of the lysergic psychoma as a possible heuristic model. According to this theory, the presence of induced psychopathological phenomena (the Psychoma) may trigger a specific reaction excepted by the not-affected part of the mind, trying to counteract the psychoma, which is perceived as a "foreign body in the mind". Of course, when the psychoma is strong and repeated in its nature, the possibility to determine a full-blown psychosis may become more concrete [93,94].

Regarding treatment options, a combination of medications may be needed according to the preceding or subsequent psychopathology. Given the limited literature about HPPD, a possible hypothesis about the pharmacotherapy of choice in relation to different etiologies has not been considered. However, the presence of psychiatric and neurological comorbidities could represent a valid criterion to address the choice. Clinical experience and an extensive and comprehensive knowledge of these phenomena are vital for successful treatment outcomes.

Controlled clinical investigations are mostly needed in order to better understand the etiology, mechanisms of action, clinical issues, and pharmacological treatment options for Hallucinogen Persisting Perception Spectrum Disorders (HPPSD).

**Author Contributions:** "G.M. and A.G.L. conceived, designed, and coordinated the review; R.S. and M.d.G. wrote the introduction and the discussion; M.C.S. and M.L. performed the database research; C.M. wrote the clinical sections; M.P. wrote the pharmacological sections.

## References


1. Abraham, H.D.; Aldridge, A.M.; Gogia, P. The psychopharmacology of hallucinogens. *Neuropsychopharmacology* **1996**, *14*, 285–298. [CrossRef]
2. Garcia-Romeu, A.; Kersgaard, B.; Addy, P.H. Clinical Applications of Hallucinogens: A Review. *Exp. Clin. Psychopharmacol.* **2016**, *24*, 229–268. [CrossRef] [PubMed]
3. Caton, C.L.M.; Drake, R.E.; Hasin, D.S.; Dominguez, B.; Shrout, P.E.; Samet, S.; Schanzer, W.B. Differences Between Early-Phase Primary Psychotic Disorders with Concurrent Substance Use and Substance-Induced Psychoses. *Arch. Gen. Psychiatry* **2005**, *62*, 137–145. [CrossRef] [PubMed]
4. Abraham, H.D.; Aldridge, A.M. Adverse consequences of lysergic acid diethylamide. *Addiction* **1993**, *88*, 1327–1334. [CrossRef] [PubMed]
5. Inaba, D.S.; Cohen, W.E.; Holstein, M.E. Uppers owners, all arounders. In *Physical and Mental Effects of Psychoactive Drugs*, 3rd ed.; CNS Publications, Inc.: Ashland, OR, USA, 1997.
6. U.S. Department of Health and Human Services, Substance Abuse and Mental Health Services Administration. Results from the 2012 National Survey on Drug Use and Health: Summary of National Findings. Available online: https://www.samhsa.gov/data/sites/default/files/NSDUHresults2012/NSDUHresults2012.pdf (accessed on 1 September 2017).
7. Schifano, F.; Orsolini, L.; Duccio Papanti, G.; Corkery, J.M. Novel psychoactive substances of interest for psychiatry. *World Psychiatry* **2015**, *14*, 15–26. [CrossRef] [PubMed]
8. Martinotti, G.; Lupi, M.; Carlucci, L.; Cinosi, E.; Santacroce, R.; Acciavatti, T.; Chillemi, E.; Bonifaci, L.; Janiri, L.; di Giannantonio, M. Novel psychoactive substances: Use and knowledge among adolescents and young adults in urban and rural areas. *Hum. Psychopharmacol.* **2015**, *30*, 295–301. [CrossRef] [PubMed]
9. Schifano, F.; Deluca, P.; Agosti, L.; Martinotti, G.; Corkery, J.M.; Alex, B.; Caterina, B.; Heikki, B.; Raffaella, B.; Anna, C.; et al. Psychonaut 2002 Research Group. New trends in the cyber and street market of recreational drugs? The case of 2C-T-7 ('Blue Mystic'). *J. Psychopharmacol.* **2005**, *19*, 675–679. [CrossRef] [PubMed]
10. Cinosi, E.; Corazza, O.; Santacroce, R.; Lupi, M.; Acciavatti, T.; Martinotti, G.; di Giannantonio, M. New drugs on the Internet: The case of Camfetamine. *BioMed Res. Int.* **2014**, *2014*, 419026. [CrossRef] [PubMed]
11. Corazza, O.; Valeriani, G.; Bersani, F.S.; Corkery, J.; Martinotti, G.; Bersani, G.; Schifano, F. "Spice", "kryptonite", "black mamba": An overview of brand names and marketing strategies of novel psychoactive substances on the web. *J. Psychoact. Drugs* **2014**, *46*, 287–294. [CrossRef] [PubMed]
12. Orsolini, L.; Francesconi, G.; Papanti, D.; Giorgetti, A.; Schifano, F. Profiling online recreational/prescription drugs' customers and overview of drug vending virtual marketplaces. *Hum. Psychopharmacol.* **2015**, *30*, 302–318. [CrossRef] [PubMed]

13. Bersani, F.S.; Corazza, O.; Albano, G.; Valeriani, G.; Santacroce, R.; Bolzan Mariotti Posocco, F.; Cinosi, E.; Simonato, P.; Martinotti, G.; Bersani, G.; et al. 25C-NBOMe: Preliminary data on pharmacology, psychoactive effects, and toxicity of a new potent and dangerous hallucinogenic drug. *BioMed Res. Int.* **2014**, *2014*, 734749. [CrossRef] [PubMed]
14. Martinotti, G.; Lupi, M.; Acciavatti, T.; Cinosi, E.; Santacroce, R.; Signorelli, M.S.; Bandini, L.; Lisi, G.; Quattrone, D.; Ciambrone, P.; et al. Novel psychoactive substances in young adults with and without psychiatric comorbidities. *BioMed Res. Int.* **2014**, *2014*, 815424. [CrossRef] [PubMed]
15. Hofmann, A. *LSD: My Problem Child*; McGraw-Hill: New York, NY, USA, 1980.
16. Halpern, J.H.; Pope, H.G. Hallucinogen persisting perception disorder: What do we know after 50 years? *Drug Alcohol Depend.* **2003**, *69*, 109–119. [CrossRef]
17. Lerner, A.G.; Gelkopf, M.; Skladman, I.; Oyffe, I. Flashback and hallucinogen persisting perception disorder: Clinical aspects and pharmacological treatment approach. *Isr. J. Psychiatry Relat. Sci.* **2002**, *39*, 92–99. [PubMed]
18. Lerner, A.G.; Rudinski, D.; Bor, O.; Goodman, C. Flashbacks and HPPD: A clinical-oriented concise review. *Isr. J. Psychiatry Relat. Sci.* **2014**, *51*, 296–302.
19. Lerner, A.G.; Goodman, C.; Rudinski, D.; Lev-Ran, S. LSD flashbacks—The appearance of new visual imagery not experienced during initial intoxication: Two case reports. *Isr. J. Psychiatry Relat. Sci.* **2014**, *51*, 307–309.
20. Lerner, A.G.; Shufman, E.; Kodesh, A.; Kretzmer, G.; Sigal, M. LSD-induced hallucinogen persisting perception disorder with depressive features treatment with reboxetine. *Isr. J. Psychiatry Relat. Sci.* **2002**, *39*, 100–103. [PubMed]
21. Espiard, M.L.; Lecardeur, L.; Abadie, P.; Halbecq, I.; Dollfus, S. Hallucinogen persisting perception disorder after psilocybin consumption: A case study. *Eur. Psychiatry* **2005**, *20*, 458–460. [CrossRef] [PubMed]
22. Michelot, D.; Melendez-Howell, L.M. Amanita Muscaria: Chemistry, Biology, Toxicology, and Ethnomycology. *Mycol. Res.* **2003**, *107*, 131–146. [CrossRef] [PubMed]
23. Lerner, A.G. Flashbacks and Hppd (Hallucinogenic Persisting Perception Disorder): Clinical Aspects and Pharmacological Treatment. In Proceedings of the First World Congress of the World Association on Dual Disorders, Madrid, Spain, 23–26 March 2017.
24. Vroegop, M.P.; Dongen, R.T.; Vantroyen, B.; Kramers, C. Ketamine as a party drug. *Ned. Tijdschr. Geneeskd.* **2007**, *151*, 2039–2042. [PubMed]
25. Ziaae, V.; Akbari, H.E.; Hosmand, A.; Amini, H.; Kebriaeizadeh, A.; Saman, K. Side effects of dextromethorphan abuse: A case series. *Addict. Behav.* **2005**, *30*, 1607–1613. [CrossRef] [PubMed]
26. Litjens, R.P.; Brunt, T.M.; Alderliefste, G.J.; Westerink, R.H. Hallucinogen persisting perception disorder and the serotonergic system: A comprehensive review including new MDMA-related clinical cases. *Eur. Neuropsychopharmacol.* **2014**, *24*, 1309–1323. [CrossRef] [PubMed]
27. Lerner, A.G.; Rudinski, D.; Bleich, A. Benign and time-limited visual disturbances (Flashbacks) in recent abstinent high-potency heavy smokers. *Isr. J. Psychiatry Relat. Sci.* **2011**, *48*, 25–29. [PubMed]
28. Schwitzer, T.; Schwan, R.; Angioi-Duprez, K.; Ingster-Moati, I.; Lalanne, L.; Giersch, A.; Laprevote, V. The cannabinoid system and visual processing: Are view on experimental findings and clinical presumptions. *Eur. Neuropsychopharmacol.* **2015**, *25*, 100–112. [CrossRef] [PubMed]
29. Zobor, D.; Strasser, T.; Zobor, G.; Schober, F.; Messias, A.; Strauss, O.; Batra, A.; Zrenner, E. Ophthalmological assessment of cannabis-induced persisting perception disorder: Is there a direct retinal effect? *Doc. Ophthalmol.* **2015**, *130*, 121–130. [CrossRef] [PubMed]
30. Ellison-Wright, Z.; Sessa, B. A persisting perception disorder after cannabis use. *Prog. Neurol. Psychiatry* **2015**, *9*, 10–13. [CrossRef]
31. Martinotti, G.; Orsolini, L.; Fornaro, M.; Vecchiotti, R.; De Berardis, D.; Iasevoli, F.; Torrens, M.; di Giannantonio, M. Aripiprazole for relapse prevention and craving in alcohol use disorder: Current evidence and future perspectives. *Expert Opin. Investig. Drugs* **2017**, *25*, 719–728. [CrossRef] [PubMed]
32. Santacroce, R.; Corazza, O.; Martinotti, G.; Bersani, F.S.; Valeriani, G.; di Giannantonio, M. Psyclones: A roller coaster of life? Hidden synthetic cannabinoids and stimulants in apparently harmless products. *Hum. Psychopharmacol.* **2015**, *30*, 265–267. [CrossRef] [PubMed]

33. Orsolini, L.; Papanti, G.D.; De Berardis, D.; Guirguis, A.; Corkery, J.M.; Schifano, F. The "Endless Trip" among the NPS Users: Psychopathology and Psychopharmacology in the Hallucinogen-Persisting Perception Disorder. A Systematic Review. *Front. Psychiatry* **2017**, *8*, 240. [CrossRef] [PubMed]
34. Abraham, H.D.; Duffy, F.H. Stable qEEG differences in post-LSD visual disorder by split half analyses: Evidence for disinhibition. *Psychiatry Res. Neuroimaging* **1996**, *67*, 173–187. [CrossRef]
35. Abraham, H.D.; Duffy, F.H. EEG coherence in post-LSD visual hallucinations. *Psychiatry Res. Neuroimaging* **2001**, *107*, 151–163. [CrossRef]
36. Garrat, J.; Alreja, M.; Aghajanian, G.K. LSD has high efficacy relative to serotonin in enhancing the cationic current ih: Intracellular studies in rat facial motorneurons. *Synapse* **1993**, *13*, 123–134. [CrossRef] [PubMed]
37. Young, C.R. Sertraline treatment of hallucinogen persisting perception disorder. *J. Clin. Psychiatry* **1997**, *58*, 85. [CrossRef] [PubMed]
38. Sander-Bush, E.; Burris, K.D.; Knoth, K. Lysergic acid diethylamide and 2,5-dimethoxy-4-methylamphetamine are partial agonists at serotonin eceptors linked to phosphoinositide hydrolysis. *J. Pharmacol. Exp. Ther.* **1988**, *246*, 924–928.
39. Stahl, S.M. *Stahl's Essential Psychopharmacology*, 1st ed.; Cambridge University Press: New York, NY, USA, 1996.
40. Halpern, J.H.; Lerner, A.G.; Passie, T. A Review of Hallucinogen Persisting Perception Disorder (HPPD) and an Exploratory Study of Subjects Claiming Symptoms of HPPD. In *Current Topics in Behavioral Neurosciences*; Springer: Berlin/Heidelberg, Germany, 2016; pp. 1–28.
41. Guillery, R.; Sherman, S.M. Thalamic relay functions and their role in corticocortical communication: Generalizations from the visual system. *Neuron* **2002**, *33*, 163–175. [CrossRef]
42. Cudeiro, J.; Sillito, A.M. Looking back: Corticothalamic feedback and early visual processing. *Trends Neurosci.* **2006**, *29*, 298–306. [CrossRef] [PubMed]
43. Xu, X.; Ichida, J.M.; Allison, J.D.; Boyd, J.D.; Bonds, A.B.; Casagrande, V.A. A comparison of koniocellular, magnocellular and parvocellular receptive field pro perties in the lateral geniculate nucleus of the owl monkey (*Aotus trivirgatus*). *J. Physiol.* **2001**, *531*, 203–218. [CrossRef] [PubMed]
44. Schankin, C.J.; Maniyar, F.H.; Sprenger, T.; Chou, D.E.; Eller, M.; Goadsby, P.J. The Relation between Migraine, Typical Migraine Aura and "Visual Snow". *Headache J. Head Face Pain* **2014**, *54*, 957–966. [CrossRef] [PubMed]
45. Holland, D.; Passie, T. *Flashback-Phaenomene als Nachwirkung von Halluzinogeneinnahme*; VWB-Verlag: Berlin, Germany, 2011.
46. Gaillard, M.C.; Borruat, F.X. Persisting visual hallucinations and illusions in previously drug-addicted patients. *Klin. Monbl. Augenheilkd.* **2003**, *220*, 176–178. [CrossRef] [PubMed]
47. Lerner, A.G.; Goodman, C.; Bor, O.; Lev-Ran, S. Synthetic Cannabis Substances (SPS) Use and Hallucinogen Persisting Perception Disorder (HPPD): Two Case Reports. *Isr. J. Psychiatry Relat. Sci.* **2014**, *51*, 277–280.
48. Anderson, L.; Lake, H.; Walterfang, M. The trip of a lifetime: Hallucinogen persisting perceptual disorder. *Australas. Psychiatry* **2017**, *26*, 11–12. [CrossRef] [PubMed]
49. Brodrick, J.; Mitchell, B.G. Hallucinogen Persisting Perception Disorder and Risk of Suicide. *J. Pharm. Pract.* **2016**, *29*, 431–434. [CrossRef] [PubMed]
50. Coppola, M.; Mondola, R. JWH-122 Consumption Adverse Effects: A Case of Hallucinogen Persisting Perception Disorder Five-Year Follow-Up. *J. Psychoact. Drugs* **2017**, *49*, 262–265. [CrossRef] [PubMed]
51. Lerner, A.G.; Gelkopf, M.; Skaldman, I.; Rudinski, D.; Nachshon, H.; Bleich, A. Clonazepam treatment of LSD-induced hallucination persisting perception disorder with anxiety features. *Int. Clin. Psychopharmacol.* **2003**, *18*, 101–105. [CrossRef] [PubMed]
52. Lerner, A.G.; Gelkopf, M.; Oyffe, I.; Finkel, B.; Katz, S.; Sigal, M.; Weizman, A. LSD-induced hallucinogen persisting perception disorder (HPPD) treatment with clonidine: An open pilot study. *Int. Clin. Psychopharmacol.* **2000**, *18*, 35–37. [CrossRef]
53. Lev-Ran, S.; Feingold, D.; Goodman, C.; Lerner, A.G. Comparing triggers to visual disturbances among individuals with positive vs. negative experiences of hallucinogen-persisting perception disorder (HPPD) following LSD use. *Am. J. Addict.* **2017**, *26*, 568–571. [CrossRef] [PubMed]
54. Hermle, L.; Simon, M.; Ruchsow, M.; Geppert, M. Hallucinogen Persisting Perception Disorder. *Ther. Adv. Psychopharmacol.* **2012**, *2*, 199–205. [CrossRef] [PubMed]
55. Lerner, A.G.; Lev-Ran, S. LSD-associated "Alice in Wonderland Syndrome" (AIWS): A Hallucinogen Persisting Perception Disorder (HPPD) case report. *Isr. J. Psychiatry Relat. Sci.* **2015**, *52*, 67–69.

56. Baggott, M.J.; Coyle, J.R.; Erowid, E.; Erowid, F.; Robertson, L.C. Abnormal visual experiences in individuals with histories of hallucinogen use: A web-based questionnaire. *Drug Alcohol Depend.* **2011**, *114*, 61–67. [CrossRef] [PubMed]
57. Lev-Ran, S.; Feingold, D.; Rudinski, D.; Katz, S.; Arturo, L.G. Schizophrenia and hallucinogen persisting perception disorder: A clinical investigation. *Am. J. Addict.* **2015**, *24*, 197–199. [CrossRef] [PubMed]
58. Lev-Ran, S.; Feingold, D.; Frenkel, A.; Lerner, A.G. Clinical characteristics of individuals suffering from schizophrenia and Hallucinogen Persisting Perceptual Disorders: A preliminary investigation. *J. Dual Diagn.* **2014**, *10*, 79–83. [CrossRef] [PubMed]
59. Lerner, A.G.; Oyffe, I.; Isaacs, G.; Sigal, M. Naltrexone treatment of hallucinogen persisting perception disorder. *Am. J. Psychiatry* **1997**, *154*, 437. [PubMed]
60. Lauterbach, E.C.; Abdelhamid, A.; Annandale, J.B. Posthallucinogen-like visual illusions (palinopsia) with risperidone in a patient without previous hallucinogen exposure: Possible relation to serotonin 5HT2a receptor blockade. *Pharmacopsychiatry* **2000**, *33*, 38–41. [CrossRef] [PubMed]
61. Goodman, C.; Bor, O.; Lev-Ran, S. Synthetic Cannabis Substances (SPS) Use and Hallucinogen Persisting Perception Disorder (HPPD): Two case reports. *Isr. J. Psychiatry Relat. Sci.* **2014**, *51*, 277–280.
62. Pettorruso, M.; De Risio, L.; Di Nicola, M.; Martinotti, G.; Conte, G.; Janiri, L. Allostasis as a Conceptual Framework Linking Bipolar Disorder and Addiction. *Front. Psychiatry* **2014**, *5*, 173. [CrossRef] [PubMed]
63. Kemph, J.P.; DeVane, L.; Levin, G.M.; Jarecke, R.; Miller, R. Treatment of aggressive children with clonidine: Results of an open pilot study. *J. Am. Acad. Child Adolesc. Psychiary* **1993**, *32*, 577–581. [CrossRef] [PubMed]
64. Kolb, L.; Burris, B.C.; Griffitshs, S. *Propanolol and Clonidine in the Treatment of Post Traumatic Disorders of War*; van der Kolk, B.A., Ed.; Post Traumatic Stress Disorder: Psychological and Biological Sequelae; American Psychiatric Press: Washington, DC, USA, 1984.
65. Gerra, G.; Zaimovic, A.; Giusti, F.; Di Gennaro, C.; Zambelli, U.; Gardini, S.; Delsignore, R. Lofexidine versus clonidine in rapid opiate detoxification. *J. Subst. Abuse Treat.* **2001**, *21*, 11–17. [CrossRef]
66. Keaney, F.; Strang, J.; Gossop, M.; Marshall, E.J.; Farrell, M.; Welch, S.; Hahn, B.; Gonzalez, A. A double-blind randomized placebo-controlled trial of lofexidine in alcohol withdrawal: Lofexidine is not a useful adjunct to chlordiazepoxide. *Alcohol Alcohol.* **2001**, *36*, 426–430. [CrossRef] [PubMed]
67. Lerner, A.G.; Skladman, I.; Kodesh, A.; Sigal, M.; Shufman, E. LSD-induced Hallucinogen Persisting Perception Disorder treated with clonazepam: Two case reports. *Isr. J. Psychiatry Relat. Sci.* **2001**, *38*, 133–136. [PubMed]
68. Noushad, F.; Al Hillawi, Q.; Siram, V.; Arif, M. 25 years of Hallucinogen Persisting Perception Disorder—A diagnostic challenge. *Br. J. Med. Pract.* **2015**, *8*, a805.
69. Moskowitz, D. Use of haloperidol to reduce LSD flashbacks. *Milit. Med.* **1971**, *136*, 754–756.
70. Anderson, W.; O'Malley, J. Trifluoperazine for the trailing phenomena. *JAMA* **1972**, *220*, 1244–1245. [PubMed]
71. Abraham, H.D.; Mamen, A. LSD-like panic from risperidone in post-LSD visual disorder. *J. Clin. Psychopharmacol.* **1996**, *16*, 238–241. [CrossRef] [PubMed]
72. Morehead, D.B. Exacerbation of hallucinogen-persisting perception disorder with risperidone. *J. Clin. Psychopharmacol.* **1997**, *17*, 327–328. [CrossRef] [PubMed]
73. Alcantara, A.G. Is there a role of alpha 2 antagonism in the exacerbation of HPPD with risperidone? *J. Clin. Psychopharmacol.* **1998**, *18*, 487–488. [CrossRef] [PubMed]
74. Martinotti, G.; Pettorruso, M.; De Berardis, D.; Varasano, P.A.; Lucidi Pressanti, G.; De Remigis, V.; Valchera, A.; Ricci, V.; Di Nicola, M.; Janiri, L.; et al. Agomelatine Increases BDNF Serum Levels in Depressed Patients in Correlation with the Improvement of Depressive Symptoms. *Int. J. Neuropsychopharmacol.* **2016**, *19*, 149–156. [CrossRef] [PubMed]
75. Thurlow, H.J.; Girvin, J.P. Use of antiepileptic medication in treating flashbacks from hallucinogenic drugs. *Can. Med. Assoc.* **1971**, *105*, 947–948.
76. Aicardi, J. *Epilepsy: A Comprehensive Textbook*, 2nd ed.; Wolters Kluwer Health/Lippincott Williams & Wilkins: Philadelphia, PA, USA, 2008.
77. Martinotti, G.; Di Nicola, M.; Romanelli, R.; Andreoli, S.; Pozzi, G.; Moroni, N.; Janiri, L. High and low dosage oxcarbazepine versus naltrexone for the prevention of relapse in alcohol-dependent patients. *Hum. Psychopharmacol.* **2007**, *22*, 149–156. [CrossRef] [PubMed]
78. Martinotti, G. Pregabalin in clinical psychiatry and addiction: Pros and cons. *Expert Opin. Investig. Drugs* **2012**, *21*, 1243–1245. [CrossRef] [PubMed]

79. Martinotti, G.; Di Nicola, M.; De Vita, O.; Hatzigiakoumis, D.S.; Guglielmo, R.; Santucci, B.; Aliotta, F.; Romanelli, R.; Verrastro, V.; Petruccelli, F.; et al. Low-dose topiramate in alcohol dependence: A single-blind, placebo-controlled study. *J. Clin. Psychopharmacol.* **2014**, *34*, 709–715. [CrossRef] [PubMed]
80. Casa, B.; Bosio, A. 1589 Levetiracetam efficacy in hallucinogen persisting perception disorders: A prospective study. *J. Neurol. Sci.* **2005**, *238*, S504.
81. Markel, H.; Lee, A.; Holmes, R.D.; Domino, E.F. LSD flashback syndrome exacerbated by selective serotonin reuptake inhibitor antidepressants in adolescents. *J. Pediatr.* **1994**, *125*, 817–819. [CrossRef]
82. Spagnolo, P.A.; Goldman, D. Neuromodulation interventions for addictive disorders: Challenges, promise, and roadmap for future research. *Brain* **2017**, *140*, 1183–1203. [CrossRef] [PubMed]
83. Moccia, L.; Pettorruso, M.; De Crescenzo, F.; De Risio, L.; di Nuzzo, L.; Martinotti, G.; Bifone, A.; Janiri, L.; Di Nicola, M. Neural correlates of cognitive control in gambling disorder: A systematic review of fMRI studies. *Neurosci. Biobehav. Rev.* **2017**, *78*, 104–116. [CrossRef] [PubMed]
84. Ghanbari, J.A.; Naji, B.; Nasr, E.M. Repetitive Transcranial Magnetic Stimulation in Resistant Visual Hallucinations in a Woman with Schizophrenia: A Case Report. *Ira. J. Psychiatry Behav. Sci.* **2016**, *10*, e3561. [CrossRef] [PubMed]
85. Merabet, L.B.; Kobayashi, M.; Barton, J.; Pascual-Leone, A. Suppression of complex visual hallucinatory experiences by occipital transcranial magnetic stimulation: A case report. *Neurocase* **2003**, *9*, 436–440. [CrossRef] [PubMed]
86. Kilpatrick, Z.P.; Bard Ermentrout, G. Hallucinogen persisting perception disorder in neuronal networks with adaptation. *J. Comput. Neurosci.* **2012**, *32*, 25–53. [CrossRef] [PubMed]
87. Jardri, R.; Pins, D.; Bubrovszky, M.; Lucas, B.; Lethuc, V.; Delmaire, C.; Vantyghem, V.; Despretz, P.; Thomas, P. Neural functional organization of hallucinations in schizophrenia: Multisensory dissolution of pathological emergence in consciousness. *Conscious. Cogn.* **2009**, *18*, 449–457. [CrossRef] [PubMed]
88. American Psychiatric Association. *Diagnostic and Statistical Manual of Mental Disorders*, 5th ed.; American Psychiatric Publishing: Arlington, VA, USA, 2013.
89. National Institute on Drug Abuse (NIDA). How do Hallucinogens (LSD and Psilocybin) Affect the Brain and Body? Available online: http://www.drugabuse.gov/publications/research-reports/hallucinogens-dissociative-drugs/where-can-i-get-more-scientific-information-hallucinogens-diss (accessed on 4 September 2017).
90. Abdulrahim, D.; Bowden-Jones, O.; NEPTUNE Expert Group. *Guidance on the Management of Acute and Chronic Harms of Club Drugs and Novel Psychoactive Substances*; Novel Psychoactive Treatment UK Network (NEPTUNE): London, UK, 2015.
91. Schifano, F.; Leoni, M.; Martinotti, G.; Rawaf, S.; Rovetto, F. Importance of cyberspace for the assessment of the drug abuse market: Preliminary results from the Psychonaut 2002 project. *Cyberpsychol. Behav.* **2003**, *6*, 405–410. [CrossRef] [PubMed]
92. Cinosi, E.; Martinotti, G.; Simonato, P.; Singh, D.; Demetrovics, Z.; Roman-Urrestarazu, A.; Bersani, F.S.; Vicknasingam, B.; Piazzon, G.; Li, J.H.; et al. Following "the Roots" of Kratom (*Mitragyna speciosa*): The Evolution of an Enhancer from a Traditional Use to Increase Work and Productivity in Southeast Asia to a Recreational Psychoactive Drug in Western Countries. *BioMed Res. Int.* **2015**, *2015*, 968786. [CrossRef] [PubMed]
93. Martinotti, G.; Di Nicola, M.; Quattrone, D.; Santacroce, R.; Schifano, F.; Murray, R.; di Giannantonio, M. Novel psychoactive substances and induced phenomena in psychopathology: The lysergic psychoma. *J. Psychopathol.* **2015**, *21*, 400–405.
94. Martinotti, G.; Ferro, F. The exogenous model of induced psychotic experience in addiction. *Res. Adv. Psychiatry* **2015**, *2*, 81–82.

# 9

# Sales and Advertising Channels of New Psychoactive Substances (NPS): Internet, Social Networks and Smartphone Apps

**Cristina Miliano [1], Giulia Margiani [1], Liana Fattore [2] and Maria Antonietta De Luca [1,*]**

1 Department of Biomedical Sciences, University of Cagliari, Cittadella Universitaria di Monserrato-SP 8, Km 0.700, 09042 Monserrato, Cagliari, Italy; cristinamiliano@hotmail.it (C.M.); giulia.margiani35@gmail.com (G.M.)

2 CNR Institute of Neuroscience-Cagliari, National Research Council, Cittadella Universitaria di Monserrato-SP 8, Km 0.700, 09042 Monserrato, Cagliari, Italy; lfattore@in.cnr.it

* Correspondence: deluca@unica.it

**Abstract:** In the last decade, the trend of drug consumption has completely changed, and several new psychoactive substances (NPS) have appeared on the drug market as legal alternatives to common drugs of abuse. Designed to reproduce the effects of illegal substances like cannabis, ecstasy, cocaine, or ketamine, NPS are only in part controlled by UN conventions and represent an emerging threat to global public health. The effects of NPS greatly differ from drug to drug and relatively scarce information is available at present about their pharmacology and potential toxic effects. Yet, compared to more traditional drugs, more dangerous short- and long-term effects have been associated with their use, and hospitalizations and fatal intoxications have also been reported after NPS use. In the era of cyberculture, the Internet acts as an ideal platform to promote and market these compounds, leading to a global phenomenon. Hidden by several aliases, these substances are sold across the web, and information about consumption is shared by online communities through drug fora, YouTube channels, social networks, and smartphone applications (apps). This review intends to provide an overview and analysis of social media that contribute to the popularity of NPS especially among young people. The possibility of using the same channels responsible for their growing diffusion to make users aware of the risks associated with NPS use is proposed.

**Keywords:** psychoactive drug marketing; sales channels; Internet; social networks; YouTube; Facebook; Twitter; Instagram

---

## 1. Introduction

In the last 10 years, an increasing number of new psychoactive substances (NPS) has flooded the drug market. NPS are drugs of misuse not included in the International United Nations Conventions, which can easily bypass the supply reduction strategies of law enforcement agencies and sanctions related to the use and sale of illicit substances. The advent of NPS has contributed to the appearance and growth of a new "drug scenario" characterized by an increased number of drug users among young people and the consumption of drugs with unknown effects or safety profiles. At the initial stage of the phenomenon, NPS are typically used by a small group of people. After the use of these substances becomes well-known, their widespread marketing through media and Internet sales begins. This sequence of events causes the beginning of an epidemic diffusion that is eventually prevented by law enforcement agencies that perform important actions and fight against the trafficking and sale of NPS. Unfortunately, the subsequent legal control of these substances only initiates the reformulation of NPS, which induces a typical loop that is highly dangerous to public health. In order to understand the full spectrum of the complex issue of NPS, we provide here an updated overview of the specific field of sales and advertising channels of NPS that represent an important ring in this chain of events.

## 2. The Complex Issue of the New Psychoactive Substances (NPS)

NPS are synthetic compounds that are very popular worldwide, as shown by the alarming number of NPS (779) reported between 2008 and 2017 by 111 countries and territories [1–4]. Designed in order to substitute classical drugs of abuse with legal surrogates, their expansion leads to an endless effort made by governments and law enforcement agencies to try to contain this phenomenon. A mix of features makes them very attractive, including the difficulty to detect them in human fluid samples by standard drug screening test, their ambiguous legal status, and, as in the case of synthetic cannabinoids, the perceived low risk despite their toxic effects and abuse liability [5,6]. Noteworthy, the exponential increase in the market size of these compounds has been facilitated by the World Wide Web (WWW), where information about their purchase and use are shared, advertised, and spread to everyone. In light of the changing scenario for drug marketing and advertising, the aim of this review is to analyze the role of the web in this emerging trend, focusing on social networks and smartphone applications (apps).

In the current world where communication is based on the Internet and social networks, online sites operate on both the surface and deep web [7–10] to supply NPS labeled as "not for human consumption" and sold as plant fertilizers, incense, bath salts, or with other aliases in order to avoid legislative controls [11]. The dark net plays a key role in this "super safe drug dealing", which buyers and sellers can access anonymously to provide drugs and pay for them with a virtual wallet [2]. Essentially, a few clicks are enough to supply highly psychoactive substances, cheaply and in a low-risk way [12,13], even through smartphone apps [14,15]. Therefore, NPS can be sold to everyone, including very young people, in complete anonymity and easily avoiding law enforcement [10,16,17]. Along with the emergence of new psychoactive drugs in the world drug market, new concepts are emerging to better describe this new, global phenomenon and its associated health consequences. That is, the term "spiceophrenia" has been proposed by Papanti and collaborators [18] to describe the psychotic symptoms (e.g., hallucinations, delusions) that likely occur in chronic users of synthetic cannabinoids. It has been reported that the use of Spice/K2 drugs may exacerbate psychotic symptoms in vulnerable individuals or trigger psychosis in individuals with no previous history of psychosis [19]. The synthetic cannabinoids present in these products may also induce important adverse neuropsychiatric consequences, including acute and lasting psychosis, since their pro-psychotic effects are likely related to the activity of the $CB_1$-receptor on dopaminergic, serotoninergic, and glutamatergic pathways [20].

Similarly, within the e-health context, the term "e-addictology" has been recently used to indicate new technologies for assessing pathological dependencies and intervening on addictive behaviors, including computerized adaptive testing, e-health programs, web-based interventions, and digital phenotyping [21]. Importantly, new technologies can profoundly change not only the way illegal drugs are supplied, but they can also improve our understanding of drug addiction and favor the development of new interventions for addictive disorders [21].

Because not everyone has the finances or the technical skills to create or manage an Internet site, Facebook is often used as an alternative channel for sales and for advertising the use of these kinds of products [8]. On several drug fora, such as www.drugs-forum.com or www.erowid.org, these compounds are promoted and their subjective effects are discussed [9], but drug-related contents also exist on virtually all social networking sites, picture- and video-sharing services, and drug-dedicated apps. Drug selling through social media has also been reported, often using drug slang and jargon [22]. The changing policy on marijuana use in some states in North America, i.e., legalization of medical cannabis, led to an increased rate of cannabis use both in young people and adults [23,24] even though the causal effect of legalization has not been firmly assessed [25]. On the other hand, for young people, is it difficult to recognize the risk of marijuana consumption if the law allows its use for medical purposes, and this might represents a "gateway of curiosity" [26].

### 3. The Deep Web and the Surface Web: Market Resilience

By typing a keyword in a search engine query such as Google, Bing, Yahoo, or others, web surfers can obtain a list of results belonging to the "surface web", while other, nonsearchable contents are referred to as the "deep web" or "invisible web" (see Figure 1). The deep web is often confused with the "dark net", but the two terms are not synonymous and overlap only partially. Basically, the deep web contains all the information stored online which is not indexed by search engines, with most information hidden simply because it is irrelevant for most users. Access to the deep web does not require special tools and a visitor can use specialized search engines or directories to locate the data for which he or she is looking. The dark web, instead, represents a small part of the deep web containing information hidden on purpose, and it typically requires special tools to enter. Like the surface web, the dark web is scattered among servers around the world and represents the portion of the Internet most frequently known for illicit activities. The most common way to access it is through The Onion Router (TOR) and the Invisible Internet Project (I2P).

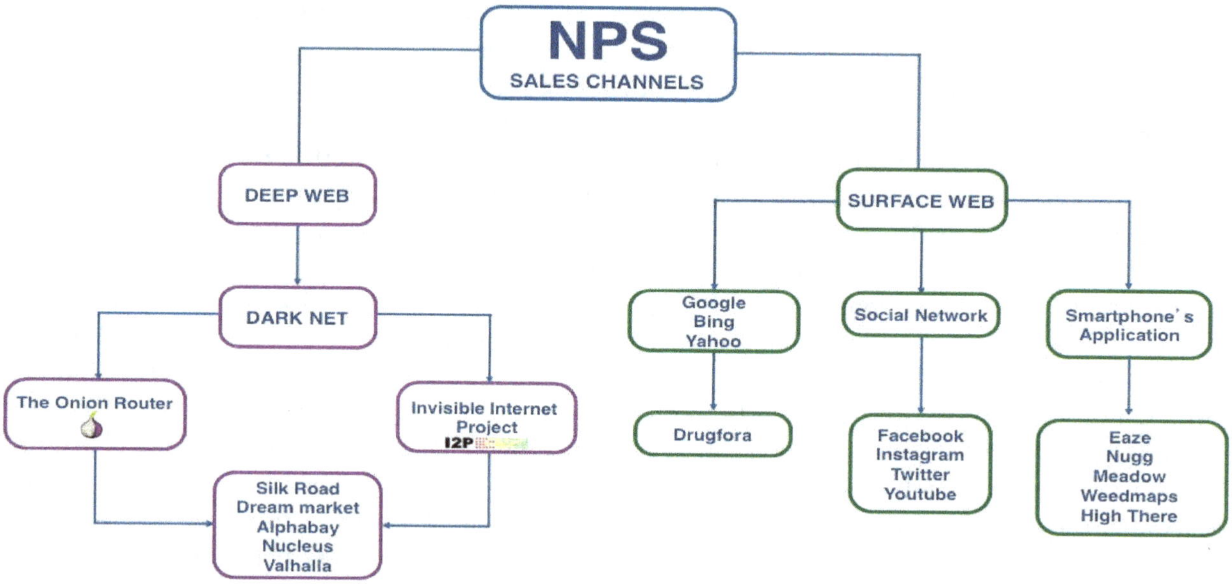


**Figure 1.** NPS marketing, advertising, and communication network.

Developed in 2010 by the U.S. Army, the TOR browser is able to encrypt a user's IP address [27], thus making all the operations untraceable. In this way, the anonymous identities of administrators, sellers, and customers are protected [28–31] and the safe payment of any illicit good is guaranteed by of the use of cryptocurrencies, mainly bitcoins and litecoins, i.e., virtual money not controlled by government [32]. The peer-to-peer software I2P, instead, was created in 2003 purposely for illegal activities [31] in order to provide anonymous access and to bypass police and law enforcement surveillance. I2P uses a ".i2p" domain, different from TOR's classic Internet domain (WWW), to allow users to host services by I2P's homepage. The anonymous status in the web is also maintained by encryption of e-mails, files, and messages using different cryptosystems such as Pretty Good Privacy (PGP), the Amnesiac Incognito Live System, and the Tails [33].

Recently, online drug dealing has started replacing the old way of supplying drugs of abuse. Surfing in both the surface and deep web, it is possible to buy traditional illicit drugs but also temporarily legal NPS [1].

In this hidden world, the most famous platform is the Silk Road hub. Born but shutdown by the Federal Bureau of Investigation (FBI) in October 2013, it impressively reappeared after a month under the name Silk Road 2.0 in order to supply to demanding customers [34]. Although Silk Road 2.0 was closed in November 2014, it got back on track in May 2016 and is now available as Silk Road 3.0. Moreover, in recent years, many cryptomarkets became available for buying and selling NPS, including Dream Market [33] and others such as Alphabay, Nucleus, and Valhalla, which were shut down in 2016 and 2017, respectively. In addition, a collection of data from drug fora and blogs on the surface web shows that people who possess the knowledge for using the deep web are also able to access drug marketplaces and buy drugs, including NPS [31]. Since the late 2000s, a number of studies have investigated the online supply of NPS through online shops, among which was the two-year, European Commission-funded "Psychonaut 2002 project", coordinated by Fabrizio Schifano, that provided a quantitative and qualitative assessment of the online supply of NPS in a time-specific context, i.e.,"snapshot" [35]. More recently, another European project, the I-TREND (Internet Tools for Research in Europe on New Drugs) project, cofinanced by the Drug Prevention and Information Programme of the European Union, monitored the evolution of online shops and online user fora, conducted an online survey focused on NPS users, and, based on the analysis of samples and the exchange of reference standards among laboratories, ultimately produced a "top list" of NPS at the national level [22].

However, since the deep web remains inaccessible to everyone, research of NPS occurs also on the surface web, where several websites are currently selling them, advertising the products as incense, bath salts, fresheners, plant fertilizers, etc. Notably, when inserting into classical searching engines, such as Google, keywords like "legal highs" or "herbal highs", many websites are listed that offer drugs which are still legal thanks to the time that typically elapses from the appearance of a new substance into the market and its introduction in the list of regulated substances [13]. Few of these websites explicitly sold NPS; gaudy pictures, reduced price for first purchase, proposals for use of new equipment (e.g., vaporizers or smoking pipes), gift ideas, and holidays sales are only some examples of the tricks they use to capture the attention of young consumers. Everyone who is looking for a new sensorial experience and willing to try a psychoactive substance is encouraged to make the purchase with guaranteed secure payment and fast shipment.

## 4. Sharing Information: Drug Fora and YouTube

A large proportion of the world's population uses social networking websites, especially young adults. Therefore, it is not unexpected that conversations about drug use have transferred onto Internet drug fora and message boards [36]. The nature of conversations on drug fora (e.g., www.drugs-forum.com, www.erowid.org) varies significantly. Indeed, drug fora are used for many purposes, including sharing methods of using drugs and learning about new drugs but also for harm reduction purposes [37]. Notably, many users declare to access drug fora primarily to learn how to handle drugs more safely. As a matter of fact, some users claim to be experts and provide detailed guidelines on doses and routes of administration for each drugs class, advising against dangerous drugs interactions as well [38]. The types of visitors and/or participants to drug fora are diverse, but many of them can be considered recreational users who do not consider themselves drug addicts, do not look for treatment, and are not planning to discontinue drug use [39,40].

Drug fora are also very popular among NPS consumers. They are used to report their experiences of the positive and negative effects of substances and to provide advice on doses, routes of administration, and on how to obtain them easily [39], frequently sharing their favorite substances using pharmacological language.

The impact of conversations on drug fora on drug-use behaviors is not known, but it is reasonable to argue that monitoring such discussions could help policy and law enforcement agencies to identify emerging trends in drug use and markets [41]. In addition to drug fora, it is very common to find trip reports on YouTube, the most popular video-sharing site used by teenagers (among other users), and also on the picture-sharing sites Flickr and Instagram. Previously used to report marijuana-, tobacco-, and alcohol-related experiences [42,43], a number of videos of various NPS are now available on YouTube, in which consumers describe in first person all proven effects including negative aspects of their experiences. Sometimes live streams after ingestion of the drug are posted. Many videos can be classified as "cautionary videos" (better known as vernacular prevention videos), others as "hedonistic/celebratory videos" (but not for crystal meth or heroin), and some are "do-it-yourself" (DIY) videos where, for example, detailed instructions on how to grow your own cannabis are provided [44]. Considering the novelty-seeking propensity of young people, this easily available online information might promote the use of these substances. Concern has been expressed for the potential negative impact of social media content depicting drug use and related behaviors [45].

## 5. Social Networks and Smartphone Apps

In these times, the way to surf the Internet has radically changed and social networks are the new leaders of this trend, with a large percentage of use by teenagers [17]. According to a recent survey from a leading global information and measurement company [46], Internet users engage longer in social media sites and apps than in activity on any other type of website. The same survey estimated that the social networking giant Facebook has currently more than 1.6 billion registered users, that the video-sharing site YouTube has more than 1 billion active users, while the social streaming site Twitter has more than 500 million registered users worldwide. Given these numbers, all these platforms have inevitably attracted the interest of drug suppliers, which strictly follow their evolution and diffusion among young people over time. In the last few years, several social networks have acquired important roles in market places for both NPS and illicit drugs [33] (see Figure 2). Simply looking on Facebook, it is now possible to find information and direct links to proceed with the purchase of several NPS or to simply share your experiences in groups created for drug-users only. Even the picture- and video-sharing service Instagram, despite its different use compared to the more famous Facebook, is used to look for new possible customers [47]. Several ambiguous profiles are used to post pictures of their products with hashtags such as #cannabiseeds, #headshop, #herbalicense, and #over18sonly. In 2014, drugabuse.com, for example, published on Instagram an infographic documenting drug-dealer activity [48].

| Facebook | Instagram | Twitter |
|---|---|---|
| legal highs | #cannabiseeds | #legalhights |
| pharmaceuticals | #headshop | #ResearchChemical |
| chemicals | #herbalicense | #syntheticdrug |
| researchchemicals | #over18sonly | |

**Figure 2.** Keywords and hashtags in social networks with explicit content on NPS.

On Twitter, by simply typing #legalhighs, it is possible to buy "the blue stuff", otherwise known as methamphetamine, of the famous *Breaking Bad* television series as well as other #ResearchChemicals, with free shipping offers and credit/debit card payments accepted. All the users, indeed, can be part of a #highsociety, allowing them to share their #proudstoners daily states of mind. Very recently, epidemiologists and linguistic scientists used Twitter to test the feasibility of producing a fully-automated "drug term discovery" system capable of tracking emerging NPS terms in real time [49], which confirms that data collected on Twitter may be used to explore trends in NPS selling and use [50]. Along with other cyber drug communities (e.g., blogs, drug fora, Facebook), Twitter allowed the identification and characterization of a new generation of NPS users, the so-called "e-psychonauts", that considered themselves as psychedelic researchers, mind navigators, or chemicals experimenters [51].

In a technological world where about 2.4 billion people use a smartphone and an increasing number of people use apps, drug dealers adapt their activity accordingly and create simple apps that make buying any kind of psychoactive substance easier, including NPS. Although some apps are designed to prevent drug use, such as "Your Face on Meth" (where you can upload your picture and see its physical degradation over time potentially resulting from using methamphetamine), many apps are created specifically to promote drug use [52].

In North America, the number of cannabis-related smartphone apps is very impressive. In 2014, the number of apps returned from searches using terms like "cannabis" and "marijuana" were 124 and 218, respectively, in Apple's Store, and 250 for both on Google Play [14]. These apps have several content codes, contain information on different cannabis strains and synthetic cannabinoids mixture (e.g., K2, Spice), advice for growing cannabis, and recipes for cooking "special meals". Several apps create a connection with medical marijuana doctors to obtain a prescription, while other apps, such as Eaze, Nugg, Meadow, and Weed Maps, offer to trace medical dispensaries of marijuana, indicating to users the closest spot based on their location in addition to finding the closest doctor that will recommend medical marijuana [14,15]. Additionally, using the app High There, for instance, it is possible to match people to smoke together, while other apps, similar to Instagram and used mostly in Europe and the United States, are utilized for posting photos, videos, or texts related to marijuana or psychoactive substances. Noteworthy, apps useful for making untraceable calls to drug dealers are becoming very popular.

## 6. Conclusions

New psychoactive substances are very popular among young people and online communities, but very little information about toxicological and side effects are available on the Internet. The web-based open sale of unregulated NPS has shown a steady increase in recent years; the easy availability of NPS and the fluctuating dynamics of this new drug market represent a public health concern and an intricate regulatory issue. Research in the field is increasing, and several groups of clinical and preclinical researchers worldwide are investigating the central and peripheral effects of synthetic cannabinoids and synthetic cathinones [1,53–58], synthetic opioids and ketamine-like compounds [59,60], and many others [61,62]. Yet, it is fundamental to share scientific evidence on risks related to the consumption of these compounds using the same channels that promote them. Analyses of social media may represent a new approach to uncover and track changes in drug terms and markets in near real time. In conclusion, the NPS phenomenon is intricate and still very difficult to control. Using the same channels responsible for their growing diffusion to disseminate information and scientific knowledge about the risks associated with their use could represent a potential new approach to limit the diffusion of these dangerous substances.

**Author Contributions:** C.M. design and wrote the first draft of the paper and carefully performed bibliography and sitography; G.M. contributed with figures and internet resources and revised the bibliography; L.F. provided useful contribution to the content and substantially revised the manuscript; M.A.D.L. conceived the topic, designed the structure of the review, supervised and coordinate the work and wrote the final version of the manuscript. All the coauthors contributed to the present piece of work before approving it for final submission.

**Acknowledgments:** All the popular and Internet sources, as well as public and private websites sponsored by organizations or dedicated to a single topic, have been contacted in order to obtain permission of citation by owners or directors. The authors thank all these sources for cooperation in the development of this scientific review article.

## References

1. Miliano, C.; Serpelloni, G.; Rimondo, C.; Mereu, M.; Marti, M.; De Luca, M.A. Neuropharmacology of New Psychoactive Substances (NPS): Focus on the Rewarding and Reinforcing Properties of Cannabimimetics and Amphetamine-Like Stimulants. *Front. Neurosci.* **2016**, *10*, 1–21. [CrossRef] [PubMed]
2. United Nations Office on Drugs and Crime (UNODC). *World Drug Report*; UNODC: Vienna, Austria, 2016; ISBN 9789211482867.
3. United Nations Office on Drugs and Crime (UNODC). *World Drug Report*; Booklet4; UNODC: Vienna, Austria, 2017; ISBN 978-92-1-148296-6.
4. Understanding the Synthetic Drug Market: The NPS Factor. Available online: https://www.unodc.org/documents/scientific/Global_Smart_Update_2018_Vol.19.pdf (accessed on 29 June 2018).
5. Seely, K.A.; Lapoint, J.; Moran, J.H.; Fattore, L. Spice drugs are more than harmless herbal blends: A review of the pharmacology and toxicology of synthetic cannabinoids. *Prog. Neuropsychopharmacol. Biol. Psychiatry* **2012**, *39*, 234–243. [CrossRef] [PubMed]
6. De Luca, M.A.; Bimpisidis, Z.; Melis, M.; Marti, M.; Caboni, P.; Valentini, V.; Margiani, G.; Pintori, N.; Polis, I.; Marsicano, G.; et al. Stimulation of in vivo dopamine transmission and intravenous self-administration in rats and mice by JWH-018, a Spice cannabinoid. *Neuropharmacology* **2015**, *99*, 705–714. [CrossRef] [PubMed]
7. Corazza, O.; Valeriani, G.; Bersani, F.S.; Corkery, J.; Martinotti, G.; Bersani, G.; Schifano, F. "Spice", "kryptonite", "black mamba": An overview of brand names and marketing strategies of novel psychoactive substances on the web. *J. Psychoact. Drugs* **2014**, *46*, 287–294. [CrossRef] [PubMed]
8. Burns, L.; Roxburgh, A.; Bruno, R.; Van Buskirk, J. Monitoring drug markets in the Internet age and the evolution of drug monitoring systems in Australia. *Drug Test Anal.* **2014**, *6*, 840–845. [CrossRef] [PubMed]
9. De Luca, M.A.; Solinas, M.; Bimpisidis, Z.; Goldberg, S.R.; Di Chiara, G. Cannabinoidfacilitation of behavioral and biochemical hedonic taste responses. *Neuropharmacology* **2012**, *63*, 161–168. [CrossRef] [PubMed]
10. Nuove Sostanze Psicoattive (NSP): Schede Tecniche Relative Alle Molecole Registrate dal Sistema Nazionale di Allerta Precoce. Available online: http://www.dronet.org/pubblicazioni_new/pubb_det.php?id=690 (accessed on 29 June 2018).
11. Smith, J.P.; Sutcliffe, O.B.; Banks, C.E. An overview of recent developments in the analytical detection of new psychoactive substances (NPSs). *Analyst* **2015**, *140*, 4932–4948. [CrossRef] [PubMed]
12. Fattore, L.; Fratta, W. Beyond THC: The New Generation of Cannabinoid Designer Drugs. *Front. Behav. Neurosci.* **2011**, *5*, 60. [CrossRef] [PubMed]
13. Schmidt, M.M.; Sharma, A.; Schifano, F.; Feinmann, C. "Legal highs" on the net-Evaluation of UK-based Websites, products and product information. *Forensic Sci. Int.* **2011**, *206*, 92–97. [CrossRef] [PubMed]
14. Ramo, D.E.; Popova, L.; Grana, R.; Zhao, S.; Chavez, K. Cannabis Mobile Apps: A Content Analysis. *JMIR mHealth uHealth* **2015**, *3*, e81. [CrossRef] [PubMed]
15. Bierut, T.; Krauss, M.J.; Sowles, S.J.; Cavazos-Rehg, P.A. Exploring Marijuana Advertising on Weedmaps, a Popular Online Directory. *Prev. Sci.* **2017**, *18*, 183–192. [CrossRef] [PubMed]
16. United Nations Office on Drugs and Crime (UNODC). *World Drug Report 2014*; UNODC: Vienna, Austria, 2014; Volume 3, ISBN 9789211482775.
17. European Monitoring Centre for Drugs and Drug Addiction (EMCDDA). *European Drug Report. Trends and Developments*; EMCDDA: Lisbon, Portugal, 2015; ISBN 9789291686117.
18. Papanti, D.; Schifano, F.; Botteon, G.; Bertossi, F.; Mannix, J.; Vidoni, D.; Impagnatiello, M.; Pascolo-Fabrici, E.; Bonavigo, T. "Spiceophrenia": A systematic overview of "spice"-related psychopathological issues and a case report. *Hum. Psychopharmacol.* **2013**. [CrossRef] [PubMed]
19. Fattore, L. Synthetic cannabinoids-further evidence supporting the relationship between cannabinoids and psychosis. *Biol. Psychiatry* **2016**, *79*, 539–548. [CrossRef] [PubMed]

20. Fantegrossi, W.E.; Wilson, C.D.; Berquist, M.D. Pro-psychotic effects of syntheticcannabinoids: Interactions with central dopamine, serotonin, and glutamate systems. *Drug Metab. Rev.* **2018**, *50*, 65–73. [CrossRef] [PubMed]
21. Ferreri, F.; Bourla, A.; Mouchabac, S.; Karila, L. E-addictology: An overview of new technologies for assessing and intervening in addictive behaviors. *Front. Psychiatry* **2018**, *9*, 51. [CrossRef] [PubMed]
22. European Monitoring Centre for Drugs and Drug Addiction (EMCDDA). *The Internet and Drug Markets*; EMCDDA: Lisbon, Portugal, 2016; ISBN 9789291688418.
23. Harper, S.; Strumpf, E.C.; Kaufman, J.S. Do Medical Marijuana Laws Increase Marijuana Use? Replication Study and Extension. *Ann. Epidemiol.* **2012**, *22*, 207–212. [CrossRef] [PubMed]
24. De Luca, M.A.; Di Chiara, G.; Cadoni, C.; Lecca, D.; Orsolini, L.; Papanti, D.; Corkery, J.; Schifano, F. Cannabis; Epidemiological, Neurobiological and Psychopathological Issues: An Update. *CNS Neurol. Disord. Drug Targets* **2017**, *16*, 598–609. [CrossRef] [PubMed]
25. Cerdá, M.; Wall, M.; Keyes, K.M.; Galea, S.; Hasin, D. Medical marijuana laws in 50 states: Investigating the relationship between state legalization of medical marijuana and marijuana use, abuse and dependence. *Drug Alcohol Depend.* **2012**, *120*, 22–27. [CrossRef] [PubMed]
26. D'Amico, E.J.; Miles, J.N.; Tucker, J.S. Gateway to curiosity: Medical marijuana adsand intention and use during middle school. *Psychol. Addict. Behav.* **2015**, *29*, 613–619. [CrossRef] [PubMed]
27. Van Hout, M.C.; Bingham, T. Responsible vendors, intelligent consumers: Silk Road, the online revolution in drug trading. *Int. J. Drug Policy* **2014**, *25*, 183–189. [CrossRef] [PubMed]
28. AlQahtani, A.A.; El-Alfy, E.-S.M. Anonymous Connections Based on Onion Routing: A Review and a Visualization Tool. *Procedia Comput. Sci.* **2015**, *52*, 121–128. [CrossRef]
29. Martin, J. *Drugs on the Dark Net*; Palgrave Macmillan UK: London, UK, 2014; ISBN 978-1-349-48566-6.
30. Christin, N. Traveling the Silk Road: A measurement analysis of a large anonymous online marketplace. *arXiv* **2012**, arXiv:1207.7139.
31. Orsolini, L.; Papanti, D.; Corkery, J.; Schifano, F. An insight into the deep web; why it matters for addiction psychiatry? *Hum. Psychopharmacol.* **2017**, *32*, 1–7. [CrossRef] [PubMed]
32. Rhumorbarbe, D.; Staehli, L.; Broséus, J.; Rossy, Q.; Esseiva, P. Buying drugs on a Darknet market: A better deal? Studying the online illicit drug market through the analysis of digital, physical and chemical data. *Forensic Sci. Int.* **2016**, *267*, 173–182. [CrossRef] [PubMed]
33. Van Hout, M.C.; Hearne, E. New psychoactive substances (NPS) on cryptomarketfora: An exploratory study of characteristics of forum activity between NPS buyers and vendors. *Int. J. Drug Policy* **2017**, *40*, 102–110. [CrossRef] [PubMed]
34. Dolliver, D.S. Evaluating drug trafficking on the Tor Network: Silk Road 2, the sequel. *Int. J. Drug Policy* **2015**, *26*, 1113–1123. [CrossRef] [PubMed]
35. Schifano, F.; Deluca, P.; Baldacchino, A.; Peltoniemi, T.; Scherbaum, N.; Torrens, M.; Farrě, M.; Flores, I.; Rossi, M.; Eastwood, D.; et al. Drugs on the web; the Psychonaut 2002 EU project. *Prog. Neuro-Psychopharmacol. Biol. Psychiatry* **2006**, *30*, 640–646. [CrossRef] [PubMed]
36. Wax, P.M. Just a click away: Recreational drug Web sites on the Internet. *Pediatrics* **2002**, *109*, e96. [CrossRef] [PubMed]
37. Marlatt, G.A.; Witkiewitz, K. Update on Harm-Reduction Policy and Intervention Research. *Annu. Rev. Clin. Psychol.* **2010**, *6*, 591–606. [CrossRef] [PubMed]
38. Chiauzzi, E.; DasMahapatra, P.; Lobo, K.; Barratt, M.J. Participatory research with an online drug forum: A survey of user characteristics, information sharing, and harm reduction views. *Subst. Use Misuse* **2013**, *48*, 661–670. [CrossRef] [PubMed]
39. Nicholson, T.; White, J.; Duncan, D.F. A Survey of adult recreational drug use via the World Wide Web: The DRUGNET Study. *J. Psychoact. Drugs* **1999**, *31*, 415–422. [CrossRef] [PubMed]
40. Baggott, M.J.; Erowid, E.; Erowid, F.; Galloway, G.P.; Mendelson, J. Use patterns and self-reported effects of *Salvia divinorum*: An internet-based survey. *Drug Alcohol Depend.* **2010**, *111*, 250–256. [CrossRef] [PubMed]
41. Davey, Z.; Schifano, F.; Corazza, O.; Deluca, P. Psychonaut Web Mapping Group e-Psychonauts: Conducting research in online drug forum communities. *J. Ment. Health* **2012**, *21*, 386–394. [CrossRef] [PubMed]
42. Krauss, M.J.; Sowles, S.J.; Mylvaganam, S.; Zewdie, K.; Bierut, L.J.; Cavazos-Rehg, P.A. Displays of dabbing marijuana extracts on YouTube. *Drug Alcohol Depend.* **2015**, *155*, 45–51. [CrossRef] [PubMed]

43. Krauss, M.J.; Sowles, S.J.; Stelzer-Monahan, H.E.; Bierut, T.; Cavazos-Rehg, P.A. "It Takes Longer, but When It Hits You It Hits You!": Videos About Marijuana Edibles on YouTube. *Subst. Use Misuse* **2017**, *52*, 709–716. [CrossRef] [PubMed]
44. Manning, P. YouTube, "drug videos" and drugs education. *Drugs Edu. Prev. Policy* **2013**, *20*, 120–130. [CrossRef]
45. Lau, A.Y.S.; Gabarron, E.; Fernandez-Luque, L.; Armayones, M. Social media in health—What are the safety concerns for health consumers? *Health Inf. Manag.* **2012**, *41*, 30–35. [CrossRef] [PubMed]
46. Nielsen. Nielsen Reports and Insights. The Social Media Report 2012. Available online: http://www.nielsen.com/us/en/insights/reports/2012/state-of-the-media-the-social-media-report-2012.html (accessed on 22 February 2018).
47. Cavazos-Rehg, P.A.; Krauss, M.J.; Sowles, S.J.; Bierut, L.J. Marijuana-Related Posts on Instagram. *Prev. Sci.* **2016**, *17*, 710–720. [CrossRef] [PubMed]
48. Drugabuse.com. Instagram Drug Dealers. Available online: https://drugabuse.com/featured/instagram-drug-dealers/ (accessed on 22 February 2018).
49. Simpson, S.S.; Adams, N.; Brugman, C.M.; Conners, T.J. Detecting Novel and Emerging Drug Terms Using Natural Language Processing: A Social Media Corpus Study. *JMIR Public Health Surveill.* **2018**, *4*, e2. [CrossRef] [PubMed]
50. Kolliakou, A.; Ball, M.; Derczynski, L.; Chandran, D.; Gkotsis, G.; Deluca, P.; Jackson, R.; Shetty, H.; Stewart, R. Novel psychoactive substances: An investigation of temporal trends in social media and electronic health records. *Eur. Psychiatry* **2016**, *38*, 15–21. [CrossRef] [PubMed]
51. Orsolini, L.; Papanti, G.D.; Francesconi, G.; Schifano, F. Mind Navigators of Chemicals' Experimenters? A Web-Based Description of E.-Psychonauts. *Cyberpsychol. Behav. Soc. Netw.* **2015**, *18*, 296–300. [CrossRef] [PubMed]
52. Bindhim, N.F.; Naicker, S.; Freeman, B.; Mcgeechan, K.; Trevena, L. Apps Promoting Illicit Drugs-A Need for Tighter Regulation? *J. Consum. Health Internet* **2014**, *18*, 31–43. [CrossRef]
53. Baumann, M.H.; Bukhari, M.O.; Lehner, K.R.; Anizan, S.; Rice, K.C.; Concheiro, M.; Huestis, M.A. Neuropharmacology of 3,4-Methylenedioxypyrovalerone (MDPV), Its Metabolites, and Related Analogs. *Curr. Top. Behav. Neurosci.* **2016**, *32*, 93–117.
54. Davidson, C.; Opacka-Juffry, J.; Arevalo-Martin, A.; Garcia-Ovejero, D.; Molina-Holgado, E.; Molina-Holgado, F. Spicing Up Pharmacology: A Review of Synthetic Cannabinoids from Structure to Adverse Events. *Adv. Pharmacol.* **2017**, *80*, 135–168. [CrossRef] [PubMed]
55. Karila, L.; Lafaye, G.; Scocard, A.; Cottencin, O.; Benyamina, A. MDPV and α-PVP use in humans: The twisted sisters. *Neuropharmacology* **2017**. [CrossRef] [PubMed]
56. Pintori, N.; Loi, B.; Mereu, M. Synthetic cannabinoids: The hidden side of Spice drugs. *J. Emerg. Nurs.* **2017**, *37*, 292–293. [CrossRef] [PubMed]
57. Weinstein, A.M.; Rosca, P.; Fattore, L.; London, E.D. Synthetic Cathinone and Cannabinoid Designer Drugs Pose a Major Risk for Public Health. *Front. Psychiatry* **2017**, *8*, 156. [CrossRef] [PubMed]
58. Zanda, M.T.; Fattore, L. Old and new synthetic cannabinoids: Lessons from animal models. *Drug Metab. Rev.* **2018**, *50*, 54–64. [CrossRef] [PubMed]
59. Zanda, M.T.; Fadda, P.; Chiamulera, C.; Fratta, W.; Fattore, L. Methoxetamine, a novel psychoactive substance with serious adverse pharmacological effects. *Behav. Pharmacol.* **2016**, *27*, 489–496. [CrossRef] [PubMed]
60. Zawilska, J.B. An Expanding World of Novel Psychoactive Substances: Opioids. *Front. Psychiatry* **2017**, *8*, 110. [CrossRef] [PubMed]
61. Loi, B.; Zloh, M.; De Luca, M.A.; Pintori, N.; Corkery, J.; Schifano, F. 4,4′-Dimethylaminorex ("4,4′-DMAR"; "Serotoni") misuse: A Web-based study. *Hum. Psychopharmacol.* **2017**, *32*. [CrossRef] [PubMed]
62. Pinterova, N.; Horsley, R.R.; Palenicek, T. Synthetic Aminoindanes: A Summary of Existing Knowledge. *Front. Psychiatry* **2017**, *8*, 236. [CrossRef] [PubMed]

# 10

# The Effects of Cannabinoids on Executive Functions: Evidence from Cannabis and Synthetic Cannabinoids

**Koby Cohen and Aviv Weinstein** *

Department of Behavioral Science, Ariel University, Ariel 40700, Israel; kbbcohen@gmail.com
* Correspondence: avivweinstein@yahoo.com

**Abstract:** Background—Cannabis is the most popular illicit drug in the Western world. Repeated cannabis use has been associated with short and long-term range of adverse effects. Recently, new types of designer-drugs containing synthetic cannabinoids have been widespread. These synthetic cannabinoid drugs are associated with undesired adverse effects similar to those seen with cannabis use, yet, in more severe and long-lasting forms. Method—A literature search was conducted using electronic bibliographic databases up to 31 December 2017. Specific search strategies were employed using multiple keywords (e.g., "synthetic cannabinoids AND cognition," "cannabis AND cognition" and "cannabinoids AND cognition"). Results—The search has yielded 160 eligible studies including 37 preclinical studies (5 attention, 25 short-term memory, 7 cognitive flexibility) and 44 human studies (16 attention, 15 working memory, 13 cognitive flexibility). Both pre-clinical and clinical studies demonstrated an association between synthetic cannabinoids and executive-function impairment either after acute or repeated consumptions. These deficits differ in severity depending on several factors including the type of drug, dose of use, quantity, age of onset and duration of use. Conclusions—Understanding the nature of the impaired executive function following consumption of synthetic cannabinoids is crucial in view of the increasing use of these drugs.

**Keywords:** cannabis; synthetic cannabinoids; executive function

---

## 1. Introduction

The most popular illicit drug of the 21st century is cannabis, in its many forms and shapes [1–5]. According to the United Nation Office on Drugs and Crime (UNODC), approximately 181 million adults have used cannabis across the globe [2]. Moreover, in many countries more than 50% of young adults have used cannabis at least once in their lifetime [3]. Recently, new types of drugs that contain Synthetic Cannabinoids (SC) have become popular among drugs users worldwide [5–7]. SC drugs are associated with severe adverse effects (Table 1), have greater harm potential and they are more addictive than the traditional organic cannabis drugs [4,6–9]. Therefore, governments and health institutions across the Western world make major efforts in order to prevent the spread of SC and to improve the knowledge regarding SC and their potential risks [5,8]. One of the most notorious adverse effects that is associated with cannabinoids consumption is impairment of cognitive function [4]. Both pre-clinical and human studies drew a link between consumption of cannabinoids and long-term deficits of cognitive functions, especially high-order cognitive functions [4,5,10–13]. The purpose of the current review is to present and describe the acute and long-term effects of SC drugs in comparison with organic cannabis on executive function (EF) based on current literature from both human and animal research. A literature search was conducted using electronic bibliographic databases (PubMed®, ScienceDirect ®and Google Scholar platforms) up to 31 December 2017. Database-specific search strategies were employed using multiple keywords (e.g., "synthetic cannabinoids AND cognition," "cannabis AND cognition" and "cannabinoids AND cognition"). The search has yielded 160 eligible studies including 37 preclinical studies (5 attention, 25 short-term memory, 7 cognitive flexibility) (Table 2) and 44 human studies (16 attention, 15 working memory, 13 cognitive flexibility). Studies were included if they stated the following inclusion criteria: use of objective measurements of specific executive function (working memory, attention and cognitive flexibility) involving cannabinoid users (regular and recreational users) or cannabinoid treatments and a control group. Exclusion criteria were: studies that involved participants who had other neurological or psychiatric disorders or individuals who met criteria for alcohol dependence or other substance use disorders (abuse or dependence) different from cannabis and nicotine.

**Table 1.** Common clinical adverse effects induced after consuming synthetic cannabinoids.

| Type of Effects | Symptoms |
|---|---|
| Psychosis | Recurrent psychosis episodes [9,14–16]. |
| Agitation | Last for several hours after intoxication of SC [16–18]. |
| Affect disturbance | Severe anxiety symptoms and panic attacks shortly after consuming SC [14,17–20]. |
| Cognitive alterations | Impairment in memory and attention deficits [14,20–22] |
| Cardiovascular effects | Both tachycardia, tachyarrhythmia and cardiotoxicity were reported after exposure to SC [14,23]. |
| Gastrointestinal effects | Nausea, vomiting and diarrhea after severe exposure to SC [14,24,25]. |

**Table 2.** Pre-clinical rodent studies of the effects of cannabinoid-agonists on executive function.

| Animals | Cannabinoids Tested | Main Findings | Reference |
|---|---|---|---|
| Male Long–Evans rats | WIN55,212-2 and Δ9-THC | Dose-related attention impairments afteracute exposure to cannabinoid $CB_1$ receptor agonist. Impairments were reduced after treatment with $CB_1$ antagonist. | [26,27] |
| Male Sprague–Dawley rats | Δ9-THC | Decreased performance on a divided attention tasklasts for 2 weeks after chronic administration withcannabinoid $CB_1$ receptor agonist. | [28] |
| Male Sprague–Dawley rats | AM-4054 | Decreased sustained attention after acute treatmentwith a cannabinoid $CB_1$ receptor agonist.Impairments were associated with task demands. | [14] |
| Male Sprague–Dawley rats | Δ9-THC | Impairments of visual attention on an operant signaldetection task after acute treatment with cannabinoid $CB_1$ receptor agonist. | [29] |
| Male Sprague–Dawley rats | WIN55,212-2 | Deficits of working memory after chronic treatmentwith a cannabinoid $CB_1$ receptor agonist. | [30] |
| Female Long–Evans rats | Δ9-THC | Repeated administration with cannabinoid $CB_1$ receptoragonist in adolescence induced persistent impairment of working memory. | [31] |
| Male Sprague–Dawley rats | WIN55,212-2 | Acute injection of cannabinoid $CB_1$ receptor agonist in late-adolescence period induced temporary impairment of short-term memory. Chronic treatment with cannabinoid $CB_1$ receptor agonist impair short-term memory for several weeks after the last administration. | [32] |
| Male Sprague–Dawley rats | Δ9-THC | Acute exposure to a cannabinoid $CB_1$ receptor agonistinduced working memory impairments | [33,34] |
| Male Sprague–Dawley rats, Lister rats and C57B16 mice | Δ9-THC | Working memory impairments were induced afterchronic treatment with a cannabinoid $CB_1$ receptor agonist. | [35,36] |
| Wild-type and $CB_1$ receptor knockout mice | JWH-081 | Acute treatment with cannabinoid $CB_1$ receptor agonist induced short-term memory deficits in wild-type mice but not in knockout mice. | [37] |
| Male Long–Evans rats | HU-210 | Acute treatment with a cannabinoid $CB_1$ receptor agonistinduced working memory deficits. | [38,39] |
| Male C57B1/6 mice | Δ9-THC | Acute injection of Δ9-THC disrupted performance of the working memory task, impairments were reversed by SR1417161A. | [40] |
| Male Wistar Rats | Δ9-THC | Acute administration induced set-shifting impairments24 h after treatment. | [41] |

**Table 2.** *Cont.*

| Animals | Cannabinoids Tested | Main Findings | Reference |
|---|---|---|---|
| Male albino Wistar rats | Δ9-THC | Acute treatment with a cannabinoid $CB_1$ receptor agonistinduced short-term memory deficits, impairments were attenuated after treatment with cannabinoid $CB_1$ antagonist. | [42] |
| Male ICR (CD-1) mice | JWH-018, JWH-018-Cl, JWH-018-Br and Δ9-THC | SCs dose-dependently impaired short- term memory. Their effects resulted more potent respect to that evoked by Δ9-THC. | [43] |
| Male Long–Evans rats | JWH-018 | Chronic exposer to cannabinoid $CB_1$ receptor agonist induced spatial learning and short-term memory alterations well after the drugs exposure period. | [44] |
| Male Lister Hooded and Wistar rats | CP55,940 | Acute administration of cannabinoid CB1 receptor agonist impaired short-term memory in both strains, yet, no long-term effects were observed. | [45] |
| Male Long–Evans rats | Δ9-THC | Acute treatment with a cannabinoid $CB_1$ receptor agonistinduced reversal learning deficits while set-shifting ability has maintained | [46] |
| Male Long–Evans rats | HU-210 | Administration of the cannabinoid $CB_1$ receptor agonistelicited dose-dependent disruptive effects on set-shiftingperformance. Impairments were diminished afteradministration of the $CB_1$ antagonist AM251. | [47] |
| Male Albino Wistar rats | AB-PINACA or AB-FUBINACA compere with Δ9-THC | Two weeks after repeated administration of cannabinoid-agonist short-term memory impairments were observed, in SCs groups the impairments were greater and last for longer time. | [48] |
| Female and Male Sprague–Dawley rats | WIN55,212-2 | Self-administration of SCs in low dosages during adolescence period improve or did not induce permanent memory impairments, while treatments of high dosages of SCs in adolescence period induced permanent short-term memory impairments. | [49,50] |

## 2. Pharmacology of Organic Cannabis

Cannabis is the generic name of the psychoactive drug that is derived from the female plant *Cannabis sativa* [51]. There are more than 400 compounds including more than 60 cannabinoids, which are aryl-substituted meroterpenes unique to *Cannabis sativa* [52,53]. The main psychoactive ingredient in cannabis is Δ9-Tetrahydrocannabinol (Δ9-THC), which is the most potent cannabinoid that is present in the organic form of cannabis [53]. Besides Δ9-THC, organic cannabis products contain additional cannabinoids which do not induce psychoactive effects, such as Cannabidiol (CBD), Δ8-Tetrahydrocannabinol and Cannabinol [54–56]. Furthermore, CBD is considered a non-psychoactive cannabinoid that also moderates the psycho tropic effects of Δ9-THC [57–60].

The psychoactive effects of cannabis are dose-dependent [58,61,62] and there is evidence that as the content of Δ9-THC increases, the psychoactive effects of cannabis drugs increase [59,62]. Cannabinoid agonists in general and specifically Δ9-THC, exert their effects by acting on at least two types of endogenous cannabinoid receptors (CB1, CB2), which are widely distributed in numerous regions within mammals' brain [52,63,64]. Pacher and Kunos (2013) suggested that endocannabinoid receptors, the two endocannabinoid ligands and their related enzymes are the components of the Endo-Cannabinoid System (ECS), which is involved in a wide range of somatic and mental functions [65].

## 3. Synthetic Cannabinoids, from Therapeutic Agents to a Global Disease

### 3.1. Old Origins, New Trends

Since the discovery of Δ9-THC and the involvement of the ECS in a wide range of health conditions, cannabinoids have been synthesized for medical research purposes as promising research and therapeutic tools [23,24]. In contrast to organic cannabinoids such as Δ9-THC, SCs selectively activate the endocannabinoid receptors [24,56,57].

In the beginning of the new millennium, a growing number of reports indicated that there were new psychoactive products which included mostly SC ingredients mixed with other herbal blends [6,66,67]. The production, distribution and use of SC drugs were initially neither controlled nor illegal, therefore they are presented as "legal-highs" [67], by various generic names such as; "Mr. Nice Guy," "Spice Gold," "Spice Diamond," "Yucatan Fire" and most commonly as "K2" or "Spice" [7,25]. These products were often sold without age restriction over multiple sources such as the internet and convenience stores [4,7–9,25,67]. As the popularity of SC drugs increased, their severe undesired adverse effects were observed; affective disorder, recurrent psychosis, tachycardia, seizures and prolonged hospitalization were not rare outcomes of SC intoxication [4,5,7–9]. Some of these adverse effects are related to the effect of additional psychoactive agents which these products contain [6,8,68].

Despite the fact that SCs are labeled as "not for human consumption" and "for aroma therapy use only," the popularity of these drugs appears to be growing [5]. SCs induce more intense effects than traditional cannabis, they are less expensive and they are undetectable in standardized drug tests. These unique features contribute to the growing numbers of recreational drug users who have used SCs [4,5].

### *3.2. The Psychoactive Ingredients of Synthetic Cannabinoid Products*

Over than 140 products containing SC have been identified, although, the main psychoactive components of these products are different types of SCs which are categorized into four major groups including; (a) Aminoalkylindole or JWH series, (b) classical cannabinoids, (c) non-classical cannabinoids and (d) fatty acid amides (e.g., oleamide) [21,22,69,70].

The first generation of SC products mostly contain the series of 1-alkyl-3-(1-naphthoyl) indoles known as JWH compounds or aminoalkylinodels. This SC series is named after John W. Huffman who developed these ligands for medical research purposes [71] The JWH series advanced from computational melding of the chemical structural structures of Δ9-THC with previously developed aminoalkylinodels [71]. One of the first SC from this series to be abused is JWH-18 (1-penthyl-3-(1-napthoyl) indole), which features as easy synthesizable and high potency contribute to its popularity [9]. Compared to Δ9-THC, JWH-018 has 4 times the affinity for CB1 receptors and 10 time the affinity for the CB2 receptors [72]. JWH series represent the main psychoactive compounds detected in SC products across many countries [9].

Additional components detected in SC products include analogues of Δ9-THC, so-called classical cannabinoids such as HU-210 and HU-211. HU-210 developed in the middle of the 20th century at the Hebrew University (HU) [73] and is a hundred times more potent than Δ9-THC binds both $CB_1$ and $CB_2$ receptors [73,74] Similar to other SC, HU-210 acts as CB1 receptors full-agonists [73].

The cyclohexylphenol (CP) is a non-classical cannabinoids series synthesized by *Pfizer labs* in the early 1970s; examples include CP 59,540, CP 47,497 and their n-alkyl homologues [71]. Similar to JWH-018, CP-47,497 is included in large numbers within SC products e [67]. In addition, SCs from the CP series act as CB1 receptors full agonists [67]. However, within any given SC products, various types of SC are found in different concentrations [9,67] accompanied by additional psychoactive compounds from synthetic opioids such as O-desmethyltramadol, harmine and harmaline, which are inhibitors of the monoamine oxidase enzyme, to benzophenone (HM-40) and even caffeine [9,11,68]. There are several common features among different compounds of SC products which can highlight the risk potential which these drugs have and their related adverse effects. Firstly, SCs act as full agonists to CB1 receptors and some also bind to CB2 receptors [7]. Secondly, SCs are much more potent, easily cross the blood-brain barrier and have more affinity compared to organic psychoactive cannabinoids like Δ9-THC [68,69]. In addition, SC drugs do not contain CBD, which has high potency as an antagonist to CB1 and CB2 receptors and therefore it is able to revert the psychotic and anxiolytic adverse effects of cannabinoid-agonists. It is suggested that the lack of CBD in SC products amplifies their psychotropic effects [4,6,75]. Moreover, SC products hold a unique characteristic, which is its ever-changing composition. The first generation of SC products commonly contain JWH-018, JWH-073 and CP-47,49, since these SCs became regulated, there has been an emergence of new types of SCs like JWH-081, JWH-210 and AM-2201, in an attempt to dodge regulations. Despite slight chemical structure modification, all of these SCs share the same main features and aim to mimic the psychoactive effects of Δ9-THC and even to transcend it [4,6,66,67,75].

## 4. Executive Function (EF) and the Long-Term Effects of Cannabinoids

### *4.1. The Three Core Factors Model of Executive Function*

Although preclinical and human studies demonstrate that endocannabinoids involve and affect cognitive function in general and specifically high-order cognitive function [12,13,51,68], there is still a debate regarding the effects of chronic consumption of cannabinoid products such as cannabis or SCs on EF [12,13,46,70] (Table 1).

The term EF refers to "high-order" cognitive functions, which involve regulation, "lower-order" cognitive process and goal-directed behaviors [76,77]. EF generally clusters various cognitive abilities such as verbal reasoning, problem-solving, planning behaviors, sequencing, multi-tasking, cognitive flexibility, sustained attention, resistance to interferences and the ability to deal with novel information [77–80]. Due to the wide range of functions which are considered as executive or high-order, there is still an ongoing debate regarding the mechanisms which underlie executive function, performances and regarding which cognitive functions should be marked as executive [76].

Diamond (2013) suggested that EF should be divided into two subgroups: core EF and higher order EF [77]. Accordingly, the three cores EFs are (a) inhibition control or attention (b) Working Memory (WM) and (c) cognitive flexibility. The basic EFs are essential for the production of higher order cognitive functions such as verbal reasoning, problem-solving, planning behaviors, sequencing and multi-tasking. Accordingly, these functions do not involve much emotional arousal and they are logic based [77].

### *4.2. Cannabinoids and Attention-Evidence from Preclinical Studies*

The ability to evaluate and allocate priority to external stimuli or internal habits and to optimize behavioral response requires attention [13,77]. These enable focus and selectively attend to desired stimuli and to inhibit response to irrelevant stimuli [77]. Studies have suggested that numerous brain regions facilitate attention performance, yet, it is mediated by the frontal lobes [81,82]. Additionally, the Anterior Cingulate Cortex (ACC) is a crucial factor in the execution of this function [82,83].

Preclinical studies provide strong evidence regarding the effects of repeated treatment with cannabinoid-agonists and impaired attention. The Lateralized Reaction Time task (LRT) of visuo-spatial attention that has been previously used in rats, is considered as a valid model for attention in rodents. In this paradigm, rodents need to attend to apparatus for the location of a visual stimulus over numbers of trails [83]. Arguello and Jentsch (2004) reported that acute treatments with the SC agonist WIN55212-2 (2.5 mg/kg) induced deficits in attention measured on the LRT task. In addition, treatment with SR141716A 1 mg/kg which is a CB1 antagonist reversed the WIN55212-2-induced attention impairment, although, when administered alone, this compound did not produce any effects on attention [26].

A further study by Verrico et al (2004) examined the effect of repeated treatments with Δ9-THC on attention using the LRT task in rats. In their study, rats that were daily treated with Δ9-THC 20 mg/kg for 2 weeks, presented attention impairments which lasted 14 days after the last treatment with Δ9-THC [28]. Later-on, Miller et al. (2013) treated rats with small doses of novel SC agonists AM-4054 before performing a two-choice reaction time task, which measures sustained attention. They reported that AM-4054 induced attention impairments which were positively correlated with task demands and harder trails were associated with poorer functions [14].

Some authors suggested that lesions of the medial prefrontal cortex or striatum can produce attention deficits similar to those presented after cannabinoid administration [84,85]. Chronic exposure to cannabinoid-agonists led to alterations within meso-limbic dopaminergic neurons [86], thus, cannabinoid-induced attention impairment might arise via continuous activation of CB1 receptors across the striatum or prefrontal cortex [83].

### 4.3. Cannabinoids and Attention-Evidence from Clinical Studies

The disruptive acute effect of cannabis on attention is widely described in clinical studies [87–90] and systematic reviews [11,70,87]. Yet, human studies failed to draw consistent evidence regarding the effect of chronic consumption of cannabinoids and impaired attention. While some studies described impairments of tasks which demand attention in chronic cannabis users [17,19,61,89,91], other studies demonstrated no differences in behavioral performance between cannabis users and non-users [22,87]. Since neuronal and functional alterations of the ACC region were consistency observed among chronic cannabis users [92] a recent review study suggested that the marginal effects that were observed in these studies are probably an outcome of a compensation mechanism that was developed among chronic users [87].

There are several tasks for measuring attention. In a paradigm such the Stroop task, a control of interference from of a pre-potent response is required [93]. Incongruent conditions of the classical Stroop color-word task contain color words written in another color. Subjects are required to ignore the semantic meaning of the word and instead attend to and report the color. Since humans are trained to read and to ignore other words' features such as font style or color, people are slower and prone to make more errors in the incongruent trials of the Stroop task [77].

On the Go/No-Go task, the participants do not inhibit natural response at the expense of another. On this task, participants are required to respond when target stimulus is presented and should not respond when a non-target stimulus appears [94]. Other tasks such as the Continuous Performance Task (CPT) are being used for measuring sustained attention. In this paradigm, participants are required to maintain attention over a continuous period in order to detect infrequent targets, thus ensuring that the goals of the behavior are kept over time [20].

Eldreth and colleagues (2004) have examined the performance on a modified Stroop task in which healthy individuals were compared with abstinent cannabis users. Although there were no behavioral differences between the groups, cannabis users had greater activation in prefrontal brain regions than non-users [95]. Similarly, Jager et al. (2006) observed moderate differences in brain activity between cannabis users and healthy individuals while performing attention and WM tasks. They reported that compared with healthy subjects, cannabis users presented hypo-activation in the left superior parietal cortex while performing the attention task [96].

Recently, Hatchard and colleagues (2014) observed a similar pattern among young cannabis users. Recreational cannabis users did not differ in performance on the modified Stroop task compared with non-users, however, differences in neuronal activity of several brain regions including the ACC and post-central gyrus were observed, suggesting that chronic consumption of cannabis affects neuronal process even in an absence of behavioral expressions [97]. In another study, Hester et al (2009) reported that alterations in attention correlated with neuronal hypo-activity of ACC in heavy cannabis users. The attention deficits expressed in performing more errors on the Go/No-go task, suggested that attention depended on cannabis consumption history, including doses, frequency and age of onset [98].

The studies described so far examined the complex association between chronic consumption of organic cannabis and impaired attention, yet, there is limited objective evidence for an association between chronic consumption of SCs and impaired attention in humans [9]. Cohen et al (2017) showed that SC users had more errors performing on the classic Stroop color-word task compared with regular cannabis users and healthy subjects [11]. Furthermore, several case reports described SC users who experienced "thinking problems" which last from days to weeks following last consumption. However, attention deficits were less common and they were accompanied with additional symptoms such as affective disturbances and cognitive dysfunction including severe alterations in short-term memory [8,99,100].

### 4.4. *Cannabinoids and Working Memory-Evidence from Preclinical Studies*

Working Memory (WM) is defined as a cognitive mechanism for the temporary storage and manipulation of stored information [101], or simply, as a cognitive system which involves holding information in mind and mentally working with it [77].

The function of WM has been associated with integration of a wide range of neural networks. WM networks are associated with frontal-parietal regions including dorso-lateral pre-frontal cortex, ventro-lateral prefrontal cortex, pre-motor cortex, lateral parietal cortex and the frontal lobe [102]. An additional brain region which is considered a major component in WM is the hippocampus, which is essential for acquiring, encoding and consolidating new types of information. This information is represented and manipulated by the WM system in the prefrontal cortex [103]. In rodent models, changes in hippocampal morphology were observed following chronic treatments of various doses with cannabinoid agonists like Δ9-THC and WIN55,212-2, these neuronal alterations correlated with behavioral dysfunction [30–32].

Preclinical studies which used rodent as animal models, utilized both maze-based and instrumental tasks for investigating the effect of cannabinoids on WM [31]. Maze-based tasks require the rodent to use spatial cues correctly. These tasks are based on the navigational behaviors of rodent for foraging or in order to escape from predators [104]. Several works have suggested that chronic treatment of Δ9-THC induced WM impairments on in different types of maze-based tasks [33,34] and in water maze tasks [35,36,38]. These impairments are dose-related, thus greater impairments were observed after exposures to more potent cannabinoid-agonists [36,41]. Therefore, it is not surprising that SC agonists such as JWH-081 and HU-210 induce similar disruptive effect on WM performances in maze-based tasks [37,39]. In addition, similar impairment is induced with anti-cholinergic agents like physostigmine, suggesting that cannabinoid-agonists induce WM impairments due to interaction with acetylcholine system [105].

Instrumental WM tasks in rodents include the delayed matching to sample (DMTS) or delayed non-matching to sample (DNMS) tasks. During these tasks, the animal is initially presented with a stimulus and following delay period, both the original stimulus and a novel stimulus are presented. The animal must indicate either the sample stimulus or the novel stimulus follow the task's rule [31]. The effects of chronic treatment with cannabinoid agonists such as WIN55212-2 and Δ9-THC on WM in DMTS or DNMS paradigms are widely observed, both in rodents [27,41,42,106] and in primate models [107,108]. Again, most of the studies report that the disruptive effects of cannabinoid agonists are dose-dependent [31].

Recently, Barbieri et al. (2016) reported that administration of a CB1 receptors antagonist AM251 to mice as pre-treatment, fully prevented the disruptive effects of cannabinoid agonists including JWH-018 and Δ9-THC on WM, thus suggesting a CB1 receptor involvement in the effect of cannabinoids on WM [43]. Other studies reported that repeated treatment with SC agonists JWH-018 and CP55,940 in the puberty period induced severe WM impairments that remained in adulthood [44,45]. These findings are consistent with previous theories which suggested the involvement of ECS in brain development and that consumption of cannabinoid agonists in adolescence alter the function of the ECS [24,32,109,110].

Interestingly, some studies report contrary results where reduced impairments following repeated treatment with cannabinoid agonists were presented [38], although, this might be a result of tolerance [31]. In addition, further preclinical research is needed to examine the degree of persistence of deficiencies induced by chronic treatments with cannabinoid agonists [31]. Yet, a growing number of publications indicate that exposures to cannabinoids in early age are associated with greater and persistent WM deficits, suggesting that the age of onset may be a mediating factor in the association between cannabinoids and WM performance [32,106,111–113].

### *4.5. Cannabinoids and Working Memory- Evidence from Clinical Studies*

The disrupted effect of acute cannabis intoxication on WM performance in humans is widely documented [33,87]; however, there is a growing debate whether chronic cannabinoid consumption induces long-term impairments of WM [87,114,115].

The most common paradigm for measuring WM performance is the n-back task. During this task a sequence of constant stimuli in form of digits, shapes or numbers are presented to the subject, who need to decide if the presented stimulus is identical to a previous stimulus from n steps earlier. The load factor n reflects different WM loads; lower n represents an easier task [116]. Kanayama and colleagues (2004) investigated WM in chronic cannabis users and used functional Magnetic Resonance Imaging (fMRI) [117]. They reported that cannabis users did not show WM dysfunction; however, increased activation of several brain regions including prefrontal-cortex, ACC and basal-ganglia regions were observed. The authors suggested that chronic consumption of cannabis induced subtle neurophysiological deficits which are compensated by hyper-activation to meet the demands of the task [117,118].

In addition, an fMRI study which focused on hippocampus activity during performance on the n-back task, compared cannabis users with two control groups of healthy individuals and tobacco smokers [119]. Poorer performance was observed in cannabis users compared with both control groups on the task's overall score. Furthermore, cannabis users presented less activity in the right hippocampus across the task's conditions contrary to both control groups [119]. In a further neuroimaging study, Jager et al. (2007) examined the effects of cannabis use on neuronal activity in abstained cannabis users and healthy control participants during performance on the n-back task consisting of encoding and recall conditions [120]. Similar to previous studies [121], there were no differences between the groups in terms of behavioral performance. Interestingly, cannabis users exhibited hypo-activation in the right dorso-lateral pre-frontal cortex and in bilateral hippocampus regions. This reduced activity in WM responsible areas were limited to the encoding phase and were not presented in the rest of the task phases' [120].

Smith and colleagues (2010) used fMRI to examine the neuronal brain activity of heavy cannabis users and control non-users while performing different loads of the n-back task. The two groups presented similar WM performance, however, in contrast to other studies, cannabis users demonstrated hyper-activity in the right frontal gyrus, left middle inferior frontal gyrus and right superior temporal gyrus [122]. In a recent systematic review, Bossong and colleagues (2014) suggested that most functional neuroimaging studies present similar pattern of hyper neuronal brain activity in cannabis users compared with control participants that were accompanied with normal WM function [123]. They support the view that increased activity reflects greater neural effort in order to maintain good task performance [123]. On the other hand, a-3-year longitudinal neuroimaging study failed to find behavioral or functional differences between cannabis users and control participants, suggesting that a moderate use of cannabis may not have substantial effects on WM neural network and behavioral performance [124]. However, WM deficits in chronic cannabis users are more likely to be elicited in complex conditions [115]. Therefore, a lack of differences in WM performance between cannabis users and control participants does not necessarily indicate a lack of association between chronic consumption of cannabis and WM [123].

Convergent evidence from structural neuroimaging studies supports the last view indicating that chronic consumption of cannabis is associated with neuronal alterations in several brain regions which are involved in WM including reduction in size of the hippocampus and amygdala. In addition, these alterations correlated with the amount of cannabis use and dependence [125]. Recently, Battistella et al. (2014) reported similar data, where neuronal alterations in several brain regions including the parahippocampal gyrus were observed in chronic cannabis users compared with occasional users.

Furthermore, these alterations are associated with age of onset and frequency of cannabis use in the last 3 months [126].

To our knowledge, there is a limited number of available laboratory human studies investigating the association between persistence consumption of SC with WM performance. Yet, Castellanos and Thornton (2011) reported that young adults who used SC drugs experienced alterations in short-term memory; however, their main symptom was a severe psychotic episode [127]. Further reports described similar clinical manifestations where SC users experienced symptoms including alterations in short-term memory [128,129]. Cohen et al. (2017) demonstrated WM impairments observed among SC users compared with non-users and recreational cannabis users [11]. These reports are not surprising since CB1 receptors are highly distributed in the hippocampus and in prefrontal cortical regions [130,131], which are associated with WM [102]. In addition, SC products contain high-potency cannabinoid agonists, therefore it is reasonable that chronic consumption of SC induces impairments in WM function in more salient forms than those which are induced by organic cannabis [66,67].

### 4.6. Cannabinoids and Cognitive Flexibility- Evidence from Preclinical Studies

Cognitive flexibility has been described as the cognitive ability to think about multiple concepts simultaneously and to be able to switch between thinking about two different concepts [18]. Miyake et al. (2000) identified cognitive flexibility as the ability to shift one's thinking and attention between unrelated tasks, typically in response to a change in environmental demands [81]. Diamond (2013) expanded the view of the term and suggested that an additional feature of cognitive flexibility is being able to change perspectives spatially or inter-personally. Accordingly, for changing perspectives, an individual needs to inhibit the last perspective and to load a new perspective into WM [77]. In that sense, cognitive flexibility builds and depends on WM and inhibition control. Other aspects of cognitive flexibility involve changing the way of thinking in response to external demands and thinking "outside the box" [77].

In rodents, variations of attention set-shifting paradigms are being used to assess behavioral flexibility. During these tasks rats are required to change behavioral responses, by learning new stimulus-reward associations through earlier learned response inhibition tendencies [13]. These paradigms differentiate between two types of behavioral flexibility; (a) for successful extra-dimensional shifts the rats need to shift attention bias between different features of stimuli, (b) reversal-learning discriminations required the rats to update relations between stimuli and rewards presentation, in this inter-dimensional discrimination based on cue from a single modality [13,83]. This differentiation is important since these two aspects of behavioral flexibility are linked with different brain regions [13], while reversal learning is associated with orbito-frontal cortex [132], extra-dimensional shifts are mediated by the medial pre-frontal cortex [133,134].

Several preclinical studies investigated the effects of cannabinoid-agonists on cognitive flexibility and indicated inconsistent results. Egerton and colleagues (2005) reported that acute administration of 5 mg/kg Δ9-THC induced impairments in reversal learning, whilst attention set shifting ability was maintained [46]. Further primate research presented similar results using smaller doses and demonstrated that an acute administration of 0.5 mg/kg Δ9-THC induced more errors in reversal learning and it did not affect attention set shifting ability [135].

However, an additional rodent study has demonstrated different findings, whereby administration of 0.2 mg/kg of the SC agonists HU-210 2 days before measuring set-shifting, induced dose-dependent impairments in extra-dimensional set shifting ability [47]. These impairments were diminished after administration of a CB1 antagonist AM251. In addition, cannabinoids did not affect inter-dimensional reversal learning [47].

Further evidence regarding the effects of cannabinoids on cognitive flexibility was demonstrated by Varvel and Lichtman (2001). Knockout mice, which lack cannabinoid CB1 receptors presented impaired reversal learning in inter-dimensional water maze reversal learning task [40]. Their findings support the view that the ECS are involved in execution of cognitive flexibility [13]. Consistent with earlier studies, Gomes and colleges (2015) recently indicated that rats which were repeatedly treated with 1.2 mg/kg of a CB1 agonist WIN55,212-2 for 2 weeks in adolescence, showed deficits in adulthood in performance of set-shifting tasks and alterations in dopamine levels in the ventral tegmental area. These alterations were present in adulthood and were similar to those which were shown in pre-clinical models of schizophrenia [136].

The conflicting results demonstrated by previous studies, reflect the need for further studies on the effect of cannabinoids on cognitive flexibility. The available evidence demonstrates that cannabinoids have indeed an effect on cognitive flexibility [13], possibly via modulation of dopamine and glutamate concentrations in several brain regions including the ACC and prefrontal cortex [13,83].

### *4.7. Cannabinoids and Cognitive Flexibility- Evidence from Clinical Studies*

Recent studies using fMRI have found a variety of brain regions that were activated while performing cognitive processes that demand flexibility, including, the pre-frontal cortex, basal ganglia, ACC and posterior parietal cortex [137]. Some of the regions which underlie cognitive flexibility are involved in WM and inhibition control and thus, the findings support the hypothesis that cognitive flexibility depends both on WM and inhibition control [81]. In addition, levels of certain neurotransmitters such as monoamines in several brain regions are associated with cognitive flexibility [138].

Paradigms for investigating cognitive flexibility include a wide array of task-switching and set-shifting tasks. One of the oldest and most common task for measuring this performance is the Wisconsin Card Sorting Task (WCST) [139]. In this task, a number of stimulus cards are sorted by color, shape or number. The participant is required to conclude the correct sorting criterion on the basis of feedback. Set-shifting ability is required when sorting criterion has been changed and perseverative errors are the outcome of failure in set-shifting [77]. Additional tasks for measuring cognitive flexibility include verbal fluency and semantic fluency. In these tasks participants are required to demonstrate unusual patterns of thinking by answering a serial of verbal questions (What is common between a fly and a tree?) in order to be successful [77].

Acute intoxication of cannabis has disruptive effects on cognitive flexibility [62,105,140]. However, the evidence on non-acute effects of cannabinoids on cognitive flexibility have been inconsistent. Bolla et al. (2002) reported dose-related effects of cannabis use on cognitive function. They have examined several aspects of cognitive function including cognitive flexibility in heavy cannabis users compared with moderate and occasional users who abstained from cannabis for 28 days. Poorer performance was positively correlated with increased frequency of cannabis consumption [61].

Later on, Pope et al. (2003) has reported similar effects, except that deficits in performance on the WCST were observed in heavy cannabis users who had started smoking cannabis during adolescence [141]. In addition, there were no differences in flexibility performance between cannabis users who had started using cannabis in adulthood compared with non-users [141]. A further study demonstrated that heavy cannabis users' performance on the WCST resemble those of schizophrenic patients; however, there was no association between frequency of cannabis use and errors on the WCST [142]. Contrary to the last results, several studies indicated that while repeated consumption of cannabis has disruptive effects on some cognitive functions, impairments in cognitive flexibility were not presented in heavy cannabis users even after controlling for demographic variables [143,144].

In a systematic meta-analysis, Grant and colleagues (2003) examined the non-acute effects of cannabis on several aspects of cognitive function using strict inclusion criteria on a limited number of studies. The authors failed to find significant non-acute effects of cannabis consumption on cognitive flexibility. However, it should be noted that cognitive flexibility was referred as a component within the factor of abstraction reasoning [145]. This methodological issue is critical since abstract reasoning and cognitive flexibility are different components of EF [77].

The evidence so far points out to a lack of available evidence regarding the effects of SC on cognitive flexibility in humans. Altintas et al. (2016) examined several cognitive domains in SC users who experienced psychotic episodes and compared their performance with hospitalized schizophrenic patients. Interestingly, there were no differences between the groups in cognitive flexibility measurement [146]. Yet, their results cannot be interpreted as an outcome of SC use exclusively since it cannot be differentiated from psychotic symptoms that were observed among SC users as well. There are two additional aspects of the association between cannabinoid abuse and cognitive flexibility which should be noted. First, impairments in cognitive flexibility have been suggested to play a major role in continuous use of cannabinoids despite negative consequences [83]. Secondly, deficits in cognitive flexibility were associated with affective alterations [147]. Both greater mood alterations and greater rates of abuse are commonly observed among SC users and heavy cannabis users [9,148].

In summary, both pre-clinical and clinical findings suggest that the ECS are involved in cognitive flexibility [13]. Although, there are inconsistent findings in human studies, the non-acute disruptive effect of cannabinoids on cognitive flexibility is probably mediated by several factors including the age of onset and the frequency of cannabinoid consumption [58,141], yet, further exploration of the last relation is required.

## 5. Conclusions

Cannabinoid drugs, in both organic and synthetic forms became increasingly popular despite the potential harms associated with their use [6,10,87]. While the main psychoactive ingredient of cannabis is the CB1 receptor partial-agonist Δ9-THC [13,51–53], SC drugs contain varied types of cannabinoid-agonists which are more potent than organic cannabinoids [65,149]. Although SC and organic cannabinoids bind to the same CB receptors, the psychotropic effects of SC are more severe, more rigid and much more unpredictable than those induced by organic cannabinoids [4,5,65,75]. Taking into account the above evidence that SC drugs do not contain CBD, their harm potential is significant [5,75,114].

Taking together the recent finding of both animal and human studies, repeated consumption of cannabinoids is associated with EF impairments, yet, there is still a gap of knowledge regarding the last of these impairments [11,114]. The available data from both animal and human studies suggest that ECS involve and effect cognitive functions in general and EF specifically [9,10,12,13,83]. The ECS has a major role in neurodevelopmental and maturational process, which are especially prevalent during adolescence. Consumption of exogenous cannabinoids affect the functioning of the ECS, it is plausible that chronic consumption during early adolescence alters the neurodevelopmental maturational process during this period [5]. Consequently, it is not surprising that current evidence suggests that exposure to cannabinoids during the adolescent period may induce severe long-lasting cognitive impairments [5,78,96,108,147,148]. Furthermore, most of the current evidence indicates an association between the amount of cannabinoid consumption with the degree of impairment; more consumption, or consumption of drugs which contain more potent cannabinoids is associated with greater impairments [5,83,87]. Accordingly, although there is a limited number of human studies which examine both the acute and long-term effect of SCs on EF, it is reasonable to assume that SC which contain extremely potent cannabinoid-agonists may induce long-term EF-impairments [5–8]. Yet, further research is needed to expend to knowledge of the last phenomena.

It is important to note some of the limitations of the current review. Most of the available evidence regarding the effects of SCs on EF is based on pre-clinical studies. When interpreting these results, it is important to take into account that the methodological limitations which animal studies naturally hold. Firstly, while cannabis or SC users mostly use these drugs by smoking or inhaling [1,3,7], most of the pre-clinical studies mentioned in this review treated animals by intraperitoneal (I.P) injection which in contrast to inhaling induce greater effect in shorter time [9,32]. Furthermore, it is important to take into account that most of the mentioned pre-clinical studies have used specific SCs or pure Δ9-THC for exploring their exclusive effect on a chosen factor [3,9,32]. In contrast to that, evidence from epidemiological data or human studies present information regarding the effects of SC or cannabis products which mostly contain a range of cannabinoids and in some cases additional psychoactive compounds [1,3,7,9,32].

Understanding the effects of cannabinoids on EF has considerable practical utility in the clinical setting. Executive function is essential to an individual's multiple abilities in daily life [77]. It has been suggested that due to impaired EF, patients may have difficulties in learning new coping behaviors and accordingly increases the likelihood of treatment dropout and poor treatment outcomes [12]. Therefore, the current review emphasizes the need of attention by the clinician regarding cognitive abilities of patients who suffer from cannabinoid abuse. In case of cognitive impairments, an alternative unique therapeutic method should be considered such as behavioral therapy [150] or introducing the patient with cognitive rehabilitation strategies [12]. This may be crucial, especially in cases of patients who are heavy cannabinoid users, or young patients who used cannabinoids in early age for persistent periods.

**Acknowledgments:** This study was partly funded by a grant from the National Institute for Psychobiology in Israel to Aviv Weinstein. The study is a part of a Ph.D thesis of Koby Cohen who is funded by a grant from Ariel University.

**Author Contributions:** Koby Cohen and Aviv Weinstein contributed substantially to the conception and design of the review. All the authors contributed to further drafts of the manuscript, critically revised and approved the final version of the manuscript.

## References

1. Hall, W.; Degenhardt, L. Adverse health effects of non-medical cannabis use. *Lancet* **2009**, *374*, 1383–1391. [CrossRef]
2. UNODC. World drug report 2014. Available online: https://www.unodc.org/documents/wdr2014/World_Drug_Report_2014_web.pdf (accessed on 28 October 2017).
3. Iversen, L. Long-term effects of exposure to cannabis. *Curr. Opin. Pharmacol.* **2005**, *5*, 69–72. [CrossRef] [PubMed]
4. Volkow, N.D.; Swanson, J.M.; Evins, A.E.; DeLisi, L.E.; Meier, M.H.; Gonzalez, R.; Baler, R. Effects of cannabis use on human behavior, including cognition, motivation and psychosis: A review. *JAMA Psychiatry* **2016**, *73*, 292–297. [CrossRef] [PubMed]
5. Curran, H.V.; Freeman, T.P.; Mokrysz, C.; Lewis, D.A.; Morgan, C.J.; Parsons, L.H. Keep off the grass? Cannabis, cognition and addiction. *Nat. Rev. Neurosci.* **2016**, *17*, 293–306. [CrossRef] [PubMed]
6. Fattore, L.; Fratta, W. Beyond THC: The new generation of cannabinoid designer drugs. *Front. Behav. Neurosci.* **2011**, *5*, 60. [CrossRef] [PubMed]
7. Spaderna, M.; Addy, P.H.; D'Souza, D.C. Spicing things up: Synthetic cannabinoids. *Psychopharmacology* **2013**, *228*, 525–540. [CrossRef] [PubMed]
8. Weinstein, A.M.; Rosca, P.; Fattore, L.; London, E.D. Synthetic Cathinone and Cannabinoid Designer Drugs Pose a Major Risk for Public Health. *Front. Psychiatry* **2017**, *8*, 156. [CrossRef] [PubMed]
9. Castaneto, M.S.; Gorelick, D.A.; Desrosiers, N.A.; Hartman, R.L.; Pirard, S.; Huestis, M.A. Synthetic cannabinoids: Epidemiology, pharmacodynamics and clinical implications. *Drug Alcohol Depend.* **2014**, *144*, 12–41. [PubMed]
10. Papanti, D.; Schifano, F.; Botteon, G.; Bertossi, F.; Mannix, J.; Vidoni, D.; Bonavigo, T. "Spiceophrenia": A systematic overview of "Spice"-related psychopathological issues and a case report. *Hum. Psychopharmacol.* **2013**, *28*, 379–389. [CrossRef] [PubMed]
11. Cohen, K.; Kapitány-Fövény, M.; Mama, Y.; Arieli, M.; Rosca, P.; Demetrovics, Z.; Weinstein, A. The effects of synthetic cannabinoids on executive function. *Psychopharmacology* **2017**, *234*, 1121–1134. [CrossRef] [PubMed]
12. Crean, R.D.; Crane, N.A.; Mason, B.J. An evidence based review of acute and long-term effects of cannabis use on executive cognitive functions. *J. Addict. Med.* **2011**, *5*, 1–8. [CrossRef] [PubMed]
13. Pattij, T.; Wiskerke, J.; Schoffelmeer, A.N.M. Cannabinoid modulation of executive functions. *Eur. J. Pharmacol.* **2008**, *585*, 458–463. [CrossRef] [PubMed]

14. Miller, R.L.A.; Thakur, G.A.; Stewart, W.N.; Bow, J.P.; Bajaj, S.; Makriyannis, A.; McLaughlin, P.J. Effects of a novel CB1 agonist on visual attention in male rats: Role of strategy and expectancy in task accuracy. *Exp. Clin. Psychopharmacol.* **2013**, *21*, 416–425. [CrossRef] [PubMed]
15. Müller, H.; Sperling, W.; Köhrmann, M.; Huttner, H.B.; Kornhuber, J.; Maler, J.M. The synthetic cannabinoid Spice as a trigger for an acute exacerbation of cannabis induced recurrent psychotic episodes. *Schizophr. Res.* **2010**, *118*, 309–310. [CrossRef] [PubMed]
16. Ustundag, M.F.; Ozhan Ibis, E.; Yucel, A.; Ozcan, H. Synthetic cannabis-induced mania. *Case Rep. Psychiatry* **2015**. [CrossRef] [PubMed]
17. Ehrenreich, H.; Rinn, T.; Kunert, H.J.; Moeller, M.R.; Poser, W.; Schilling, L.; Hoehe, M.R. Specific attentional dysfunction in adults following early start of cannabis use. *Psychopharmacology* **1999**, *142*, 295–301. [CrossRef] [PubMed]
18. Scott, W.A. Cognitive complexity and cognitive flexibility. *Sociometry* **1962**, *25*, 405–414. [CrossRef]
19. Thames, A.D.; Arbid, N.; Sayegh, P. Cannabis use and neurocognitive functioning in a non-clinical sample of users. *Addict. Behav.* **2014**, *39*, 994–999. [CrossRef] [PubMed]
20. Solowij, N.; Michie, P.T. Cannabis and cognitive dysfunction: Parallels with endophenotypes of schizophrenia? *J. Psychiatry Neurosci.* **2007**, *32*, 30. [PubMed]
21. Howlett, A.C.; Barth, F.; Bonner, T.I.; Cabral, G.; Casellas, P.; Devane, W.A.; Martin, B.R. International Union of Pharmacology. XXVII. Classification of cannabinoid receptors. *Pharmacol. Rev.* **2002**, *54*, 161–202. [CrossRef] [PubMed]
22. Lewin, A.H.; Seltzman, H.H.; Carroll, F.I.; Mascarella, S.W.; Reddy, P.A. Emergence and properties of spice and bath salts: A medicinal chemistry perspective. *Life Sci.* **2014**, *97*, 9–19. [CrossRef] [PubMed]
23. Di Marzo, V.; Petrocellis, L.D. Plant, synthetic and endogenous cannabinoids in medicine. *Ann. Rev. Med.* **2006**, *57*, 553–574. [CrossRef] [PubMed]
24. Pacher, P.; Bátkai, S.; Kunos, G. The endocannabinoid system as an emerging target of pharmacotherapy. *Pharmacol. Rev.* **2006**, *58*, 389–462. [CrossRef] [PubMed]
25. Zawilska, J.B. Legal highs": New players in the old drama. *Curr. Drug Abuse. Rev.* **2011**, *4*, 122–130. [CrossRef] [PubMed]
26. Arguello, P.A.; Jentsch, J.D. Cannabinoid CB1 receptor-mediated impairment of visuospatial attention in the rat. *Psychopharmacology* **2004**, *177*, 141–150. [CrossRef] [PubMed]
27. Hampson, R.E.; Deadwyler, S.A. Cannabinoids reveal the necessity of hippocampal neural encoding for short-term memory in rats. *J. Neurosci.* **2000**, *20*, 8932–8942. [PubMed]
28. Verrico, C.D.; Jentsch, J.D.; Roth, R.H.; Taylor, J.R. Repeated, Intermittent-Tetrahydrocannabinol Administration to Rats Impairs Acquisition and Performance of a Test of Visuospatial Divided Attention. *Neuropsychopharmacology* **2004**, *29*, 522–529. [CrossRef] [PubMed]
29. Presburger, G.; Robinson, J.K. Spatial signal detection in rats is differentially disrupted by Δ-9-tetrahydrocannabinol, scopolamine and MK-801. *Behav. Brain Res.* **1999**, *99*, 27–34. [CrossRef]
30. Lawston, J.; Borella, A.; Robinson, J.K.; Whitaker-Azmitia, P.M. Changes in hippocampal morphology following chronic treatment with the synthetic cannabinoid WIN 55,212-2. *Brain Res.* **2000**, *877*, 407–410. [CrossRef]
31. Winsauer, P.J.; Daniel, J.M.; Filipeanu, C.M.; Leonard, S.T.; Hulst, J.L.; Rodgers, S.P.; Sutton, J.L. Long-term behavioral and pharmacodynamic effects of delta-9-tetrahydrocannabinol in female rats depend on ovarian hormone status. *Addict. Biol.* **2011**, *16*, 64–81. [CrossRef] [PubMed]
32. Abush, H.; Akirav, I. Short- and Long-Term Cognitive Effects of Chronic Cannabinoids Administration in Late-Adolescence Rats. *PLoS ONE* **2012**, *7*, e31731. [CrossRef] [PubMed]
33. Jentsch, J.D.; Andrusiak, E.; Tran, A.; Bowers, M.B.; Roth, R.H. Δ 9-Tetrahydrocannabinol increases prefrontal cortical catecholaminergic utilization and impairs spatial working memory in the rat: Blockade of dopaminergic effects with HA966. *Neuropsychopharmacology* **1997**, *16*, 426–432. [CrossRef]
34. Nava, F.; Carta, G.; Battasi, A.M.; Gessa, G.L. D2 dopamine receptors enable Δ9-tetrahydrocannabinol induced memory impairment and reduction of hippocampal extracellular acetylcholine concentration. *Br. J. Pharmacol.* **2000**, *130*, 1201–1210. [CrossRef] [PubMed]
35. Nava, F.; Carta, G.; Colombo, G.; Gessa, G.L. Effects of chronic Δ 9-tetrahydrocannabinol treatment on hippocampal extracellular acetylcholine concentration and alternation performance in the T-maze. *Neuropharmacology* **2001**, *41*, 392–399. [CrossRef]

36. Fadda, P.; Robinson, L.; Fratta, W.; Pertwee, R.G.; Riedel, G. Differential effects of THC-or CBD-rich cannabis extracts on working memory in rats. *Neuropharmacology* **2004**, *47*, 1170–1179. [CrossRef] [PubMed]
37. Basavarajappa, B.S.; Subbanna, S. CB1 receptor-mediated signaling underlies the hippocampal synaptic, learning and memory deficits following treatment with JWH-081, a new component of spice/K2 preparations. *Hippocampus* **2014**, *24*, 178–188. [CrossRef] [PubMed]
38. Hill, M.N.; Froc, D.J.; Fox, C.J.; Gorzalka, B.B.; Christie, B.R. Prolonged cannabinoid treatment results in spatial working memory deficits and impaired long-term potentiation in the CA1 region of the hippocampus in vivo. *Eur. J. Neurosci.* **2004**, *20*, 859–863. [CrossRef] [PubMed]
39. Ferrari, F.; Ottani, A.; Vivoli, R.; Giuliani, D. Learning impairment produced in rats by the cannabinoid agonist HU 210 in a water-maze task. *Pharmacol. Biochem. Behav.* **1999**, *64*, 555–561. [CrossRef]
40. Varvel, S.; Hamm, R.; Martin, B.; Lichtman, A. Differential effects of Δ9-THC on spatial reference and working memory in mice. *Psychopharmacology* **2001**, *157*, 142–150. [PubMed]
41. Miyamoto, A.; Yamamoto, T.; Watanabe, S. Effect of repeated administration of Δ 9-tetrahydrocannabinol on delayed matching-to-sample performance in rats. *Neurosci. Lett.* **1995**, *201*, 139–142. [CrossRef]
42. Mallet, P.E.; Beninger, R.J. The cannabinoid CB1 receptor antagonist SR141716A attenuates the memory impairment produced by Δ9-tetrahydrocannabinol or anandamide. *Psychopharmacology* **1998**, *140*, 11–19. [CrossRef] [PubMed]
43. Barbieri, M.; Ossato, A.; Canazza, I.; Trapella, C.; Borelli, A.C.; Beggiato, S.; Marti, M. Synthetic cannabinoid JWH-018 and its halogenated derivatives JWH-018-Cl and JWH-018-Br impair novel object recognition in mice: Behavioral, electrophysiological and neurochemical evidence. *Neuropharmacology* **2016**, *109*, 254–269. [CrossRef] [PubMed]
44. Compton, D.M.; Megan, S.; Grant, P.; Brian, G.; Chris, W.; Ross, D. Adolescent exposure of JWH-018 "Spice" produces subtle effects on learning and memory performance in adulthood. *J. Behav. Brain Sci.* **2012**, *2*, 146–155. [CrossRef]
45. Renard, J.; Krebs, M.O.; Jay, T.M.; Le Pen, G. Long-term cognitive impairments induced by chronic cannabinoid exposure during adolescence in rats: A strain comparison. *Psychopharmacology* **2013**, *225*, 781–790. [CrossRef] [PubMed]
46. Egerton, A.; Brett, R.R.; Pratt, J.A. Acute Δ9-tetrahydrocannabinol-induced deficits in reversal learning: Neural correlates of affective inflexibility. *Neuropsychopharmacology* **2005**, *30*, 1895–1905. [CrossRef] [PubMed]
47. Hill, M.N.; Froese, L.M.; Morrish, A.C.; Sun, J.C.; Floresco, S.B. Alterations in behavioral flexibility by cannabinoid CB1 receptor agonists and antagonists. *Psychopharmacology* **2006**, *187*, 245–259. [CrossRef] [PubMed]
48. Kevin, R.C.; Wood, K.E.; Stuart, J.; Mitchell, A.J.; Moir, M.; Banister, S.D.; McGregor, I.S. Acute and residual effects in adolescent rats resulting from exposure to the novel synthetic cannabinoids AB-PINACA and AB-FUBINACA. *J. Psychopharmacol.* **2017**, *31*, 757–769. [CrossRef] [PubMed]
49. Kirschmann, E.K.; McCalley, D.M.; Edwards, C.M.; Torregrossa, M.M. Consequences of Adolescent Exposure to the Cannabinoid Receptor Agonist WIN55, 212-2 on Working Memory in Female Rats. *Front. Behav. Neurosci.* **2017**, *11*, 137. [CrossRef] [PubMed]
50. Kirschmann, E.K.; Pollock, M.W.; Nagarajan, V.; Torregrossa, M.M. Effects of adolescent cannabinoid self-administration in rats on addiction-related behaviors and working memory. *Neuropsychopharmacology* **2017**, *42*, 989. [CrossRef] [PubMed]
51. Hall, W.; Solowij, N. Adverse effects of cannabis. *Lancet* **1998**, *352*, 1611–1616. [CrossRef]
52. Ashton, C.H. Pharmacology and effects of cannabis: A brief review. *Br. J. Psychiatry* **2001**, *178*, 101–106. [CrossRef]
53. Gaoni, Y.; Mechoulam, R. Isolation, structure and partial synthesis of an active constituent of hashish. *J. Am. Chem. Soc.* **1964**, *86*, 1646–1647. [CrossRef]
54. Huffman, J.W.; Bushell, S.M.; Miller, J.R.A.; Wiley, J.L.; Martin, B.R. 1-Methoxy-, 1-deoxy-11-hydroxy-and 11-hydroxy-1-methoxy-Δ 8-tetrahydrocannabinols: New selective ligands for the CB 2 receptor. *Bioorgan. Med. Chem.* **2002**, *10*, 4119–4129. [CrossRef]
55. Pertwee, R.G. Pharmacological actions of cannabinoids. In *Handbook of Experimental Pharmacology*; Pertwee, R.G., Ed.; Springer: New York, NY, USA, 2005; Volume 168, pp. 1–51.

56. Rhee, M.H.; Vogel, Z.; Barg, J.; Bayewitch, M.; Levy, R.; Hanuš, L.; Mechoulam, R. Cannabinol derivatives: Binding to cannabinoid receptors and inhibition of adenylylcyclase. *J. Med. Chem.* **1997**, *40*, 3228–3233. [CrossRef] [PubMed]
57. Lorenzetti, V.; Solowij, N.; Yücel, M. The role of cannabinoids on neuroanatomical alterations in cannabis users. *Biol. Psychiatry* **2015**, *79*, 17–31. [CrossRef] [PubMed]
58. Mechoulam, R.; Peters, M.; Murillo-Rodriguez, E.; Hanuš, L.O. Cannabidiol–recent advances. *Chem. Biodivers.* **2007**, *4*, 1678–1692. [CrossRef] [PubMed]
59. Iseger, T.A.; Bossong, M.G. A systematic review of the antipsychotic properties of cannabidiol in humans. *Schizophr. Res.* **2015**, *162*, 153–161. [CrossRef] [PubMed]
60. Colizzi, M.; Bhattacharyya, S. Does Cannabis Composition Matter? Differential Effects of Delta-9-tetrahydrocannabinol and Cannabidiol on Human Cognition. *Curr. Addict. Rep.* **2017**, *4*, 62–74. [CrossRef] [PubMed]
61. Bolla, K.I.; Brown, K.; Eldreth, D.; Tate, K.; Cadet, J.L. Dose-related neurocognitive effects of marijuana use. *Neurology* **2002**, *59*, 1337–1343. [CrossRef] [PubMed]
62. Curran, V.H.; Brignell, C.; Fletcher, S.; Middleton, P.; Henry, J. Cognitive and subjective dose-response effects of acute oral Δ9-tetrahydrocannabinol (THC) in infrequent cannabis users. *Psychopharmacology* **2002**, *164*, 61–70. [CrossRef] [PubMed]
63. D'Souza, D.C.; Fridberg, D.J.; Skosnik, P.D.; Williams, A.; Roach, B.; Singh, N.; Pittman, B. Dose-related modulation of event-related potentials to novel and target stimuli by intravenous Δ9-THC in humans. *Neuropsychopharmacology* **2012**, *37*, 1632–1646. [CrossRef] [PubMed]
64. Adams, I.B.; Martin, B.R. Cannabis: Pharmacology and toxicology in animals and humans. *Addiction* **1996**, *91*, 1585–1614. [CrossRef] [PubMed]
65. Pacher, P.; Kunos, G. Modulating the endocannabinoid system in human health and disease–successes and failures. *FEBS J.* **2013**, *280*, 1918–1943. [CrossRef] [PubMed]
66. Seely, K.A.; Lapoint, J.; Moran, J.H.; Fattore, L. Spice drugs are more than harmless herbal blends: A review of the pharmacology and toxicology of synthetic cannabinoids. *Prog. Neuro-Psychopharmacol. Biol. Psychiatry* **2012**, *39*, 234–243. [CrossRef] [PubMed]
67. Seely, K.A.; Prather, P.L.; James, L.P.; Moran, J.H. Marijuana-based drugs: Innovative therapeutics or designer drugs of abuse? *Mol. Interv.* **2011**, *11*, 36. [CrossRef] [PubMed]
68. Fattore, L. Synthetic cannabinoids—further evidence supporting the relationship between cannabinoids and psychosis. *Biol. Psychiatry* **2016**, *79*, 539–548. [CrossRef] [PubMed]
69. Pertwee, R.G. Novel pharmacological targets for cannabinoids. *Curr. Neuropharmacol.* **2004**, *2*, 9–29. [CrossRef]
70. Weinstein, A.; Livny, A.; Weizman, A. Brain imaging studies on the cognitive, pharmacological and neurobiological effects of cannabis in humans: Evidence from studies of adult users. *Curr. Pharm. Design* **2016**, *22*, 6366–6379. [CrossRef] [PubMed]
71. Huffman, J.W.; Dai, D.; Martin, B.R.; Compton, D.R. Design, synthesis and pharmacology of cannabimimetic indoles. *Bioorg. Med. Chem. Lett.* **1994**, *4*, 563–566. [CrossRef]
72. Loeffler, G.; Hurst, D.; Penn, A.; Yung, K. Spice, bath salts and the US military: The emergence of synthetic cannabinoid receptor agonists and cathinones in the US Armed Forces. *Milit. Med.* **2012**, *177*, 1041–1048. [CrossRef]
73. Hazekamp, A.; Ware, M.A.; Muller-Vahl, K.R.; Abrams, D.; Grotenhermen, F. The medicinal use of cannabis and cannabinoids—an international cross-sectional survey on administration forms. *J. Psychoact. Drugs* **2013**, *45*, 199–210. [CrossRef] [PubMed]
74. Mechoulam, R.; Feigenbaum, J.J.; Lander, N.; Segal, M.; Järbe, T.U.C.; Hiltunen, A.J.; Consroe, P. Enantiomeric cannabinoids: Stereospecificity of psychotropic activity. *Cell. Mol. Life Sci.* **1988**, *44*, 762–764. [CrossRef]
75. Van Amsterdam, J.; Brunt, T.; van den Brink, W. The adverse health effects of synthetic cannabinoids with emphasis on psychosis-like effects. *J. Psychopharmacol.* **2015**, *29*, 254–263. [CrossRef] [PubMed]
76. Snyder, H.R.; Miyake, A.; Hankin, B.L. Advancing understanding of executive function impairments and psychopathology: Bridging the gap between clinical and cognitive approaches. *Front. Psychol.* **2015**, *6*, 1–24. [CrossRef] [PubMed]
77. Diamond, A. Executive functions. *Ann. Rev. Psychol.* **2013**, *64*, 135–168. [CrossRef] [PubMed]
78. Burgess, P.W.; Veitch, E.; Costello, A.D.; Shallice, T. The cognitive and neuroanatomical correlates of multitasking. *Neuropsychologia* **2000**, *38*, 848–863. [CrossRef]

79. Chan, R.C.K.; Shum, D.; Toulopoulou, T.; Chen, E.Y.H. Assessment of executive functions: Review of instruments and identification of critical issues. *Arch. Clin. Neuropsychol.* **2008**, *23*, 201–216. [CrossRef] [PubMed]
80. Hofmann, W.; Schmeichel, B.J.; Baddeley, A.D. Executive functions and self-regulation. *Trends Cogn. Sci.* **2012**, *16*, 174–180. [CrossRef] [PubMed]
81. Miyake, A.; Friedman, N.P.; Emerson, M.J.; Witzki, A.H.; Howerter, A.; Wager, T.D. The unity and diversity of executive functions and their contributions to complex "frontal lobe" tasks: A latent variable analysis. *Cogn. Psychol.* **2000**, *41*, 49–100. [CrossRef] [PubMed]
82. Funahashi, S. Neuronal mechanisms of executive control by the prefrontal cortex. *Neurosci. Res.* **2001**, *39*, 147–165. [CrossRef]
83. Egerton, A.; Allison, C.; Brett, R.R.; Pratt, J.A. Cannabinoids and prefrontal cortical function: Insights from preclinical studies. *Neurosci. Biobehav. Rev.* **2006**, *30*, 680–695. [CrossRef] [PubMed]
84. Burk, J.A.; Mair, R.G. Effects of intralaminar thalamic lesions on sensory attention and motor intention in the rat: A comparison with lesions involving frontal cortex and hippocampus. *Behav. Brain Res.* **2001**, *123*, 49–63. [CrossRef]
85. Christakou, A.; Robbins, T.W.; Everitt, B.J. Functional disconnection of a prefrontal cortical–dorsal striatal system disrupts choice reaction time performance: Implications for attentional function. *Behav. Neurosci.* **2001**, *115*, 812. [CrossRef] [PubMed]
86. Diana, M.; Melis, M.; Muntoni, A.L.; Gessa, G.L. Mesolimbic dopaminergic decline after cannabinoid withdrawal. *Proc. Natl. Acad. Sci. USA* **1998**, *95*, 10269–10273. [CrossRef] [PubMed]
87. Broyd, S.J.; van Hell, H.H.; Beale, C.; Yücel, M.; & Solowij, N. Acute and chronic effects of cannabinoids on human cognition—a systematic review. *Biol. Psychiatry* **2016**, *79*, 557–567. [CrossRef] [PubMed]
88. Ramaekers, J.G.; Kauert, G.; van Ruitenbeek, P.; Theunissen, E.L.; Schneider, E.; Moeller, M.R. High-potency marijuana impairs executive function and inhibitory motor control. *Neuropsychopharmacology* **2006**, *31*, 2296–2303. [CrossRef] [PubMed]
89. Dougherty, D.M.; Mathias, C.W.; Dawes, M.A.; Furr, R.M.; Charles, N.E.; Liguori, A.; Acheson, A. Impulsivity, attention, memory and decision-making among adolescent marijuana users. *Psychopharmacology* **2013**, *226*, 307–319. [CrossRef] [PubMed]
90. Lisdahl, K.M.; Price, J.S. Increased marijuana use and gender predict poorer cognitive functioning in adolescents and emerging adults. *J. Int. Neuropsychol. Soc.* **2012**, *18*, 678–688. [CrossRef] [PubMed]
91. Battisti, R.A.; Roodenrys, S.; Johnstone, S.J.; Pesa, N.; Hermens, D.F.; Solowij, N. Chronic cannabis users show altered neurophysiological functioning on Stroop task conflict resolution. *Psychopharmacology* **2010**, *212*, 613–624. [CrossRef] [PubMed]
92. Batalla, A.; Bhattacharyya, S.; Yücel, M.; Fusar-Poli, P.; Crippa, J.A.; Nogué, S.; Martin-Santos, R. Structural and functional imaging studies in chronic cannabis users: A systematic review of adolescent and adult findings. *PLoS ONE* **2013**, *8*, e55821. [CrossRef] [PubMed]
93. MacLeod, C.M. Half a century of research on the Stroop effect: An integrative review. *Psychol. Bull.* **1991**, *109*, 163–203. [CrossRef] [PubMed]
94. Nosek, B.A.; Banaji, M.R. The go/no-go association task. *Soc. Cogn.* **2001**, *19*, 625–666. [CrossRef]
95. Eldreth, D.A.; Matochik, J.A.; Cadet, J.L.; Bolla, K.I. Abnormal brain activity in prefrontal brain regions in abstinent marijuana users. *Neuroimage* **2004**, *23*, 914–920. [CrossRef] [PubMed]
96. Jager, G.; Kahn, R.S.; Van Den Brink, W.; Van Ree, J.M.; Ramsey, N.F. Long-term effects of frequent cannabis use on working memory and attention: An fMRI study. *Psychopharmacology* **2006**, *185*, 358–368. [CrossRef] [PubMed]
97. Hatchard, T.; Fried, P.A.; Hogan, M.J.; Cameron, I.; Smith, A.M. Marijuana Use Impacts Cognitive Interference: An fMRI Investigation in Young Adults Performing the Counting Stroop Task. *J. Addict. Res. Therapy* **2014**, *5*, 197–203. [CrossRef]
98. Hester, R.; Nestor, L.; Garavan, H. Impaired error awareness and anterior cingulate cortex hypoactivity in chronic cannabis users. *Neuropsychopharmacology* **2009**, *34*, 2450–2458. [CrossRef] [PubMed]
99. Zimmermann, U.S.; Winkelmann, P.R.; Pilhatsch, M.; Nees, J.A.; Spanagel, R.; Schulz, K. Withdrawal phenomena and dependence syndrome after the consumption of "spice gold". *Dtsch. Arztebl. Int.* **2009**, *106*, 464–467. [PubMed]
100. Nacca, N.; Vatti, D.; Sullivan, R.; Sud, P.; Su, M.; Marraffa, J. The synthetic cannabinoid withdrawal syndrome. *J. Addict. Med.* **2013**, *7*, 296–298. [CrossRef] [PubMed]

101. Baddeley, A.D.; Hitch, G.J. Working memory. In *The psychology of learning and motivation*; Bower, G.H., Ed.; Academic Press: New York, NY, USA, 1974; Volume 8, pp. 47–89.
102. Owen, A.M.; McMillan, K.M.; Laird, A.R.; Bullmore, E. N-back working memory paradigm: A meta-analysis of normative functional neuroimaging studies. *Hum. Brain Mapp.* **2005**, *25*, 46–59. [CrossRef] [PubMed]
103. Goldman-Rakic, P.S. Architecture of the prefrontal cortex and the central executive. *Ann. N. Y. Acad. Sci.* **1995**, *769*, 71–83. [CrossRef] [PubMed]
104. Olton, D.S. The radial arm maze as a tool in behavioral pharmacology. *Physiol. Behav.* **1987**, *40*, 793–797. [CrossRef]
105. Weinstein, A.; Brickner, O.; Lerman, H.; Greemland, M.; Bloch, M.; Lester, H.; Bar-Hamburger, R. A study investigating the acute dose—response effects of 13 mg and 17 mg Δ 9-tetrahydrocannabinol on cognitive—motor skills, subjective and autonomic measures in regular users of marijuana. *J. Psychopharmacol.* **2008**, *22*, 441–451. [CrossRef] [PubMed]
106. Kevin, R.C.; Lefever, T.W.; Snyder, R.W.; Patel, P.R.; Fennell, T.R.; Wiley, J.L.; Thomas, B.F. In vitro and in vivo pharmacokinetics and metabolism of synthetic cannabinoids CUMYL-PICA and 5F-CUMYL-PICA. *Forensic Toxicol.* **2017**, *35*, 333–347. [CrossRef] [PubMed]
107. Schulze, G.E.; McMillan, D.E.; Bailey, J.R.; Scallet, A.; Ali, S.F.; Slikker, W.; Paule, M.G. Acute effects of delta-9-tetrahydrocannabinol in rhesus monkeys as measured by performance in a battery of complex operant tests. *J. Pharmacol. Exp. Ther.* **1988**, *245*, 178–186. [PubMed]
108. Winsauer, P.J.; Lambert, P.; Moerschbaecher, J.M. Cannabinoid ligands and their effects on learning and performance in rhesus monkeys. *Behavi. Pharmacol.* **1999**, *10*, 497–511. [CrossRef]
109. Devane, W.A.; Dysarz, F.A.; Johnson, M.R.; Melvin, L.S.; Howlett, A.C. Determination and characterization of a cannabinoid receptor in rat brain. *Mol. Pharmacol.* **1988**, *34*, 605–613. [PubMed]
110. Burns, J.K. Pathways from cannabis to psychosis: A review of the evidence. *Front. Psychiatry* **2012**, *4*, 1–12. [CrossRef] [PubMed]
111. Castellanos, D.; Gralnik, L.M. Synthetic cannabinoids 2015: An update for pediatricians in clinical practice. *World J. Clin. Pediatr.* **2016**, *5*, 16. [CrossRef] [PubMed]
112. Kirschmann, E.; Pollock, M.; Nagarajan, V.; Torregrossa, M.M. Addiction-like and cognitive effects of adolescent cannabinoid self-administration in rats. *Drug Alcohol Depend.* **2017**, *171*, e105. [CrossRef]
113. Tomas-Roig, J.; Benito, E.; Agis-Balboa, R.C.; Piscitelli, F.; Hoyer-Fender, S.; Di Marzo, V.; Havemann-Reinecke, U. Chronic exposure to cannabinoids during adolescence causes long-lasting behavioral deficits in adult mice. *Addict. Biol.* **2016**. [CrossRef] [PubMed]
114. Lorenzetti, V.; Alonso-Lana, S.; J Youssef, G.; Verdejo-Garcia, A.; Suo, C.; Cousijn, J.; Solowij, N. Adolescent cannabis use: What is the evidence for functional brain alteration? *Curr. Pharm. Design* **2016**, *22*, 6353–6365. [CrossRef] [PubMed]
115. Solowij, N.; Battisti, R. The chronic effects of cannabis on memory in humans: A review. *Curr. Drug Abuse Rev.* **2008**, *1*, 81–98. [CrossRef] [PubMed]
116. Jaeggi, S.M.; Buschkuehl, M.; Perrig, W.J.; Meier, B. The concurrent validity of the N-back task as a working memory measure. *Memory* **2010**, *18*, 394–412. [CrossRef] [PubMed]
117. Kanayama, G.; Rogowska, J.; Pope, H.G.; Gruber, S.A.; Yurgelun-Todd, D.A. Spatial working memory in heavy cannabis users: A functional magnetic resonance imaging study. *Psychopharmacology* **2004**, *176*, 239–247. [CrossRef] [PubMed]
118. Jacobsen, L.K.; Mencl, W.E.; Westerveld, M.; Pugh, K.R. Impact of cannabis use on brain function in adolescents. *Ann. N. Y. Acad. Sci.* **2004**, *1021*, 384–390. [CrossRef] [PubMed]
119. D'Souza, D.C.; Perry, E.; MacDougall, L.; Ammerman, Y.; Cooper, T.; Wu, Y.T.; Krystal, J.H. The psychotomimetic effects of intravenous delta-9-tetrahydrocannabinol in healthy individuals: Implications for psychosis. *Neuropsychopharmacology* **2004**, *29*, 1558. [CrossRef] [PubMed]
120. Jager, G.; Van Hell, H.H.; De Win, M.M.L.; Kahn, R.S.; Van Den Brink, W.; Van Ree, J.M.; Ramsey, N.F. Effects of frequent cannabis use on hippocampal activity during an associative memory task. *Eur. Neuropsychopharmacol.* **2007**, *17*, 289–297. [CrossRef] [PubMed]
121. Cousijn, J.; Wiers, R.W.; Ridderinkhof, K.R.; Van, D.B.W.; Veltman, D.J.; Goudriaan, A.E. Working-memory network function in heavy cannabis users predicts changes in cannabis use: A prospective fMRI study. *Hum. Brain Mapp.* **2014**, *5*, 2470–2482. [CrossRef] [PubMed]

122. Smith, A.M.; Longo, C.A.; Fried, P.A.; Hogan, M.J.; Cameron, I. Effects of marijuana on visuospatial working memory: An fMRI study in young adults. *Psychopharmacology* **2010**, *210*, 429–438. [CrossRef] [PubMed]
123. Bossong, G.M.; Jager, G.; Bhattacharyya, S.; Allen, P. Acute and non-acute effects of cannabis on human memory function: A critical review of neuroimaging studies. *Curr. Pharm. Design* **2014**, *20*, 2114–2125. [CrossRef]
124. Cousijn, J.; Wiers, R.W.; Ridderinkhof, K.R.; van den Brink, W.; Veltman, D.J.; Goudriaan, A.E. Effect of baseline cannabis use and working-memory network function on changes in cannabis use in heavy cannabis users: A prospective fMRI study. *Hum. Brain Mapp.* **2014**, *35*, 2470–2482. [CrossRef] [PubMed]
125. Cousijn, J.; Wiers, R.W.; Ridderinkhof, K.R.; van den Brink, W.; Veltman, D.J.; Goudriaan, A.E. Grey matter alterations associated with cannabis use: Results of a VBM study in heavy cannabis users and healthy controls. *Neuroimage* **2012**, *59*, 3845–3851. [CrossRef] [PubMed]
126. Battistella, G.; Fornari, E.; Annoni, J.M.; Chtioui, H.; Dao, K.; Fabritius, M.; Giroud, C. Long-term effects of cannabis on brain structure. *Neuropsychopharmacology* **2014**, *39*, 2041–2048. [CrossRef] [PubMed]
127. Castellanos, D.; Thornton, G. Synthetic cannabinoid use: Recognition and management. *J Psychiatr. Pract.* **2012**, *18*, 86–93. [CrossRef] [PubMed]
128. Bebarta, V.S.; Ramirez, S.; Varney, S.M. Spice: A new "legal" herbal mixture abused by young active duty military personnel. *Subst. Abuse* **2012**, *33*, 191–194. [CrossRef] [PubMed]
129. Simmons, J.R.; Skinner, C.G.; Williams, J.; Kang, C.S.; Schwartz, M.D.; Wills, B.K. Intoxication from smoking "spice. " *Ann. Emerg. Med.* **2011**, *57*, 187–188. [CrossRef] [PubMed]
130. Herkenham, M.; Lynn, A.B.; Little, M.D.; Johnson, M.R.; Melvin, L.S.; De Costa, B.R.; Rice, K.C. Cannabinoid receptor localization in brain. *Proc. Natl. Acad. Sci. USA* **1990**, *87*, 1932–1936. [CrossRef] [PubMed]
131. Matyas, F.; Yanovsky, Y.; Mackie, K.; Kelsch, W.; Misgeld, U.; Freund, T.F. Subcellular localization of type 1 cannabinoid receptors in the rat basal ganglia. *Neuroscience* **2006**, *137*, 337–361. [CrossRef] [PubMed]
132. McAlonan, K.; Brown, V.J. Orbital prefrontal cortex mediates reversal learning and not attentional set shifting in the rat. *Behav. Brain Rese.* **2003**, *146*, 97–103. [CrossRef]
133. Birrell, J.M.; Brown, V.J. Medial frontal cortex mediates perceptual attentional set shifting in the rat. *J. Neurosci.* **2000**, *20*, 4320–4324. [PubMed]
134. Floresco, S.B.; Magyar, O.; Ghods-Sharifi, S.; Vexelman, C.; Maric, T.L. Multiple dopamine receptor subtypes in the medial prefrontal cortex of the rat regulate set-shifting. *Neuropsychopharmacology* **2006**, *31*, 297–309. [CrossRef] [PubMed]
135. Wright, M.J.; Vandewater, S.A.; Parsons, L.H.; Taffe, M.A. Δ 9 Tetrahydrocannabinol impairs reversal learning but not extra-dimensional shifts in rhesus macaques. *Neuroscience* **2013**, *235*, 51–58. [CrossRef] [PubMed]
136. Gomes, F.V.; Guimarães, F.S.; Grace, A.A. Effects of pubertal cannabinoid administration on attentional set-shifting and dopaminergic hyper-responsivity in a developmental disruption model of schizophrenia. *Int. J. Neuropsychopharmacol.* **2015**, *18*, 1–10. [CrossRef] [PubMed]
137. Leber, A.B.; Turk-Browne, N.B.; Chun, M.M. Neural predictors of moment-to-moment fluctuations in cognitive flexibility. *Proc. Natl. Acad. Sci. USA* **2008**, *105*, 13592–13597. [CrossRef] [PubMed]
138. Kehagia, A.A.; Murray, G.K.; Robbins, T.W. Learning and cognitive flexibility: Frontostriatal function and monoaminergic modulation. *Curr. Opin. Neurobiol.* **2010**, *20*, 199–204. [CrossRef] [PubMed]
139. Milner, B. Some cognitive effects of frontal-lobe lesions in man. *Philos. Trans. R. Soc. Lond. B Biol. Sci.* **1982**, *298*, 211–226. [CrossRef] [PubMed]
140. Morrison, P.D.; Zois, V.; McKeown, D.A.; Lee, T.D.; Holt, D.W.; Powell, J.F.; Murray, R.M. The acute effects of synthetic intravenous Delta9-tetrahydrocannabinol on psychosis, mood and cognitive functioning. *Psychol. Med.* **2009**, *39*, 1607–1616. [CrossRef] [PubMed]
141. Pope, H.G.; Gruber, A.J.; Hudson, J.I.; Cohane, G.; Huestis, M.A.; Yurgelun-Todd, D. Early-onset cannabis use and cognitive deficits: What is the nature of the association? *Drug Alcohol Depend.* **2003**, *69*, 303–310. [CrossRef]
142. Scholes, K.E.; Martin-Iverson, M.T. Cannabis use and neuropsychological performance in healthy individuals and patients with schizophrenia. *Psychol. Med.* **2010**, *40*, 1635–1646. [CrossRef] [PubMed]
143. Pope, H.G.; Gruber, A.J.; Hudson, J.I.; Huestis, M.A.; Yurgelun-Todd, D. Neuropsychological performance in long-term cannabis users. *Arch. Gen. Psychiat.* **2001**, *58*, 909–915. [CrossRef] [PubMed]
144. Solowij, N.; Stephens, R.S.; Roffman, R.A.; Babor, T.; Kadden, R.; Miller, M.; Vendetti, J. Cognitive functioning of long-term heavy cannabis users seeking treatment. *Jama* **2002**, *287*, 1123–1131. [CrossRef] [PubMed]

145. Grant, I.; Gonzalez, R.; Carey, C.L.; Natarajan, L.; Wolfson, T. Non-acute (residual) neurocognitive effects of cannabis use: A meta-analytic study. *J. Int. Neuropsychol. Soc.* **2003**, *9*, 679–689. [CrossRef] [PubMed]
146. Altintas, M.; Inanc, L.; Oruc, G.A.; Arpacioglu, S.; Gulec, H. Clinical characteristics of synthetic cannabinoid-induced psychosis in relation to schizophrenia: A single-center cross-sectional analysis of concurrently hospitalized patients. *Neuropsychiat. Dis. Treat.* **2016**, *12*, 1893. [CrossRef] [PubMed]
147. Milders, M.; Ietswaart, M.; Crawford, J.R.; Currie, D. Social behavior following traumatic brain injury and its association with emotion recognition, understanding of intentions and cognitive flexibility. *J. Int. Neuropsychol. Soc.* **2008**, *14*, 318–326. [CrossRef] [PubMed]
148. Radhakrishnan, R.; Wilkinson, S.T.; D'Souza, D.C. Gone to pot–a review of the association between cannabis and psychosis. *Front. Psychiatry.* **2014**, *5*, 54. [CrossRef] [PubMed]
149. Wiley, J.L.; Marusich, J.A.; Huffman, J.W. Moving around the molecule: Relationship between chemical structure and in vivo activity of synthetic cannabinoids. *Life Sci.* **2014**, *97*, 55–63. [CrossRef] [PubMed]
150. Ghitza, U.E.; Epstein, D.H.; Schmittner, J.; Vahabzadeh, M.; Lin, J.L.; Preston, K.L. Randomized trial of prize-based reinforcement density for simultaneous abstinence from cocaine and heroin. *J. Consult. Clin. Psychol.* **2007**, *75*, 765. [CrossRef] [PubMed]

# 11

# The Dynamic Environment of Crypto Markets: The Lifespan of New Psychoactive Substances (NPS) and Vendors Selling NPS

**Elle Wadsworth [1,*], Colin Drummond [2,3] and Paolo Deluca [2]**

1 School of Public Health and Health Systems, University of Waterloo, Waterloo, ON N2L 3G1, Canada
2 National Addiction Centre, Institute of Psychiatry, Psychology & Neuroscience, King's College London, London SE5 8BB, UK; colin.drummond@kcl.ac.uk (C.D.); paolo.deluca@kcl.ac.uk (P.D.)
3 South London and Maudsley NHS Foundation Trust, Maudsley Hospital, London SE5 8AZ, UK
* Correspondence: ewadsworth@uwaterloo.ca

**Abstract:** The Internet has played a major role in the distribution of New Psychoactive Substances (NPS), and crypto markets are increasingly used for the anonymous sale of drugs, including NPS. This study explores the availability of individual NPS and vendors on the crypto markets and considers whether crypto markets are a reliable platform for the sale of NPS. Data was collected from 22 crypto markets that were accessed through the hidden web using the Onion Router (Tor). Data collection took place bimonthly from October 2015 to October 2016 as part of the CASSANDRA (Computer **A**ssisted **S**olutions for **S**tudying the **A**vailability a**N**d **D**ist**R**ibution of novel psycho**A**ctive substances) project. In seven snapshots over 12 months, 808 unique vendors were found selling 256 unique NPS. The total number of individual NPS and vendors increased across the data collection period (increase of 93.6% and 71.6%, respectively). Only 24% ($n$ = 61) of the total number of NPS and 4% ($n$ = 31) of vendors appeared in every snapshot over the 12 months, whereas 21% ($n$ = 54) of NPS and 45% ($n$ = 365) of vendors only appeared once throughout the data collection. The individual NPS and vendors did not remain the same over the 12 months. However, the availability of NPS and vendors selling NPS grew. NPS consistently available on crypto markets could indicate popular substances.

**Keywords:** new psychoactive substances; legal highs; darknet; hidden web; crypto market

---

## 1. Introduction

New psychoactive substances (NPS) are an emerging phenomenon, and their representation on the hidden web (also known as the darknet) is under-researched. The Internet has played a major role in the distribution of NPS, and drug marketplaces (also known as crypto markets) on the hidden web are increasingly used for the anonymous sale of drugs, including NPS [1–3].

The European Union (EU) Early Warning System currently monitors over 650 substances [4]. However, not all substances are a cause of concern, and NPS rise and fall in popularity. Only a few have had sizable prevalence or media attention [5], and research has shown that the legal status of a substance is one of the factors determining why some NPS become popular and others do not [6]. Various legislations have been created to tackle NPS diffusion across Europe and the world. For example, the UK introduced the Psychoactive Substances Act in May 2016, which prohibited the import, export, and supply of psychoactive substances (with some exemptions) but permitted possession [7]. The Act achieved a reduction in UK-based online stores and offline retail stores [8]. As more countries seek to restrict access to NPS, the legal markets could be displaced by alternative routes such as street-level drug dealing or crypto markets [3]. However, movement to the illicit market is dependent on its popularity, and therefore only those NPS with sufficient demand will transition into it [9].

On the hidden web, drugs can be sold and purchased anonymously through crypto markets that use an "eBay"-style system where buyers can publicly review the sellers and therefore build their reputation, attracting future transactions [10–14]. Conversely, negative reviews can discourage buyers and shun unworthy vendors from the crypto markets [11,15]. It is argued that this feedback mechanism and creation of a reputation are vital to the continuing function of the market and also represent an explanation for a vendor's lifespan [15,16]. To date, the majority of crypto market research has been conducted on the Silk Road [13,17–21], which was closed by law enforcement in 2013 [22]. Christin [20] found that most sellers disappeared before three months, and most items sold for less than three weeks. Christin [20] proposed the theory that short vendor lifespans could be due to lack of stock or to vendors using the "stealth mode". The stealth mode consists in vendors removing their listings or only selling their listings to a specific customer base [13]. Potentially, the turnover of vendors is a product of the instability of the crypto markets; individual crypto markets are said to be unpredictable and have a frequent turnover, causing instability in the community [23]. Law enforcements have succeeded in closing crypto markets in the past [14,22,24]. However, all successful operations have not stopped the online trade of drugs [25], and the number of vendors has increased [3]. Previous research on crypto markets have shown a small yet definite presence of NPS. Barratt, Ferris, and Winstock [18] examined the use of Silk Road in a sample from the UK, US, and Australia and found that out of the top 20 substances that were purchased, four of these were NPS. In addition, Van Buskirk et al. [3] explored crypto markets in 2015 and concluded that around one-fifth of vendors offered NPS.

Crypto markets are increasingly being used for the sale and purchase of drugs, regardless of the instability both the markets and the vendors show. To date, research has not focussed specifically on the lifespan of vendors selling NPS, substances whose popularity and availability are unpredictable. This paper, therefore, aims to explore the lifespan of individual NPS sold on the crypto markets, explore the lifespan of individual vendors selling NPS on the crypto markets, and consider whether crypto markets are a reliable platform for the sale of NPS.

## 2. Methods

The study was part of the CASSANDRA (**C**omputer **A**ssisted **S**olutions for **S**tudying the **A**vailability a**N**d **D**ist**R**ibution of novel psycho**A**ctive substances) project [26]. The crypto markets on the hidden web were accessed through Tor (torproject.org, 501(c)(3), The Tor Project, Inc., Cambridge, MA, USA), and the data were collected bimonthly over 12 months in October, December (2015), February, April, June, August, and October (2016). The data were collected over two days in each of the seven snapshots. The crypto markets that were included sold NPS, were conducted in English, and had an open registration at the time of collection. The crypto markets present over the 12 months of data collection fluctuated because of crypto markets opening, adding NPS to their sales, or closing following exit scams or law enforcement. A table of the crypto markets included in this study can be found elsewhere [27].

Data were collected on each crypto market for NPS being sold that was visible to the researchers. The data collected were: name of the NPS (not including conventional illicit drugs, steroids, or prescription drugs), name of the vendor selling NPS, and name of the crypto market used by the vendor. Some NPS were sold under various aliases; these were categorised by their most common name. Furthermore, branded NPS that were commonly found on the visible Internet were categorised according to their contents. All analyses were performed using Microsoft Excel 2016 (Microsoft Office 2016, Microsoft, Redmond, WA, United States), unless otherwise specified.

All users on crypto markets were anonymous. The research was purely observational and did not involve interaction with either buyers or sellers. The study was approved by King's College London PNM Research Ethics reference number: LRS-15/16-3084 as part of the CASSANDRA project.

## 3. Results

The total number of individual NPS and vendors increased across the seven snapshots in the data collection period (increase of 93.6% and 71.6%, respectively) (Figure 1). Over 12 months, a total of 808 individual vendors were found selling 256 individual NPS.

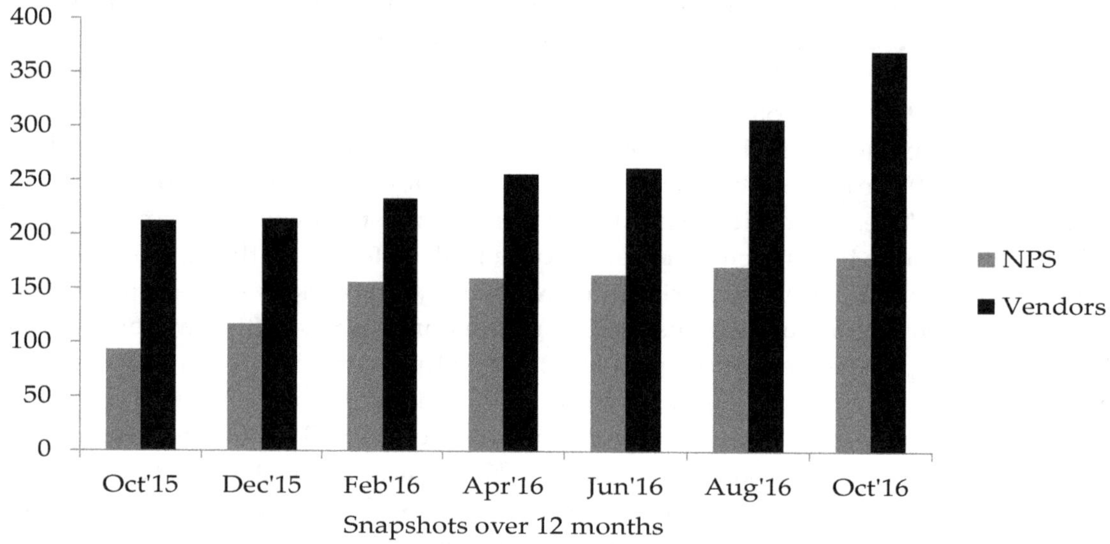


**Figure 1.** Number of NPS and vendors in each month of data collection (seven snapshots in 12 months). NPS: New Psychoactive Substances.

A total corresponding to 21% ($n$ = 54) of the NPS reported over the 12-month period only appeared in one snapshot (Figure 2). Fourteen percent ($n$ = 36) of the total number of NPS appeared in two of the seven snapshots. Ten percent ($n$ = 26) appeared in three of the seven snapshots, 7% ($n$ = 18) appeared in four of the seven snapshots, 11% ($n$ = 29) appeared in five of the seven snapshots, and 13% ($n$ = 32) appeared in six of the seven snapshots. In addition, 24% ($n$ = 61) of the total number of NPS appeared in each of the seven snapshots over the 12-month period (Table 1).

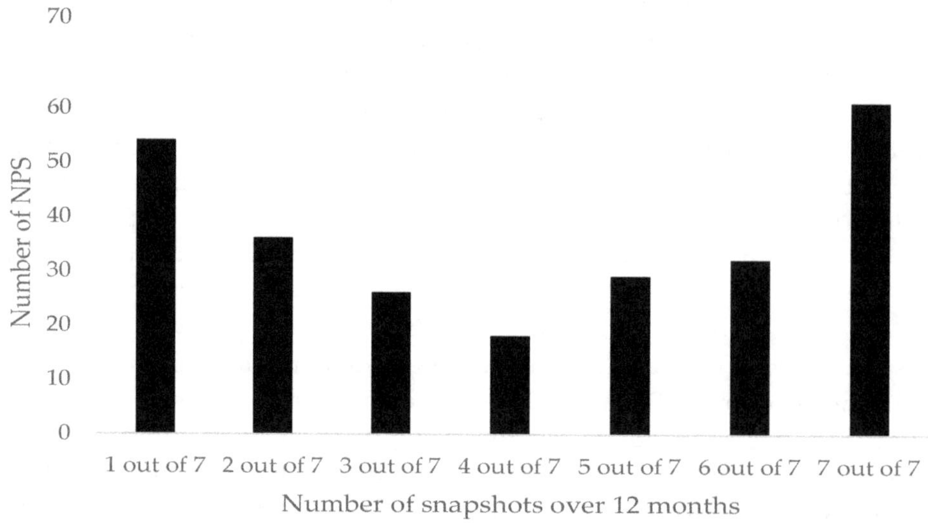


**Figure 2.** The number of NPS available across the seven snapshots (12 months) of data collection. NPS: New Psychoactive Substances.

**Table 1.** New Psychoactive Substances that were available in every snapshot over 12 months of data collection ($n = 61$).

| Benzodiazepine Analogue | Cathinone | Dissociative | Opioids | Phenethylamine | Synthetic Cannabinoid | Tryptamine | Other |
|---|---|---|---|---|---|---|---|
| Etizolam (Etilaam, Etizola, Eticalm) | 3-CMC (3-chloromethcathinone) | 3-MeO-PCP (3-methoxyphencyclidine) | Fu-F (furanylfentanyl) | 25B-NBOMe (N-bombs, cimbi-36) | AB-CHMINACA (AB-C) | 4-AcO-DMT (o-acetylpsilocin, psilacetin) | 1P-LSD (NP-LAD, 1-Propionyl-d-lysergic acid diethylamide) |
| | 3-MMC (3-methylmethcathinone, 3-mephedrone) | DXE (deschloroketamine, DCK, 2′oxo-PCM) | Kratom (ketum, kratum) | 25C-NBOMe (N-bombs, cimbi-82) | MAM-2201 (4′-methyl-AM-2201, 5″-fluoro-JWH-122) | 4-HO-MET (metocin, methylcybin) | AL-LAD (6-allyl-6-nor-LSD) |
| | 4-CMC (4-chloromethcathinone, clephedrone) | | W-18 (4-chloro-*N*-[1-[2-(4-nitrophenyl)ethyl]-2piperidinylidene] benzenesulfonamide) | 25D-NBOMe (N-bombs) | NM-2201 (CBL-2201) | 4-HO-MiPT (miprocin) | LSA (ergine, d-lyseramide, LAA, LA-111) |
| | 4-EMC (4-ethylmethcathinone) | | | 25i-NBOMe (N-bombs, cimbi-5) | "Spice" | 5-MeO-DALT (*N*,*N*-Diallyl-5-methoxytryptamine, Foxtrot) | MPA (methylthienylpropamine, methiopropamine, methedrene, syndrax) |
| | 4-FMC (4-fluoromethcathinone, flephedrone) | | | 2CB (Tripstacy) | | 5-MeO-MiPT (5-Methoxy-*N*-methyl-*N*-isopropyltryptamine, Moxy) | MXP (methoxphenidine, 2-MeO-diphenidine) |
| | 4F-PV8 (4-Fluoro-α-PHPP, para-fluoro-PV8) | | | 2CE (Tripstacy) | | | Salvia |
| | 4-MEC (4-methylethcathinone) | | | 2CI (Tripstacy) | | | |
| | 4-MMC (mephedrone, Mcat, meowmeow, bubble, drone) | | | 2CP (Tripstacy) | | | |
| | 5-ME (5-methyl-ethylone) | | | 2FA (2-fluoroamphetamine, PAL-353) | | | |
| | a-PHP (alpha-PHP, PV7, a-pyrrolidinohexiophenone) | | | 2FMA (2-fluoromethamphetamine) | | | |
| | a-PVP (a-pyrrolidinopentiophenone, flakka, k-prolintane, O-2387) | | | 3-FPM (3-fluorophenmetrazine, PAL-593) | | | |
| | Dibutylone (bk-DMBDB, booty) | | | 4FA (4-FMP, PAL-303, Flux, PFA) | | | |
| | Dimethocaine (DMC, larocaine) | | | 5-EAPB (1-(benzofuran-5-yl)-*N*-ethylpropan-2-amine) | | | |

**Table 1.** *Cont.*

| Benzodiazepine Analogue | Cathinone | Dissociative | Opioids | Phenethylamine | Synthetic Cannabinoid | Tryptamine | Other |
|---|---|---|---|---|---|---|---|
| | Ethylone | | | 5-MAPB (1-(benzofuran-5-yl)-*N*-methylpropan-2-amine) | | | |
| | MDPV (NRG-1, methylenedioxypyrovalerone) | | | 6-APB (6-(2-aminopropyl) benzofuran) | | | |
| | Methylone (M1, MDMC, bk-MDMA) | | | DOC (4-Chloro-2,5-dimethoxyamphetamine) | | | |
| | PV9 (a-POP, alpha-POP) | | | DOM (2,5-Dimethoxy-4-methylamphetamine) | | | |
| | TH-PVP (3′,4′-tetramethylene-α-Pyrrolidinovalerophenone) | | | ephedrine | | | |
| | | | | Ethylphenidate (EPH) | | | |
| | | | | MAL (methallylescaline) | | | |
| | | | | MDA (3,4-Methylenedioxyamphetamine) | | | |

Almost half of all vendors (45%, $n = 365$) appeared only once over the 12-month period (Figure 3). Twenty-three percent ($n = 184$) of the total number of vendors appeared in two snapshots over the 12-month period, 13% ($n = 103$) appeared in three snapshots, 8% ($n = 63$) appeared in four snapshots, 4% ($n = 30$) appeared in five snapshots, 4% ($n = 32$) appeared in six snapshots, and only 4% ($n = 31$) of the total number of vendors appeared in all seven snapshots.

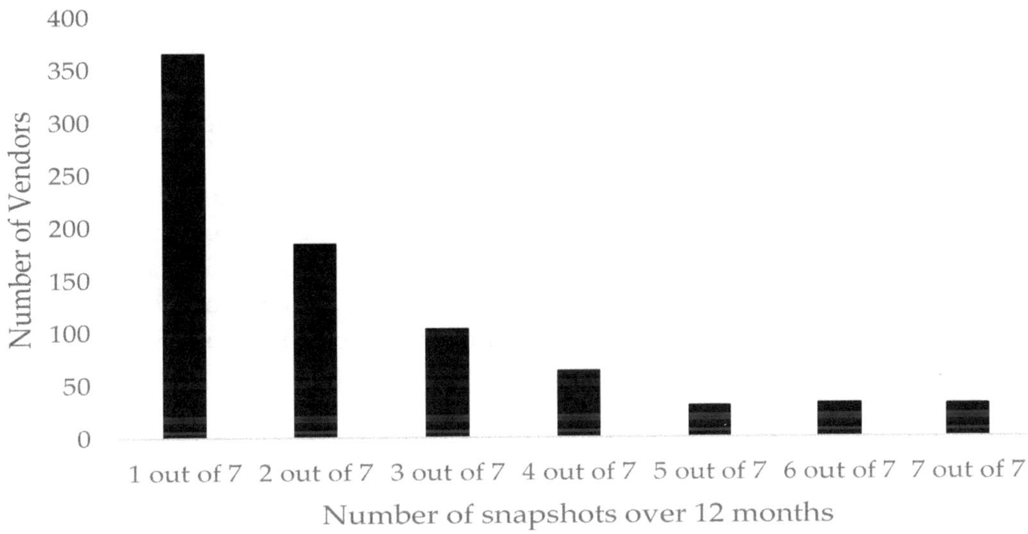


**Figure 3.** The number of vendors available across the seven snapshots (12 months) of data collection.

## 4. Discussion

The total number of individual NPS and vendors increased over the 12-month duration of the study. Almost half of the total number of vendors had a lifespan of only a few months, and the NPS advertised fluctuated over the study. One-fifth of NPS were available for the entirety of the study, whereas just under one-quarter were only available for a few months before disappearing. From the results of this study, the contents of the NPS market on the crypto markets varied, but a market was consistently available.

Research has shown that the use of crypto markets and the availability of substances including NPS have increased in recent years [3,20,24]. The results from this study complement these findings as the availability of NPS increased over the data collection period. The increased availability of NPS on the crypto markets suggests that NPS are being purchased via this method and that crypto markets are seen as a viable platform for the sale of NPS. This is necessary to observe because of the changing legislations surrounding these substances in countries around the globe, such as the ban in the UK that was implemented during this study [7]. Legal markets will look to migrate to other platforms.

This study found that 256 different NPS were available for purchase over the 12 months of the study, and nearly one-quarter of NPS remained available on the crypto markets, suggesting that these substances could be the most popular NPS. The majority of the NPS that were available in every snapshot were cathinones and phenethylamines (categorised according to [5]). However, there was frequent turnover throughout the study, whereby some NPS were available for purchase for a few months and then disappeared from availability. This pattern may have mirrored changes in popularity within the overall NPS market, fluctuating because of legality, ease of access, or similarities to traditional drugs [4,9]. It is possible that certain NPS were removed from the market because limited stocks were available to the vendors or because the demand of a specific NPS did not match up to its availability. Another possibility is that the feedback from the customers about the NPS was negative, and the stock was removed [15].

Almost half of the vendors were only captured in one snapshot over the course of the data collection, and the number of vendors who appeared in the data reduced as the snapshots increased (Figure 3). These findings show that the lifespan of the vendors was relatively short, and just under half of the vendors were available for under four months, mirroring what was found in the literature [20,28]. There are potential reasons for a short lifespan; research has suggested that vendors could only be selling their limited stock, or that vendors move into stealth mode after they have gathered a sufficient client base [13,20]. Furthermore, the crypto market system is built on trust and reputation; if vendors do not build an adequate reputation, they may remove themselves from the market either indefinitely or only apparently by setting up new accounts [15,28]. Only 4% of vendors remained available in every snapshot over the 12 months of this study. Perhaps, these consistent vendors were highly reputable vendors or vendors with a loyal customer base [28].

This study has several limitations. As this study was exploratory and lacked contact with the vendors, we were unable to verify whether the substances advertised were the same substances being purchased and received by the customers. Because of anonymity, another limitation is that studies like the present one are unable to capture how many vendor profiles are controlled by one person or if the number of vendors that are only available for a few months before disappearing are, in fact, opening and closing various accounts [29].

## 5. Conclusions

Online sales hold a predominant portion of the NPS market, and crypto markets are an emerging source of sale. NPS sold on crypto markets should be monitored to track the popularity and availability of specific substances. Our study found that vendors selling NPS had short lifespans, with half of the vendors only appearing once in the data collection. Individual NPS had longer lifespans, however not all NPS were available over the study period; only a quarter of the total NPS were available in all snapshots over the year. Regardless of the fluctuation of the vendors in the NPS market on the crypto markets, the number of NPS and vendors selling NPS increased over the year. The NPS that consistently appeared across the 12 months of data collection may suggest what substances are popular with the consumers. Crypto markets are therefore to be monitored for the sale of NPS, especially in light of the tightening regulations being applied in various countries.

**Acknowledgments:** This publication arises from the project "CASSANDRA, (Computer Assisted Solutions for Studying the Availability and Distribution of novel psychoactive substances)", which has received funding from the European Union under the ISEC programme Prevention of and fight against crime (JUST2013/ISEC/DRUGS/AG/6414). Colin Drummond was partly funded by the National Institute for Health Research (NIHR) Specialist Biomedical Research Centre at South London and Maudsley National Health Service (NHS) Foundation Trust and King's College London, the NIHR Collaboration for Leadership in Applied Health Research and Care South London at King's College Hospital NHS Foundation Trust, and an NIHR Senior Investigator Award. The views expressed are those of the authors and not necessarily those of the NHS, NIHR, or Department of Health and Social Care.

**Author Contributions:** All authors contributed to, reviewed, and approved the final manuscript and provided feedback with regard to both content and style. E.W. is the primary author and led the data collection, analysis, and writing of the manuscript; P.D. is the lead on the paper and was involved in the study design and implementation, and the preparation and review of this manuscript; C.D. provided input and feedback on the manuscript.

## References

1. Global Drug Survey. Global Drug Survey 2016. Available online: https://www.globaldrugsurvey.com/past-findings/the-global-drug-survey-2016-findings/ (accessed on 9 January 2018).
2. Walsh, C. Drugs, the Internet and change. *J. Psychoact. Drugs* **2011**, *43*, 55–63. [CrossRef] [PubMed]
3. Van Buskirk, J.; Griffiths, P.; Farrell, M.; Degenhardt, L. Trends in new psychoactive substances from surface and "dark" net monitoring. *Lancet Psychiatry* **2017**, *4*, 16–18. [CrossRef]
4. European Monitoring Centre for Drugs and Drug Addiction (EMCDDA); Europol. *EU Drug Markets Report: In-Depth Analysis*; Publications Office of the European Union: Luxembourg, Luxembourg, 2016.

5. EMCDDA. *European Drug Report: Trends and Developments*; Publications Office of the European Union: Luxembourg, Luxembourg, 2015.
6. Ledberg, A. The interest in eight new psychoactive substances before and after scheduling. *Drug Alcohol Depend.* **2015**, *152*, 73–78. [CrossRef] [PubMed]
7. UK Government. Psychoactive Substances Act. Available online: http://www.legislation.gov.uk/ukpga/2016/2/contents/enacted (accessed on 9 September 2017).
8. Wadsworth, E.; Drummond, C.; Deluca, P. The adherence to UK legislation by online shops selling new psychoactive substances. *Drugs Educ. Prev. Policy* **2018**, *25*, 97–100. [CrossRef]
9. Home Office. New Psychoactive Substances in England: A Review of the Evidence. Available online: https://www.gov.uk/government/publications/new-psychoactive-substances-in-england-a-review-of-the-evidence (accessed on 9 September 2017).
10. Barratt, M.J. Silk Road: EBay for drugs. *Addiction* **2012**, *107*, 683. [CrossRef] [PubMed]
11. Seddon, T. Drug policy and global regulatory capitalism: The case of new psychoactive substances (NPS). *Int. J. Drug Policy* **2014**, *25*, 1019–1024. [CrossRef] [PubMed]
12. Tzanetakis, M.; Kamphausen, G.; Werse, B.; von Laufenberg, R. The transparency paradox. Building trust, resolving disputes and optimising logistics on conventional and online drugs markets. *Int. J. Drug Policy* **2016**, *35*, 58–68. [CrossRef] [PubMed]
13. Van Hout, M.C.; Bingham, T. Responsible vendors, intelligent consumers: Silk Road, the online revolution in drug trading. *Int. J. Drug Policy* **2014**, *25*, 183–189. [CrossRef] [PubMed]
14. Van Hout, M.C.; Hearne, E. New psychoactive substances (NPS) on cryptomarket fora: An exploratory study of characteristics of forum activity between NPS buyers and vendors. *Int. J. Drug Policy* **2017**, *40*, 102–110. [CrossRef] [PubMed]
15. Cox, J. Reputation is everything: The role of ratings, feedback and reviews in Cryptomarkets. In *Internet and Drug Markets, EMCDDA Insights 21*; European Monitoring Centre for Drugs and Drug Addiction (EMCDDA), Ed.; Publications Office of the European Union: Luxembourg City, Luxembourg, 2016; pp. 49–54.
16. Hardy, R.A.; Norgaard, J.R. Reputation in the Internet black market: An empirical and theoretical analysis of the Deep Web. *J. Inst. Econ.* **2016**, *12*, 515–539. [CrossRef]
17. Aldridge, J.; Décary-Hétu, D. Hidden wholesale: The drug diffusing capacity of online drug cryptomarkets. *Int. J. Drug Policy* **2016**, *35*, 7–15. [CrossRef] [PubMed]
18. Barratt, M.J.; Ferris, J.A.; Winstock, A.R. Use of Silk Road, the online drug marketplace, in the United Kingdom, Australia and the United States. *Addiction* **2014**, *109*, 774–783. [CrossRef] [PubMed]
19. Barratt, M.J.; Lenton, S.; Maddox, A.; Allen, M. 'What if you live on top of a bakery and you like cakes?'—Drug use and harm trajectories before, during and after the emergence of Silk Road. *Int. J. Drug Policy* **2016**, *35*, 50–57. [CrossRef] [PubMed]
20. Christin, N. Traveling the Silk Road: A Measurement Analysis of a Large Anonymous On-Line Marketplace. Available online: https://www.andrew.cmu.edu/user/nicolasc/publications/Christin-WWW13.pdf (accessed on 9 March 2018).
21. Martin, J. Lost on the Silk Road: Online drug distribution and the 'cryptomarket'. *Criminol. Crim. Justice* **2014**, *14*, 351–367. [CrossRef]
22. Drug Enforcement Agency. Manhattan U.S. Attorney Announces Seizure of Additional $28 Million Worth of Bitcoins Belonging to Ross William Ulbricht, Alleged Owner and Operator of "Silk Road" Website. Available online: www.dea.gov/divisions/nyc/2013/nyc102513.shtml (accessed on 6 May 2017).
23. Van Buskirk, J.; Roxburgh, A.; Bruno, R.; Burns, L. *Drugs and the Internet, Issue 5, October 2015*; National Drug and Alcohol Research Centre: Sydney, Australia, 2015.
24. Kruithof, K.; Aldridge, J.; Décary-Hétu, D.; Sim, M.; Dujso, E.; Hoorens, S. Internet-Facilitated Drugs Trade: An Analysis of the Size, Scope and the Role of The Netherlands. WODC, Ministerie van Veiligheid en Justitie. 2016. Available online: https://www.rand.org/pubs/research_reports/RR1607.html (accessed on 6 May 2017).
25. Van Buskirk, J.; Roxburgh, A.; Farrell, M.; Burns, L. The closure of the Silk Road: What has this meant for online drug trading? *Addiction* **2014**, *109*, 517–518. [CrossRef] [PubMed]
26. CASSANDRA. Cassandra: Computer Assisted Solutions for Studying the Availability aNd Distribution of Novel Psycho Active Substances. Available online: www.projectcassandra.eu (accessed on 14 January 2018).
27. Wadsworth, E.; Drummond, C.; Kimergård, A.; Deluca, P. A market on both "sides" of the law: The use of the hidden web for the sale of new psychoactive substances. *Hum. Psychopharm. Clin.* **2017**, *32*. [CrossRef] [PubMed]

# 12

# Transitioning Bodies: The Case of Self-Prescribing Sexual Hormones in Gender Affirmation in Individuals Attending Psychiatric Services

**Antonio Metastasio [1,2,*], Attilio Negri [2], Giovanni Martinotti [2,3] and Ornella Corazza [2]**

1 Camden and Islington NHS Foundation Trust, London NW1 0PE, UK
2 Centre for Clinical & Health Research Services, School of Life and Medical Sciences, University of Hertfordshire, Hatfield AL10 9AB, UK; ngrttl@gmail.com (A.N.); giovanni.martinotti@gmail.com (G.M.); o.corazza@herts.ac.uk (O.C.)
3 Department of Neuroscience, Imaging, and Clinical Science, "G. d'Annunzio" University of Chieti-Pescara, 66100 Chieti, Italy
* Correspondence: antonio.metastasio@candi.nhs.uk

**Abstract:** Self-prescribing of sexual hormones for gender affirmation is a potentially widespread and poorly studied phenomenon that many clinicians are unaware of. The uncontrolled use of hormones poses significant health hazards, which have not been previously reported in the literature. We have collected seven clinical cases in general adult psychiatry settings (both inpatient and outpatients), describing transgender and gender non-conforming individuals' (TGNC) self-prescribing and self-administering hormones bought from the Internet without any medical consultation. Among these cases, two were taking androgens, and the rest were taking oestrogens. The main reason for self-administration of hormones seems to be the lack of access to specialised care due to discrimination and long waiting lists. We advocate for clinicians to be aware of the phenomenon and proactively help TGNC individuals by enquiring about self-prescribing of hormones, providing information and referring to the most appropriate treatment centre as well as encourage a public debate on the discrimination and the stigma that TGNC population suffer from. Overall, there is an urgent need for the implementation of different and innovative health care services for TGNC individuals as well as more targeted prevention strategies on such underreported and highly risky behaviours. Furthermore, it is necessary for every clinician involved in the care for TGNC people to be aware of their special needs and be able to be an allied and an advocate to help in reducing stigma and discrimination that affect the access to care for this often underserved population.

**Keywords:** transgender; gender reassignment; gender affirmation; self-medication; hormonal replacement therapy (HRT); LGTBQ health; gender dysphoria; do it yoursfelf (DIY); identity; barriers to care; discrimination

---

## 1. Introduction

A significant proportion of the population defines themselves as transgender, intersex non-binary or gender non-conforming (in this paper, we will use "TGNC" for "transgender and gender nonconforming" people as recommended by the American Psychological Association (APA) guidelines [1]). A recent demographic study estimates that in the USA 0.39% (about one million people) of the population define themselves as TGNC [2]. The exact number, however, might be bigger, and it is very difficult to quantify the precise number due to the complex methodology in estimating the numbers when gender non-conforming individuals are also considered in the statistics [3]. To estimate the same data in the UK, it is more difficult because the Office for National Statistics (ONS) does not produce estimates of the number of TGNC people living in the United Kingdom (Office for National Statistics [4]). The Gender Identity Research and Education Society (GIRES) estimates a prevalence of 1% TGNC individuals in the UK adult population [5]. TGNC people are individuals that do not identify or exclusively identify with the sex assigned to them at birth. Intersex individuals are people with a less common combination of hormones, chromosomes, and anatomy that are used to assign sex at birth. There are many examples such as Klinefelter Syndrome, Androgen Insensitivity Syndrome, and Congenital Adrenal Hyperplasia. Non Binary people are individuals that do not identify themselves completely as female/male or woman/man. Gender non-conforming people are, according to the American Psychological Association "those who have a gender identity that is not fully aligned with their sex assigned at birth" [1].

A significant number of these individuals often decide to undergo a gender affirmation process. This process consists of using sexual hormones and often undergoing surgery to affirm to the gender that they belong to. In the UK, the prevalence of the population that has sought medical care is estimated to be 0.025%, and about 0.015% are likely to have undergone a transition [5].

A recent survey made by the University of California, Los Angeles (UCLA) Centre for Health Policy and Research showed that 27% of youth between 12 and 17 in California are gender non-conforming [6]. According to another document from the same institution, such a population typically presents a "*conflict between a person's physical or assigned gender and the gender with which he/she/they identify. People with gender dysphoria may be very uncomfortable with the gender they were assigned, sometimes described as being uncomfortable with their body (particularly developments during puberty) or being uncomfortable with the expected roles of their assigned gender*" [7].

It could be, therefore, be argued that gender affirmation is a very important procedure to improve the quality of life and mental wellbeing of TGNC individuals. However, very little attention has been paid to this phenomenon.

A recent prospective study [8] assessing the psychopathology during the gender affirmation process has shown that the psychoneurotic distress measured with the Symptom Checklist-90 Revised SCL-90-R, improves after the start of the hormonal treatment, and anxiety, depression, interpersonal sensitivity, and hostility also tend to improve. This progress is so important that after the completion of the gender affirmation procedure via hormonal treatment and surgery, the psychopathology (assessed with a specific scale) is comparable to the one of the general population [8]. Another prospective study has also demonstrated that people with gender dysphoria treated with hormones presented a significant improvement at the Body Uneasiness Test (BUT) compared to the non-treated condition [9].

The use of hormones, however, might have significant side-effects or may lead to severe medical complications [10]. In particular, Cross-sex Hormone Therapy (CHT) female to male has been associated with a potential risk of cardiovascular disease, cancer (breast, ovarian and endometrial), osteoporosis; in the case of male to female therapy, there is a risk of venous thromboembolism, and potentially cardiovascular disease and cancer [10].

In clinical settings, gender affirmation is a complex and long-lasting procedure, involving many different healthcare professionals including psychiatrists, psychologists, endocrinologists, plastic surgeons, speech and language therapists, and counsellors. This procedure also needs a multidisciplinary approach with a schedule that allows time for physical and social transition [11–13]. The World Professional Association for Transgender Health (WPATH) published the most commonly accepted clinical guidelines and 'Standards of Care' for TGNC [14], including established general eligibility criteria for feminising or masculinising hormone therapy. These include (a) persistent, well-documented gender dysphoria; (b) capacity to make a fully informed decision and to consent for treatment; (c) age of majority in a given country; (d) if significant medical or mental concerns are present, they must be reasonably well-controlled.

The aim of this article is to raise awareness among mental health professionals about a phenomenon that is already known in specialist settings (e.g., gender affirmation clinics and substance misuse services) but less well known in different settings. Central to this paper is a collection of different clinical cases collected in inpatients and outpatients National Health Service (NHS) clinics in Suffolk (a rural county north east of London) and London (Camden and Islington Boroughs). It is also desirable that by raising awareness, TGNC patients will find that mental health clinicians are not only therapists but also advocates and allied in their gender affirmation journey. In response to the existing lack of knowledge among the health professionals, NHS England recently released [15] a document assessing the individual suitability for endocrine and other pharmacological treatments. Suggested arrangements for medical practitioners include: (a) prescription of endocrine and other pharmacological interventions for the purpose of harm reduction and acting in the best interest for reducing gender dysphoria; (b) the assessment of risks, benefits and limitations of such a pharmacological intervention and the assurance that the individual meets the relevant eligibility criteria set out by the World Professional Association for Transgender Health Standards of Care (2011); (c) the provision of patient-specific prescribing guidance to the General Practitioner (GP), including adequately-detailed information about the necessary pre-treatment assessments, and advice on dosages, administration, initiation, duration of treatment among others; (d) the preparation of written advice to the GP when the individual is discharged. Further details on specific treatments have been outlined in Table 1. An additional statement by the General Medical Council (GMC) clarifies that GPs can prescribe hormones to TGNC individuals [16].

**Table 1.** Types of treatment for masculinisation and feminisation [15]

| Aim | Type of Preparation | Notes | Recommendations |
|---|---|---|---|
| Medications for masculinisation | Testosterone preparations | Include testosterone injections and transdermal gels | Avoid smoking (risk of thrombosis) |
| | Medications to suppress hyptolamic-pituitary-gonadal activity | | Avoid smoking (risk of thrombosis) |
| Medications for feminisation | Estradiol preparations | Doses necessary to achieve serum estradiol levels typical of pre-menopausal woman. Include oral estradiol and transdermal estradiol as patches and gels (for people over 40 years old). Ethinylestradiol will not be recommended | Avoid if Body Mass Index > 40; avoid smoking (risk of thrombosis) |
| | Medications to suppress hypothalamic-pituitary-gonadal activity and endogenous testosterone release | Include gonadotropin releasing hormone analogues and 5-alpha reductase inhibitors | Avoid if Body Mass Index > 40; avoid smoking (risk of thrombosis) |
| | Ornithine decarboxylase inhibitors | May be recommended as an adjunct to facial hair reduction interventions | Avoid smoking (risk of thrombosis) |

Despite the availability of such clinical guidance and advice, TGNC individuals still do not receive the care they often need because of stigma, discrimination, and lack of awareness in health care settings [17,18]. A large population study from the 2014-5 Behavioural Risk Factor Surveillance System by Gonzales et al. found that "TGNC adults were more likely to be uninsured and have unmet health care needs and were less likely to have routine care, compared to cisgender (non-transgender) women". Reasons for such barriers to health care included discrimination in health care, health insurance policies, employment and inadequate health policy and regulations [19]. Although very few population surveys of this kind have been carried out, another study in Ontario confirmed that 43.9% of TGNC individuals experienced inequalities in the access to healthcare and remained medically unsupervised [20].

An additional element of concern to this phenomenon is the self-administration of CHT without clinical supervision. Evidence of such hazardous behaviour emerged from studies among TGNC population in Canada [21] and from patients attending gender reassignment clinics in the United Kingdom. In the latter case, it has been estimated that 23% of individuals referred to gender reassignment clinic were self-administering hormones, mainly bought online (70%). Such behaviour appeared to be more common among trans women, as 32% of the female sample was using hormones at the moment of referral. Alarmingly, individuals that were purchasing hormones online appeared to be less informed about the risks and the side effects of hormonal therapy [22].

The growing number of illicit online pharmacies selling counterfeited products, including "Performance and Image-Enhancing Drugs" (PIEDs) and sexual enhancers [23] taken to enhance human abilities in a myriad of spheres, is another important emerging faucet within this [24–27]. PIEDs include substances with a perceived ability to enhance physical performance, psychological status and appearance, cognitive abilities and social relations, and as such, are sometimes referred to as 'lifestyle drugs'. It has been estimated that approximately 97% of websites selling pharmaceutical products are of illicit nature [26]. Individuals can purchase a wide range of unregulated and untested medicines in these websites which are freely sold without a prescription, and at discounted prices [27,28].

## 2. Clinical Cases

A number of TGNC patients cases that have started the gender affirmation process without any medical/specialist support were collected in two general adult psychiatry assessment clinics (outpatients) in London and Suffolk between 2014 and 2018. Information was obtained as part of the routine history taking during a psychiatric assessment and no specific questionnaire was designed for the psychiatry interview. The patients were informed at the moment of the assessment that some of the information given in an anonymised version would be used for a case presentation and a case report article. The patients that were included in the article were requested to give informed consent. The assessment clinics are the first point of contact with mental health where new referrals from GPs and other health professionals are seen. Suffolk is a rural county, predominantly a white English population, with chronic lack of access to mental health and other specialist health services that are conversely available in London, where most of the specialist and national health services are located. Consulted patients were either attending the clinics, or inpatient in psychiatric wards for the assessment and treatment of mental health conditions unrelated to their gender definition. The clinics and the wards were for general adult patients only. During the psychiatric interview, it emerged, worryingly that a certain number of TGNC individuals were purchasing hormones through illegal on-line pharmacies and were using them without any medical advice or monitoring (not even at General Practitioner level) using CHT protocols that were available online or receiving advice from online forums and blogs.

The length of the current clinical procedure, which involves long waiting lists, various passages of assessment and treatment, was criticized and perceived as a barrier for receiving the standard treatment. Patients preferred to purchase the hormones online and advocated a quick and easy CHT while trusting unsolicited online protocols from non-medical professionals for a faster result. Mistrust of medical professionals has also been previously reported as a potential cause [29]. Resilience on the Internet for medical advice concerning injecting practices and dosages among other features also indicates an underlying lack of engagement with medical professionals and limited practitioner knowledge regarding these patterns of use [30].

Hormone therapy in gender affirmation may affect different organs and systems [31]. For this reason, any hormonal treatment should be prescribed and supervised by a specialist and should also be discussed in depth with the patient to prepare him/her for the treatment. In this way, it is possible to monitor and manage the treatment effectively as well as to address any of the side effects described above. Hormonal treatment with oestrogens also requires diuretics to counteract the water retention associated with their use. Diuretics should also be used under medical supervision, and the renal function and electrolytes of the patients should be checked regularly to prevent, especially in summer, potentially dangerous dehydration and electrolytes imbalances.

In this paper, seven cases of TGNC individuals are described. They were assessed in a psychiatric clinic or admitted onto a psychiatric ward for different reasons, and they were using hormones and other drugs for gender affirmation without any medical supervision and purchasing all these medications through unlicensed online dealers.

### 2.1. Oestrogens

Case 1 is a 24-year-old trans woman, working as a plumber, and single. She was referred for a psychiatric screening as the first step for the referral pathway to the Gender Identity Clinic after she disclosed to her GP that she was using hormones purchased online. The patient has no previous history of mental or physical illness, she described herself as TGNC since age 14 and started the transition, without medical supervision two years before the assessment. The patient joined on line forums where she received the information regarding the hormonal protocols and the websites selling hormones. She started the treatment on her own and subsequently asked the GP to be referred for gender reassignment/gender affirmation. At the time of the assessment, the patient did not present any comorbid psychiatric or physical conditions.

Case 2 is a 22-year-old trans woman with a previous history of depression at the age of 14 that was successfully treated with a Serotonin Reuptake Inhibitor (SSRI). The patient stated that she felt like a person "trapped in the wrong body" ever since she could remember. She complained of being bullied at school for this reason, and she thinks that the bullying and the non-acceptance from her friends caused the depressive episodes in her teens. She started the protocol online and asked the GP to continue prescribing, and the GP asked for a psychiatric opinion before proceeding. She had been using oestrogens, finasteride, and spironolactone intermittently in the last two years. The patient also has type I diabetes, treated with insulin. According to the GPs notes, the compliance with the insulin treatment and the control of his diabetes is not optimal. The mental state examination was unremarkable; the patient presented, however, traits of emotionally unstable personality disorder.

Case 3 is a 19-year-old trans woman, a college student, and single. She was referred by the GP for a psychiatric assessment following numerous suicidal attempts and self-harm episodes. She had a provisional psychiatric diagnosis of Emotionally Unstable Personality Disorder—Borderline type. During the psychiatric assessment, she disclosed using oestrogens and finasteride purchased online in order to proceed with the transition. She also reported that since she started using these hormones the emotional instability became more severe and was partly responsible for the deterioration of her clinical presentation.

Case 4 is a 26-year-old trans woman, living with a partner and working as an administrator. She was referred by her GP for psychiatric assessment as part of the procedure for a referral to the Gender Identity Clinic. The patient had no previous history of mental illness, no medical comorbidity. During the interview she disclosed using oestrogen cream and finasteride tablets purchased online although she did not disclose it before (even with the GP). The mental state examination was unremarkable.

Case 5 is a 36-year-old TGNC woman, single and unemployed. She was referred by the GP for a psychiatric assessment due to low mood and polysubstance misuse (cocaine, cannabis, amphetamine and gamma-Hidroxybutyric acid (GHB). During the interview, the patient stated that she has been taking oestrogen, spironolactone and finasteride for 15 years. A year ago, she was referred to the gender reassignment clinic where she was diagnosed with moderate depression and generalised anxiety disorder, but she was asked to see a general adult psychiatrist for the treatment. The patient complained that the main contributing factors to her depression were the stigmatisation and the lack of acceptance, in which she felt that she was victimised mainly by members of her family and her community. She also was frustrated with the length of the waiting list.

### 2.2. Androgens

Case 6 is a 25-year-old TGNC man, unemployed, living with his partner. The patient was referred for a psychiatric assessment after he disclosed to the GP about using androgens without medical advice and supervision. The patient complained of The Gender Identity Research and Education Society feeling "uneasy with his body" since the age of 12. He started to purchase androgens online, 2 years before the psychiatric assessment, following a protocol available online. The patient also has stage 4 renal failure, and he was under the care of the renal team.

Case 7 is a 27-years-old TGNC man and a university student. He was admitted to an inpatient psychiatric unit after a suicidal attempt. The patient was presenting with moderate depression, on admission, he reported of using androgens purchased online while on the waiting list for an assessment by the Gender Reassignment Clinic. The patient was using the hormones without any medical advice or supervision. The low mood and the suicidal attempt were linked to his stressful situation at the university (where he struggled to cope with academic pressure) rather than to the hormonal treatment, that he also stated that he found the hormones to be beneficial. He was also frustrated by the long waiting list before he was able to start his gender affirmation process.

## 3. Discussion and Conclusions

In our paper, we discussed the clinical cases collected by the same clinician in his clinical practice in different settings, over the span of 4 years. We are aware that it is a very limited picture and we do not think that it is necessarily representative of the entire United Kingdom. We think, however, that this raises the question of access to gender affirmation treatment and the role of every clinician as an advocate for our patients. We are aware that this phenomenon has been described before, but we believe that many clinicians are not aware of it.

Self-prescribing of sexual hormones is a widespread, but poorly studied phenomenon. As highlighted in our work, the lack of access to specialised centres, stigmatisation and marginalisation of the TGNC population as well as the motivations underlying DIY hormonal treatment, deserve further consideration.

To the best of our knowledge, this is the first report of DIY hormonal treatment in general adult psychiatric settings. Previous articles that have described the trend of self-prescribing and administrations of hormones came from sexual health clinics and gender affirmation clinics [19,20]. Psychiatric assessment clinics and psychiatric inpatient wards are often the first port of call of individuals in distress. It is very important, therefore, that the staff working in these services are aware of the particular needs of the TGNC individuals. In particular, the need to establish an environment of respect and non-stigmatisation is very important in developing an effective therapeutic relationship. It is important that the terminology used is appropriate and respectful. This applies particularly to the pronouns and it is always important to check with the patients which pronouns they prefer. It is also important to tactfully ask if they have started the gender affirmation process on their own without any clinical supervision. Psychiatrists, GPs, Sexually Transmitted Diseases' (STD) specialists and all other clinicians should be informed about this under reported trend while encouraging the safe prescribing practice of sexual hormones.

As suggested by NHS England [15], the current assessment needs to be improved by proactively asking TGNC patients whether they are taking hormones and where they are sourcing them from.

The role of mental health services is particularly important because, before the gender affirmation process, TGNC individuals suffer from a higher rate of mental illnesses and mental discomfort (often due to stigma, discrimination and non-acceptance by family and society). For this reason, mental health professionals are more likely to encounter TGNC individuals in need of support but also have a crucial role to play as an advocate. It is, therefore, important when assessing TGNC individuals to respectfully enquire whether they have started the transition and if this is happening under medical care or not. If not, it is necessary to ask if they are sourcing hormones and other medications online or from other unlicensed sources. If this is the case, clinicians have the duty not only to inform the patients of the risk but also to suggest safer alternatives and support if necessary, the individuals in this process.

A common theme that emerged from our case studies was the use of hormones purchased online without any clinical guidance or supervision before and during the treatment. As previously argued [28,32], the Internet often provides a channel for accessing peer-group experiences and disseminating such risky behaviours. The underlying interpersonal trust embedded in such sub-cultural groups, as seen for instance on discussion fora or social networking, can reinforce the establishment of risk taking norms, especially among early adopters. In addition, the intake of previously untested and unregulated medicinal products can expose users to a series of unwanted side-effects, especially in potentially risky, if unsupervised, medical practices such as intramuscular (IM) injections [33,34]. The shipping process is also questionable with the risk that even where the product is genuine, it may arrive in a condition that renders it unsafe for use. Buyers may also receive counterfeited products and, therefore, using compounds that may be toxic or even lethal. It is also concerning that substances like hormones which have a significant effect on the body and the mind, are used without guidance and monitoring of the side effects. Furthermore, the route of administration (e.g., IM) can lead to additional health risks, both chronic and acute [33].

Further studies need to be carried out to evaluate the motivation underlying such a poorly researched trend. The main reason for such behaviours seems to be due to the difficulty in accessing gender reassignment/gender affirmation treatments, leaving a significant part of the TGNC population in a condition of discomfort that make them more vulnerable to the onset of psychiatric illnesses (depression, anxiety) as well as other unhealthy conditions or practices (e.g., smoking, drug intake) [18,35,36]. Furthermore, as their need for medical assistance may grow [36], trans individuals often experience problematic accesses to healthcare in terms of professionals' education and discriminatory practices [37]. This is also due to the length of the waiting lists (up to three years) that pushes TGNC individuals into obtaining hormones online [38]. Despite the various efforts made by NHS England, the GMC and the Royal Colleges to improve the situation, a significant group of individuals still do not receive the care that they need and deserve in the United Kingdom. This may also be due to the chronic lack of funds for these services despite recent years' additional funding [39]. Gender affirmation is not the treatment of an illness but is a procedure that improves the wellbeing of TGNC and non-binary individuals and, therefore, should be appropriately funded and supported by every clinician [40].

It is necessary, therefore, to address such gaps in public health policy and clinical practice knowledge regarding gender affirmation and establish alternative services. Local clinic services, complementary to the NHS provided treatment, may be crucial to the wellbeing of individuals who are feeling disenfranchised and are not attending the gender reassignment/gender affirmation clinics while considering the treatment [41]. Examples of such services can be found in the United States with the Transgender Health Services program (STRIDE) based in San Francisco, which is structured as a peer-based model providing hormone therapy and support for the general and the psychological health of TGNC individuals [42]. Different gender reassignment/gender affirmation programs are also available in Canada. In British Columbia and Ontario projects like Trans Care BC (British Columbia) and Trans Health Connection (Ontario) aim to facilitate the access to care for TGNC by providing information and support for the TGNC community [43,44].

In summary, we believe that increasing the access to gender affirmation services alone, however, is not enough and it is necessary to raise awareness among every clinician about the special needs that TGNC individuals have when accessing healthcare. It would be necessary, to achieve this goal, to design and disseminate among all clinicians, a questionnaire regarding their attitude towards TGNC individuals, their knowledge about the gender affirmation process and the specific clinical needs that the TGNC population has. In this way, it would be possible to establish the educational needs that clinicians have and, therefore, consider specific training. This would enable improvement of access to care for TGNC individuals by fighting stigma and creating a more inclusive service. This approach should be across all the services that might care for TGNC individuals. Furthermore, disseminating knowledge and raising awareness might have another beneficial effect by transforming conscious clinicians in health to advocate for the TGNC population. In this way, it may be possible to address not only the problem highlighted in this article (the difficulty of accessing gender affirmation clinics) but also the more widespread discrimination that TGNC individuals face when accessing various health care services.

As we have seen in our study, the implementation of such different and innovative health care services for TGNC individuals as well as more targeted prevention strategies on such underreported and highly risky behaviours have become a necessity in the United Kingdom and elsewhere. Closer attention should also be paid to the online market of DIY hormones, and an open dialogue with LGBTQ organisations should be established to support TGNC individuals and better understand their unmet needs.

**Author Contributions:** A.M. designed the study and collected the case studies. He also wrote the first draft of the paper. A.N. contributed to the manuscript's preparation and submission. G.M. and O.C. supported the study design and revised the paper at various stages during its preparation.

## References

1. American Psychological Association. Guidelines for Psychological Practice with Transgender and Gender Nonconforming People. Available online: http://www.apa.org/practice/guidelines/transgender.pdf (accessed on 13 May 2018).
2. Meerwijk, E.L.; Sevelius, J.M. Transgender Population Size in the United States: A Meta-Regression of Population-Based Probability Samples. *Am. J. Public Health* **2017**, *107*, e1–e8. [CrossRef] [PubMed]
3. Deutsch, M.B. Making It Count: Improving Estimates of the Size of Transgender and Gender Nonconforming Populations. *LGBT Health* **2016**, *3*, 181–185. [CrossRef] [PubMed]
4. Office for National Statistics. Transparency and Governance. Available online: https://www.ons.gov.uk/aboutus/transparencyandgovernance/freedomofinformationfoi/transgenderpopulationfigures (accessed on 13 May 2018).
5. The Gender Identity Research and Education Society. Available online: http://www.gires.org.uk/wp-content/uploads/2014/10/Prevalence2011.pdf (accessed on 13 May 2018).
6. Williams Institute UCLA. Available online: https://williamsinstitute.law.ucla.edu/wp-content/uploads/CHIS-Transgender-Teens-FINAL.pdf (accessed on 13 May 2018).
7. Flores, A.R.; Herman, J.L.; Gates, G.J.; Brown, T.N.T. *How Many Adults Identify as Transgender in the United States?* The Williams Institute: Los Angeles, CA, USA, 2016. Available online: http://williamsinstitute.law.ucla.edu/wp-content/uploads/How-Many-Adults-Identify-as-Transgender-in-the-United-States.pdf (accessed on 30 January 2018).
8. Heylens, G.; Verroken, C.; De Cock, S.; T'Sjoen, G.; De Cuypere, G. Effects of different steps in gender reassignment therapy on psychopathology: A prospective study of persons with a gender identity disorder. *J. Sex. Med.* **2014**, *11*, 119–126. [CrossRef] [PubMed]
9. Fisher, A.D.; Castellini, G.; Bandini, E.; Casale, H.; Fanni, E.; Benni, L.; Ferruccio, N.; Meriggiola, M.C.; Manieri, C.; Gualerzi, A.; et al. Cross-sex hormonal treatment and body uneasiness in individuals with gender dysphoria. *J. Sex. Med.* **2014**, *11*, 709–719. [CrossRef] [PubMed]
10. Fabris, B.; Bernardi, S.; Trombetta, C. Cross-sex hormone therapy for gender dysphoria. *J. Endocrinol. Investig.* **2015**, *38*, 269–282. [CrossRef] [PubMed]
11. Deutsch, M.B. Guidelines for the Primary and Gender-Affirming Care for Transgender and Gender Nonbinary People. Available online: http://transhealth.ucsf.edu/pdf/Transgender-PGACG-6-17-16.pdf (accessed on 30 January 2018).
12. NHS England. Interim Gender Dysphoria Protocol and Service Guideline 2013/14. Available online: https://www.england.nhs.uk/wp-content/uploads/2013/10/int-gend-proto.pdf (accessed on 30 January 2018).
13. Royal College of Psychiatrist. Good Practice Guidelines for the Assessment and Treatment of Adults with Gender Dysphoria. Available online: http://www.rcpsych.ac.uk/files/pdfversion/CR181_Nov15.pdf (accessed on 30 January 2018).
14. World Professional Association for Transgender Health (WPATH). Standards of Care V7. Available online: https://s3.amazonaws.com/amo_hub_content/Association140/files/Standards%20of%20Care%20V7%20-%202011%20WPATH%20 (accessed on 30 January 2018).

15. National Health Service (NHS). Gender Identity Services for Adults. Available online: https://www.engage.england.nhs.uk/survey/gender-identity-services-for-adults/user_uploads/gender-identity-non-surgical-specification.pdf (accessed on 30 January 2018).
16. General Medical Council (GMC). Advice for Doctors Treating Trans Patients. Available online: https://www.gmc-uk.org/guidance/28851.asp (accessed on 30 January 2018).
17. Gonzales, G.; Henning-Smith, C. Barriers to Care among Transgender and Gender Nonconforming Adults. *Milbank Q.* **2017**, *95*, 726–748. [CrossRef] [PubMed]
18. Giblon, R.; Bauer, G.R. Health care availability, quality, and unmet need: A comparison of transgender and cisgender residents of Ontario, Canada. *BMC Health Serv. Res.* **2017**, *17*, 283. [CrossRef] [PubMed]
19. Rotondi, N.K.; Bauer, G.R.; Scanlon, K.; Kaay, M.; Travers, R.; Travers, A. Nonprescribed hormone use and self-performed surgeries: "do-it-yourself" transition in transgender communities in Ontario, Canada. *Am. J. Public Health* **2013**, *103*, 1830–1836. [CrossRef] [PubMed]
20. Mepham, N.; Bouman, W.P.; Arcelus, J.; Hayter, M.; Wylie, K.R. People with gender dysphoria who self-prescribe cross-sex hormones: Prevalence, sources, and side effects knowledge. *J. Sex. Med.* **2014**, *11*, 2995–3001. [CrossRef] [PubMed]
21. Corazza, O.; Martinotti, G.; Santacroce, R.; Chillemi, E.; Di Giannantonio, M.; Schifano, F.; Cellek, S. Sexual enhancement products for sale online: Raising awareness of the psychoactive effects of yohimbine, maca, horny goat weed, and *Ginkgo biloba*. *BioMed Res. Int.* **2014**, *2014*, 841798. [CrossRef] [PubMed]
22. Mooney, R.; Simonato, P.; Ruparelia, R.; Roman-Urrestarazu, A.; Martinotti, G.; Corazza, O. The use of supplements and performance and image enhancing drugs in fitness settings: A exploratory cross-sectional investigation in the United Kingdom. *Hum. Psychopharmacol. Clin. Exp.* **2017**, *32*. [CrossRef] [PubMed]
23. Schifano, F.; Ricciardi, A.; Corazza, O.; Deluca, P.; Davey, Z.; Rafanelli, C. New drugs of abuse on the Web: The role of Psychonaut Web Mapping Project. *Riv. Psichiatr.* **2010**, *45*, 88–93. [PubMed]
24. Corazza, O.; Parrott, A.C.; Demetrovics, Z. Novel psychoactive substances: Shedding new lights on the ever-changing drug scenario and the associated health risks. *Hum. Psychopharmacol. Clin. Exp.* **2017**, *32*. [CrossRef] [PubMed]
25. Corazza, O.; Bersani, F.S.; Brunoro, R.; Valeriani, G.; Martinotti, G.; Schifano, F. The diffusion of performance and image enhancing drugs (PIEDs) on the internet: The abuse of the cognitive enhancer piracetam. *Subst. Use Misuse* **2014**, *49*, 1849–1856. [CrossRef] [PubMed]
26. Di Nicola, A.; Martini, E. *FAKECARE—Developing Expertise against the Online Trade of Fake Medicines by Producing and Disseminating Knowledge, Counterstrategies and Tools across the EU*; eCrime Research Report; University if Trento: Trento, Italy, 2015.
27. Orizio, G.; Schulz, P.; Domenighini, S.; Bressanelli, M.; Rubinelli, S.; Caimi, L.; Gelatti, U. Online Consultations in Cyberpharmacies: Completeness and Patient Safety. *Telemed. J. E-Health* **2009**, *15*, 1022–1025. [CrossRef] [PubMed]
28. Littlejohn, C.; Baldacchino, A.; Schifano, F.; DeLuca, P. Internet pharmacies and online prescription drug sales: A cross-sectional study. *Drugs Educ. Prev. Policy* **2005**, *12*, 75–80. [CrossRef]
29. Chandler, M.; McVeigh, J. *Steroid and Image Enhancing Drugs. 2013 Survey Results*; Centre for Public Health, Liverpool John Moores University: Liverpool, UK, 2013. Available online: http://www.drugs.ie/resourcesfiles/ResearchDocs/Europe/Research/2015/Steroids_and_Image_Steroid_Image_Enhancing_Drugs_2013_Survey_Results_FINAL.pdf (accessed on 30 January 2018).
30. Brennan, R. An Ethno-Pharmacological Study of the Injecting Use of Performance and Image Enhancing Drugs (PIED). Ph.D. Thesis, Waterford Institute of Technology, Waterford, Ireland, 2018.
31. Imborek, K.L.; Graf, E.M.; McCune, K. Preventive health for transgender men and women. *Semin. Reprod. Med.* **2017**, *35*, 426–433. [PubMed]
32. Valeriani, G.; Corazza, O.; Bersani, F.S.; Melcore, C.; Metastasio, A.; Bersani, G.; Schifano, F. Olanzapine as the ideal "trip terminator"? Analysis of online reports relating to antipsychotics' use and misuse following occurence of novel psychoactive substance-related psychotic symptoms. *Hum. Psychopharmacol.* **2015**, *30*, 249–254. [CrossRef] [PubMed]
33. Gordon, R.J.; Lowy, F.D. Bacterial Infections in Drug Users. *N. Engl. J. Med.* **2005**, *353*, 1945–1954. [CrossRef] [PubMed]
34. Ebright, J.R.; Pieper, B. Skin and soft tissue infections in injection drug users. *Infect. Dis. Clin. N. Am.* **2002**, *16*, 697–712. [CrossRef]

35. Colizzi, M.; Costa, R.; Todarello, O. Transsexual patients' psychiatric comorbidity and positive effect of cross-sex hormonal treatment on mental health: Results from a longitudinal study. *Psychoneuroendocrinology* **2014**, *39*, 65–73. [CrossRef] [PubMed]
36. Sperber, J.; Landers, S.; Lawrence, S. Access to health care for transgendered persons: Results of a needs assessment in Boston. *Int. J. Transgenderism* **2008**, *8*, 75–91. [CrossRef]
37. Bauer, G.R.; Scheim, A.I.; Deutsch, M.B.; Massarella, C. Reported emergency department avoidance, use, and experiences of transgender persons in Ontario, Canada: Results from a respondent-driven sampling survey. *Ann. Emerg. Med.* **2014**, *63*, 713–720. [CrossRef] [PubMed]
38. The Indipendent. Patients 'Waiting Three Years for Gender Identity Clinic Consultation'. Available online: http://www.independent.co.uk/news/uk/home-news/patients-waiting-three-years-for-gender-identity-clinic-consultations-a6770971.html (accessed on 30 January 2018).
39. The Guardian. Gender Identity Clinic Services under Strain as Referral Rates Soar. Available online: https://www.theguardian.com/society/2016/jul/10/transgender-clinic-waiting-times-patient-numbers-soar-gender-identity-services (accessed on 30 January 2018).
40. Richards, C.; Arcelus, J.; Barrett, J.; Bouman, W.P.; Lenihan, P.; Lorimer, S.; Murjan, S.; Seal, L. Trans is not a disorder—But should still receive funding. *Sex. Relatsh. Ther.* **2015**, *30*, 309–313. [CrossRef]
41. Crall, C.S.; Jackson, R.K. Should psychiatrists prescribe gender-affirming hormone therapy to transgender adolescents? *AMA J. Ethics* **2016**, *18*, 1086–1094. [PubMed]
42. St. James Infirmary. STRIDE: Transgender Hormone Therapy Program. Available online: http://stjamesinfirmary.org/wordpress/?page_id=16 (accessed on 30 January 2018).
43. Provincial Health Services Authority. Trans Care British Columbia. Available online: http://www.phsa.ca/our-services/programs-services/trans-care-bc (accessed on 30 January 2018).
44. Rainbow Health Ontario. Trans Health Connection. Available online: https://www.rainbowhealthontario.ca/trans-health-connection/ (accessed on 30 January 2018).

# 13

# Mood Fluctuation and Psychobiological Instability: The Same Core Functions are Disrupted by Novel Psychoactive Substances and Established Recreational Drugs

**Andrew C. Parrott** [1,2]

[1] Department of Psychology, Swansea University, Swansea SA2 8PP, South Wales, UK; a.c.parrott@swansea.ac.uk

[2] Centre for Human Psychopharmacology, Swinburne University, Melbourne, VIC 3122, Australia

**Abstract:** Many novel psychoactive substances (NPS) have entered the recreational drug scene in recent years, yet the problems they cause are similar to those found with established drugs. This article will debate the psychobiological effects of these newer and more traditional substances. It will show how they disrupt the same core psychobiological functions, so damaging well-being in similar ways. Every psychoactive drug causes mood states to fluctuate. Users feel better on-drug, then feel worse off-drug. The strength of these mood fluctuations is closely related to their addiction potential. Cyclical changes can occur with many other core psychobiological functions, such as information processing and psychomotor speed. Hence the list of drug-related impairments can include: homeostatic imbalance, HPA axis disruption, increased stress, altered sleep patterns, neurohormonal changes, modified brain rhythms, neurocognitive impairments, and greater psychiatric vulnerability. Similar patterns of deficit are found with older drugs such as cocaine, nicotine and cannabis, and newer substances such as 3,4-methylenedioxymethamphetamine (MDMA), mephedrone and spice. All psychoactive drugs damage human well-being through similar basic neuropsychobiological mechanisms.

**Keywords:** amphetamine; cocaine; mephedrone; cannabis; spice; drug; mood; homeostasis

---

## 1. Mood State Fluctuations

Psychoactive drugs, by definition, cause mood states to change and fluctuate. Hence an important factor for drug-induced distress is mood instability. This is found with sedative drugs such as alcohol or cannabis, and stimulant drugs such as cocaine or methamphetamine [1–6]. Indeed, the main reason that psychoactive drugs are used recreationally is for their "positive" mood effects, such as feelings of relaxation and pleasure [4]. Novel psychoactive substances (NPS) such as mephedrone and spice cannabinoids are very similar in this regard [6–9]. Although one of the paradoxes of drug taking is that many of the apparent mood gains represent the reversal of unpleasant abstinence feelings. Nicotine is a prime example of this pattern [10–12], although it also occurs with other substances [4].

Psychoactive drugs can also produce undesirable mood state changes. For instance, recreational cannabis, whether herbal or spice, can lead to feelings of tension and suspiciousness [2,13]. Stimulants such as cocaine, methamphetamine and mephedrone can also lead to feelings of anxiety and paranoia [1,14,15]. The acute mood effects of all psychoactive drugs can be highly variable and may differ considerably between individuals. On alcohol some users become happy and jovial, while others become moody and aggressive, especially after excess levels of consumption [5,16,17]. In a similar way, Le Strat et al. [18] documented a wide range of responses to an acute dose of cannabis. Furthermore, those with positive initial mood reactions were most likely to become regular cannabis users, whereas those with negative or neutral mood reactions to cannabis tended not to persevere with its usage. Similar differences in mood response have also been empirically demonstrated with the methamphetamine derivative MDMA (3,4-methylenedioxymethamphetamine or "Ecstasy"). This drug is often described as the most euphoriant of all the recreational stimulants. Yet acute MDMA can release a wide range of feelings and cognitions-both positive and negative. Liechti et al. [19] found that an acute dose of MDMA in the laboratory led to significant increases in feelings of both introversion and extraversion, while feelings of happiness and depression were also significantly intensified. In a comprehensive review of the acute-dose MDMA mood literature, it was found that a wide range of positive and negative psychological material could be released/intensified [20]. For instance, psychotherapists who have incorporated MDMA into their therapy sessions have noted that the emergent psychological material can be difficult and stressful for the client to handle, although its release may also be important for potential therapeutic gains [20–24]. In positive environmental situations, the positive mood effects of MDMA predominate, whereas in neutral situations its mood effects can be more variable and less positive [14,15]. These adverse mood abreactions to MDMA can be more frequent than is commonly portrayed. In an article entitled: "Hug drug or thug drug", Reid et al. [25] noted that MDMA often generated feelings of anger and aggression. Rugani et al. [26] noted that acute psychotic patients who had used MDMA for recreational purposes demonstrated heightened levels of hostility, physical violence, and verbal aggression than non-users. The authors noted that this finding "surely runs counter to the expected entactogenic effects of Ecstasy" (for further debate, see [27]).

In a large Internet study of mephedrone and MDMA users, the acute mood effects of each drug were broadly similar, although some intriguing differences in pharmacodynamic tolerance were apparent [9]. A mixture of positive and negative mood changes is also found with established recreational stimulants such as cocaine [28], and laboratory doses of methamphetamine [14,15]. The effects of high doses of amphetamine and cocaine can be very strong, with reports of a physical rush or hit. These high doses can lead to intensely negative moods, with very severe feelings of suspiciousness, or clinical paranoia. Spice cannabinoids can also have far stronger effects that herbal cannabis, in both positive and negative ways [29]. The more extreme mood reactions of the more powerful drugs can lead to changeable and unpredictable patterns of behavior. However, these abreactions can occur with any psychoactive drug, irrespective of whether they are established or novel.

### *1.1. Drug Withdrawal and Repetitive Mood Vacillation*

One of the main problems with every psychoactive drug is that the brief period of on-drug mood gains is followed by a period of neurochemical depletion afterwards, when the opposite mood states develop. These rebound moods are typically negative and aversive, and are readily reversed by taking the drug again. Hence every mood-altering drug has addiction potential. Indeed, the essence of addiction is these repetitive mood vacillations [4,30]. This pattern can be illustrated by legal stimulants such as nicotine, illicit drugs such as cocaine, or novel substances such as MDMA or mephedrone. The former two drugs have been extensively studied, with nicotine showing many pharmacokinetic and pharmacodynamic similarities to cocaine [31]. Both drugs are powerful Central Nervous System (CNS) stimulants, with the first cigarette of the day increasing heart rate substantially [32,33], which is one of the reasons tobacco smokers develop hypertension. In mood terms, tobacco smokers feel more alert after the first cigarette of the day, but soon this activation is lost, and after 20–60 min the regular smoker needs yet another cigarette. This mood fluctuation repeats over the rest of the day and recurs every day for the rest of their lives—until they quit or prematurely die [10,11,34].

Similar patterns of mood fluctuation occur with cocaine, since nasal snorting leads to a rapid hit, followed by a low-mood comedown, and the urgent need for another drug hit. Cocaine therefore displays high addiction potential, with crack cocaine being even more troublesome and addictive, due its extreme rapidity of action [4,35,36]. Khat leaf chewing occurs in many countries around the Horn of

Africa [37,38], with cathinone being slowly released into the systemic circulation. Cathinone displays weaker stimulant properties than cocaine. Yet Khat chewers also report acute mood gains, followed by negative moods on withdrawal, in a pattern identical to that found with other stimulants [37]. This is also evident with MDMA, although over a longer time period. Hence the acute moods peak after a couple of hours, while the recovery period can last for several days [28,39–42]. This long pharmacodynamic profile explains why Ecstasy/MDMA is only taken intermittently and displays lower addiction potential than most other stimulants [43,44].

Cannabis may be a sedative drug, but it shows a similar pattern of mood vacillation to the stimulant drug nicotine. Vandrey et al. [45] compared the mood changes found during withdrawal from cannabis and tobacco, and concluded that they were very similar. For instance, the unpleasant mood effects of cannabis withdrawal could include feelings of irritability, anger, and depression (i.e., very similar to tobacco), along with other problems such as impaired sleep, altered circadian rhythms, changed appetite, and drug cravings [45,46]. These symptoms of cannabis withdrawal have been formalized in standardized questionnaires such as the Cannabis Withdrawal Discomfort Scale [47], and the Marijuana Craving Questionnaire [48]. The high addictiveness of cannabis does make it difficult to understand current movements to make its usage legal [49].

### *1.2. Related Psychobiological Problems*

Many other psychological skills and abilities may also fluctuate during drug stimulation and drug withdrawal. For instance, tobacco smokers display worse memories than non-smokers [50]. The reason for this is that new information is being laid down in memory and is being stored under a constantly changing background of nicotine levels. Hence memory storage and retrieval are both adversely affected by nicotine addiction [12]. Sleep is also adversely affected by nicotine addiction, while it improves to normal following smoking cessation [12]. The many psychobiological problems found in recreational stimulant users have been described in numerous comprehensive reviews [1,3,36,51,52].

Similarly, the addictiveness of herbal cannabis was noted earlier, while the stronger skunk varieties of herbal cannabis display greater potential [53]. Artificial spice cannabinoids are even stronger, and hence more damaging. Some of the artificial spices are full agonists for the cannabinoid receptor, whereas herbal cannabis is a weak partial agonist [54]. Hence spice displays far greater addictiveness, with some users committing suicide when they cannot access their normal drug supplies [6,29,55–58]. The practical consequences of cannabis dependency can be severe [49]. In the USA around 300,000 individuals approach professional drug addiction services for cannabis dependency every year [59]. Clinically disabling dependency occurs in around 10% of those who have ever tried the drug [60], while 65% of cannabis ever-users report some aspects of drug dependency [61], with young initiates the most vulnerable [62]. In summary, the core problems related to drug dependency are similar for stimulants and depressant drugs, and for older and newer psychoactive substances.

## 2. Homeostasis

One fundamental index of psychological balance and health is homeostasis. When the organism is well adapted to its environment, its daily rhythms of behavioral and physiological activity occur smoothly and efficiently. Selye [63] noted that disruption to homeostasis led to psychological imbalance, increased bio-physiological stress, and led to excessive energy expenditure. Furthermore, the repeated experience of acute stress led to cumulative chronic stress and this caused physical and psychological ill-health. Selye [63] showed that the Hypothalamic-Pituitary-Adrenal (HPA) axis was crucial for psychophysiological stability, with cortisol being the key neurohormone for maintaining homeostatic balance [64]. Healthy individuals showed regular circadian rhythms of cortisol secretion, and this master hormone helped to maintain the optimal secretion patterns for other important neurohormones [63,65,66].

Many psychoactive drugs affect neurohormonal secretions acutely, and when these drugs are taken repeatedly, they can lead to chronic stress. This may be illustrated with the recreational stimulant

MDMA [65,66]. In placebo-controlled laboratory trials, an acute dose of MDMA can generate a cortisol increase of around 150% [67]. Recreational Ecstasy/MDMA users show peak cortisol increases of around 800%, probably due to the combined effects of taking a stimulant drug in a stimulating environment [42,68]. The Cortisol Awakening Response can also be affected in recreational Ecstasy/MDMA users [69], with around 70% of recreational users complaining of disrupted sleep, even when drug-free [70]. Body temperatures can also change, with MDMA showing well-documented patterns of thermal change [71–73]. Synthetic cannabinoids such as AKB48 can induce hypothermia [74], while synthetic cathinones such as mephedrone can also affect thermal reactivity [75]. Returning to chronic stress, regular MDMA users show strong longer-term neurohormonal changes. When cortisol was measured in 3-month hair samples, the regular Ecstasy/MDMA users displayed 400% higher cortisol levels than non-user controls, while the light Ecstasy/MDMA users showed intermediate cortisol values [76]. MDMA is not the only recreational drug which can affect cortisol. Raganathan et al. [77] showed that acute tetrahydrocannabinol (THC) led to a significant increase in cortisol secretion. King et al. [78] found that chronic cannabis users had significantly higher salivary cortisol levels than non-user controls. Currently there is a paucity of empirical evidence on the neurohormonal effects of Novel Psychoactive Substances, and empirical studies in this area are therefore needed.

*Psychiatric Aspects*

All psychiatric disorders are dimensional, with symptoms ranging on a continuum from low to high. This core notion may seem rather obvious, but it needs to be stated since it can help explain how psychoactive drugs contribute to mental distress. The core processes described earlier, of mood state vacillation and homeostatic imbalance, can each contribute to mental instability, while those individuals with a predisposition to mental distress may be particularly vulnerable to the destabilizing effects of psychoactive drugs. For an example of this interactive psychiatric model applied to recreational MDMA, see Parrott [79].

The first written report of psychiatric problems being caused by any psychoactive drug were present in the world's oldest pharmacopoeia, attributed to Emperor Shen Nung in bronze-age China. This noted that when cannabis was taken in excess, it could produce "visions of devils" [80]. Modern research has confirmed that cannabis may cause a form of psychosis, with many similarities to classic schizophrenia [13]. Hence an acute dose of cannabis can induce bizarre thoughts and cognitions [81]. D'Souza and colleagues [82] administered THC and placebo to recreational cannabis users without any prior psychiatric history. The active cannabis condition led to significant increases in scores on the Positive and Negative Symptom Scale (PANSS), the standard rating scale for clinical symptoms of schizophrenia. Individual subjective experiences under the acute influence of THC included the following: "I thought I could see into the future" ... "I thought you were trying to program me" ... "I thought you could read my mind" ... "I thought I was god". These delusional thoughts as measured by raised PANSS positive symptom scores, can also correlate with changed patterns of brain activity [83].

When used regularly, cannabis can lead to both clinical psychosis, and other forms of psychiatric disorder [84]. The Swedish Conscript study was the first prospective investigation to demonstrate an association between cannabis and schizophrenia [85]. This finding has been replicated in further prospective studies, where regular cannabis use led to an increased risk of psychotic breakdown in later years. Le Bec et al. [86] undertook a comprehensive review and concluded that every published study showed a significant link between recreational cannabis and the later emergence of psychosis. One crucial factor is that the drug needs to be taken repeatedly and regularly. In one prospective study, Henquet et al. [87] found that occasional cannabis users showed no increase in risk, weekly-users showed a slightly increased risk, while daily-cannabis users showed a highly significant increase in later psychosis. Regular cannabis use is also associated with an increased risk for other mental health problems, such as depression and mania [88,89].

Recreational CNS stimulants can also cause greater psychiatric distress. Feyissa and Kelly [90] noted that Khat chewing could lead to a range of mental health problems including depression and hypomania; hence even weaker drugs such as cathinone can lead to psychiatric problems, while regular users of stronger stimulants such as amphetamine, cocaine or methamphetamine can experience a wide range of problems, including psychosis, depression, paranoia, psychomotor tics/tremors, eating disorders, and aggression [1,3,4,35,51,91]. Recreational MDMA is also associated with a wide range of adverse psychiatric consequences, such as clinical depression, aggression, problems with weight control, eating/food intake, and some of these issues may endure for years after drug cessation [26,76,92–99].

## 3. Neurocognitive Deficits

Cognitive skills are an important focus for most areas of applied psychology, and psychopharmacology is no exception. The extensive empirical literature demonstrates both acute and chronic drug influences. By definition, any drug which is psychoactive will affect not only mood states (see Section 1), but many other psychological functions including neurocognition. CNS stimulants such as cocaine or mephedrone will speed information processing, but also increase errors through increased carelessness and impulsivity. CNS depressants will generally lengthen reaction times but may increase errors through reduced alertness and vigilance/attention. When combined with drug-induced feelings of confidence, these changes can make any psychoactive drug dangerous for practical skills such as car driving [4,55,100]. Their chronic use can also be damaging. In an extensive review, Cruickshank and Dyer [1] noted that methamphetamine led to impairments in executive functioning, learning, memory, and motor skills. Other reviews have generated similar lists of neurocognitive impairments following other stimulants such as cocaine [52,101], or Ecstasy/MDMA [27,44,102–108]. Cannabis can lead to acute deficits in memory, learning, sustained attention, and higher cognitive skills, while its chronic use can lead to a wide range of cognitive deficits, even including a decline in general intelligence, with reduced IQ test scores [109–114]. Neuroimaging studies of regular cannabis users indicate deficits in various brain regions, such as the hippocampus and amygdala [114], with white matter degeneration and de-myelination [115].

## 4. Final Overview

Psychoactive drugs can damage human well-being simply by being psychoactive! In acute terms they may boost activity for a short period, but this is soon followed by a period of neurochemical recovery, when the opposite psychological states develop. These psychological fluctuations are readily seen in mood state changes of daily tobacco smokers (see Figure 1 in Parrott, [10]). However, moods and feelings provide just one index for other more general changes in psychological status. Many different psychological functions can be affected—in different ways by different drugs. They also affect many different neurotransmitter systems. Yet despite the multitude and variety of their neurotransmitter actions, in psychobiological terms these drugs all display the same underlying pattern of disrupted balance and equilibrium [4,11,30,38]. These core biological factors also explain why every psychoactive drug displays addiction potential. Regular users suffer from negative states off-drug, and feel better when on-drug, hence the "need" to take the drug repeatedly [10]. As novice users, the more they succumb to their new habit, the stronger their drug dependency becomes.

Psychoactive drugs also affect the HPA axis, causing hormonal dysregulation, and increasing the susceptibility for stress [4,66]. The healthy human organism displays a natural balance between sympathetic and parasympathetic nervous system activity. So, when humans take recreational drugs, they disturb this natural balance, and this leads to adverse consequences [4]. Proponents for drug use typically only talk about the short-term drug gains, and with this narrow focus, any psychoactive drug can be miss-described as beneficial. It is only by covering all aspects of their acute and chronic usage that a more complete picture of their damaging effects can emerge.

## References


1. Cruickshank, C.C.; Dyer, K.R. A review of the clinical pharmacology of methamphetamine. *Addiction* **2009**, *104*, 1085–1099. [CrossRef] [PubMed]
2. Hall, W. What has research over the past two decades revealed about the adverse health effects of recreational cannabis use? *Addiction* **2015**, *110*, 19–35. [CrossRef] [PubMed]
3. Panenka, W.K.; Procyshyn, R.M.; Lecomte, T.; MacEwan, G.W.; Flynn, S.W.; Honer, W.G.; Barr, A.M. Methamphetamine use: A comprehensive review of molecular, preclinical and clinical findings. *Drug Alcohol Depend.* **2013**, *129*, 167–179. [CrossRef] [PubMed]
4. Parrott, A.C. Why all stimulant drugs are damaging to recreational users: An empirical overview and psychobiological explanation. *Hum. Psychopharmacol.* **2015**, *30*, 213–224. [CrossRef] [PubMed]
5. Parrott, A.; Morinan, A.; Moss, M.; Scholey, A. *Understanding Drugs and Behaviour*; John Wiley & Sons: Chichester, UK, 2004.
6. Schifano, F.; Albanese, A.; Fergus, S.; Stair, J.L.; Deluca, P.; Corraza, O. Mephedrone (4-methylmethcathinone; 'meow meow'): Chemical, pharmacological and clinical issues. *Psychopharmacology* **2011**, *214*, 593–602. [CrossRef] [PubMed]
7. Freeman, T.P.; Morgan, C.J.A.; Vaughn-Jones, J.; Hussain, N.; Karimi, K.; Curran, V.H. Cognitive and subjective effects of mephedrone and factors influencing use of a new 'legal high'. *Addiction* **2011**, *107*, 792–800. [CrossRef] [PubMed]
8. Gurney, S.M.; Scott, K.S.; Kacinko, S.L.; Presley, B.C.; Logan, B.K. Pharmacology, Toxicology, and Adverse Effects of Synthetic Cannabinoid Drugs. *Forensic. Sci. Rev.* **2014**, *26*, 53–78. [PubMed]
9. Jones, L.; Reed, P.; Parrott, A.C. Mephedrone and MDMA: A comparison of their acute and chronic effects, as described by young recreational polydrug users. *J. Psychopharmacol.* **2016**, in press.
10. Parrott, A.C. Individual differences in stress and arousal during cigarette smoking. *Psychopharmacology* **1994**, *115*, 389–396. [CrossRef] [PubMed]
11. Parrott, A.C. Does cigarette smoking cause stress? *Am. Psychol.* **1999**, *54*, 817–820. [CrossRef] [PubMed]
12. Parrott, A.C. Nicotine psychobiology: How chronic-dose prospective studies can illuminate some of the theoretical issues from acute-dose research. *Psychopharmacology* **2006**, *184*, 567–576. [CrossRef] [PubMed]
13. Volkow, N.D.; Baler, R.D.; Compton, W.M.; Weiss, S.R.B. Adverse Health Effects of Marijuana Use. *N. Engl. J. Med.* **2014**, *370*, 2219–2227. [CrossRef] [PubMed]
14. Kirkpatrick, M.G.; Gunderson, E.W.; Perez, A.Y.; Haney, M.; Foltin, R.W.; Hart, C.L. A direct comparison of the behavioral and physiological effects of methamphetamine and 3,4-methylenedioxymethamphetamine (MDMA) in humans. *Psychopharmacology* **2012**, *219*, 109–122. [CrossRef] [PubMed]
15. Parrott, A.C.; Gibbs, A.; Scholey, A.B.; King, R.; Owens, K.; Swann, P.; Ogden, E.; Stough, C. MDMA and methamphetamine: Some paradoxical negative and positive mood changes in an acute dose laboratory study. *Psychopharmacology* **2011**, *215*, 527–536. [CrossRef] [PubMed]
16. Murgraff, V.; Parrott, A.C.; Bennett, P. Risky single occasion drinking amongst young people: Definition, correlates, policy and intervention. A broad overview of research findings. *Alcohol Alcohol.* **1998**, *33*, 3–14. [CrossRef]
17. Parrott, A.C.; Drayson, R.; Henry, L.A. Alcohol: Drink less and live more. *J. Alcohol Drug Depend. Subst. Abuse* **2016**, *2*, 4.
18. Le Strat, Y.; Ramoz, N.; Horwood, J.; Falissard, B.; Hassler, C.; Romo, L.; Gorwood, P. First positive reactions to cannabis constitute a priority risk factor for cannabis dependence. *Addiction* **2009**, *104*, 1710–1717. [CrossRef] [PubMed]
19. Liechti, M.E.; Gamma, A.; Vollenweider, F.X. Gender differences in the subjective effects of MDMA. *Psychopharmacology* **2001**, *154*, 161–168. [CrossRef] [PubMed]
20. Parrott, A.C. The psychotherapeutic potential of MDMA (3,4-methylenedioxymethamphetamine): An evidence-based review. *Psychopharmacology* **2007**, *191*, 181–193. [CrossRef] [PubMed]
21. Bouso, J.C. Using MDMA in the treatment of post-traumatic stress disorder. In *Ecstasy: The Complete Guide*; Holland, J., Ed.; Park Street Press: Rochester, NY, USA, 2001.

22. Greer, G.; Tolbert, R. Subjective reports of the effects of MDMA in a clinical setting. *J. Psychoact. Drugs* **1986**, *18*, 319–327. [CrossRef] [PubMed]
23. Parrott, A.C. MDMA assisted psychotherapy—A psychobiological perspective and critique. In *International Handbook of Psychobiology*; Murphy, P., Ed.; Routledge: Abingdon-on-Thames, UK, 2018.
24. Parrott, A.C. The potential dangers of using MDMA for psychotherapy. *J. Psychoactive Drugs* **2014**, *46*, 37–43. [CrossRef] [PubMed]
25. Reid, L.W.; Elifson, K.W.; Sterk, C.E. Hug drug or thug drug? Ecstasy use and aggressive behavior. *Violence Vict.* **2007**, *22*, 104–119. [CrossRef] [PubMed]
26. Rugani, F.; Bacciardi, S.; Rovai, L.; Pacini, M.; Maremmani, A.G.I.; Deltito, J.; Dell'Osso, L.; Maremmani, I. Symptomatological features of patients with and without ecstasy use during their first psychotic episode. *Int. J. Environ. Res. Pub. Health* **2012**, *9*, 2283–2292. [CrossRef] [PubMed]
27. Parrott, A.C. Human psychobiology of MDMA or 'Ecstasy': An overview of 25 years of empirical research. *Hum. Psychopharmacol.* **2013**, *28*, 289–307. [CrossRef] [PubMed]
28. Parrott, A.C.; Evans, L.J.; Howells, J.; Robart, R. Cocaine versus Ecstasy/MDMA: Comparative effects on mood and cognition in recreational users. *Open Addict. J.* **2011**, *4*, 36–37. [CrossRef]
29. Seely, K.A.; Lapoint, J.; Moran, J.H.; Fattore, L. Spice drugs are more than harmless herbal blends: A review of the pharmacology and toxicology of synthetic cannabinoids. *Prog. Neuro-Psychopharmacol. Biol. Psychiatry* **2012**, *39*, 234–243. [CrossRef] [PubMed]
30. Parrott, A.C. Drug taking–for better or for worse? *Psychologist* **2008**, *21*, 924–927.
31. Mello, N.K. Hormones, nicotine, and cocaine: Clinical studies. *Hormones Behav.* **2010**, *58*, 57–71. [CrossRef] [PubMed]
32. Mangan, G.L.; Golding, J.F. *The Psychopharmacology of Smoking*; Oxford University Press: Oxford, UK, 1986.
33. Parrott, A.C.; Winder, G. Nicotine chewing gum (2 mg, 4 mg) and cigarette smoking: Comparative effects upon vigilance and heart rate. *Psychopharmacology* **1989**, *97*, 257–261. [CrossRef] [PubMed]
34. Parrott, A.C. Nesbitt's Paradox resolved? Stress and arousal modulation during cigarette smoking. *Addiction* **1998**, *93*, 27–39. [CrossRef] [PubMed]
35. Cadet, J.L.; Krasnova, I.; Jayanthi, S.; Lyles, J. Neurotoxicity of substituted amphetamines: Molecular and cellular mechanisms. *Neurotox. Res.* **2007**, *11*, 183–202. [CrossRef] [PubMed]
36. Carvalho, M.; Carmo, H.; Costa, V.M.; Capela, J.P.; Pontes, H.; Remiao, F. Toxicology of amphetamines: An update. *Arch. Toxicol.* **2013**, *86*, 1167–1231. [CrossRef] [PubMed]
37. Aden, A.; Dimba, E.A.; Neola, U.M.; Chindia, M.L. Socio-economic effects of khat chewing in north eastern Kenya. *East Afr. Med. J.* **2006**, *83*, 69–73. [PubMed]
38. Parrott, A.C. Drug related harm: A complex and difficult concept to scale. *Hum. Psychopharmacol.* **2007**, *22*, 423–425. [CrossRef] [PubMed]
39. Curran, H.V.; Travill, R.A. Mood and cognitive effects of 3,4-methylenedioxymethamphetamine (MDMA, "ecstasy"): Weekend "high" followed by mid-week "low". *Addiction* **1997**, *92*, 821–831. [PubMed]
40. Curran, H.V.; Rees, H.; Hoare, T.; Hoshi, R.; Bond, A. Empathy and aggression: Two faces of ecstasy? A study of interpretive cognitive bias and mood change in ecstasy users. *Psychopharmacology* **2004**, *173*, 425–433. [CrossRef] [PubMed]
41. Parrott, A.C.; Lasky, J. Ecstasy (MDMA) effects upon mood and cognition; before, during, and after a Saturday night dance. *Psychopharmacology* **1998**, *139*, 261–268. [CrossRef] [PubMed]
42. Parrott, A.C.; Lock, J.; Conner, A.C.; Kissling, C.; Thome, J. Dance clubbing on MDMA and during abstinence from Ecstasy/MDMA: Prospective neuroendocrine and psychobiological changes. *Neuropsychobiology* **2008**, *57*, 165–180. [CrossRef] [PubMed]
43. Parrott, A.C. Chronic tolerance to recreational MDMA (3,4-methylenedioxymethamphetamine) or Ecstasy. *J. Psychopharmacol.* **2005**, *19*, 71–83. [CrossRef] [PubMed]
44. Parrott, A.C. MDMA, serotonergic neurotoxicity, and the diverse functional deficits of recreational 'Ecstasy' users. *Neurosci. Biobehav. Rev.* **2013**, *37*, 1466–1484. [CrossRef] [PubMed]
45. Vandrey, R.G.; Budney, A.J.; Moore, B.A.; Hughes, J.R. A cross-study comparison of cannabis and tobacco withdrawal. *Am. J. Addict.* **2005**, *14*, 54–63. [CrossRef] [PubMed]
46. Budney, A.J.; Hughes, J.R.; Moore, B.A.; Novy, P.L. Marijuana abstinence effects in marijuana smokers maintained in their home environment. *Arch. Gen. Psychiatry* **2001**, *58*, 917–924. [CrossRef] [PubMed]

47. Budney, A.J.; Novy, P.L.; Hughes, J.R. Marijuana withdrawal among adults seeking treatment for marijuana dependence. *Addiction* **1999**, *94*, 1311–1322. [CrossRef] [PubMed]
48. Heishman, S.J.; Singleton, E.G.; Liguori, A. Marijuana Craving Questionnaire: Development and initial validation of a self-report instrument. *Addiction* **2001**, *96*, 1023–1034. [CrossRef] [PubMed]
49. Parrott, A.C.; Hayley, A.; Downey, L. Recreational stimulants, herbal and spice cannabis: The core psychobiological processes that underlie their damaging effects. *Hum. Psychopharmacol.* **2017**, *32*, E2594. [CrossRef] [PubMed]
50. Heffernan, T.M.; Ling, J.; Parrott, A.C.; Buchanan, T.; Scholey, A.B.; Rodgers, J. Self-rated everyday and prospective memory abilities of cigarette smokers and non-smokers: A web based study. *Drug Alcohol Depend.* **2005**, *78*, 235–241. [CrossRef] [PubMed]
51. Glasner-Edwards, S.; Mooney, L.J. Methamphetamine psychosis: Epidemiology and management. *CNS Drugs* **2014**, *28*, 1115–1126. [CrossRef] [PubMed]
52. Soar, K.; Mason, C.; Potton, A.; Dawkins, L. Neuropsychological effects associated with recreational cocaine use. *Psychopharmacology* **2012**, *222*, 633–643. [CrossRef] [PubMed]
53. Copeland, J.; Clement, N.; Swift, W. Cannabis use, harms and the management of cannabis use disorder. *Neuropsychiatry* **2014**, *4*, 55–63. [CrossRef]
54. De Luca, M.A.; Castelli, M.P.; Loi, B.; Porcu, A.; Martorelli, M.; Miliano, C.; Kellett, K.; Davidson, C.; Stair, J.L.; Schifano, F.; et al. Native CB1 receptor affinity, intrinsic activity and accumbens shell dopamine stimulant properties of third generation SPICE/K2 cannabinoids: BB-22, 5F-PB-22, 5F-AKB-48 and STS-135. *Neuropharmacology* **2015**, *105*, 630–638. [CrossRef] [PubMed]
55. Downey, L.A.; Verster, J.C. Cannabis Concerns: Increased potency, availability and synthetic analogues. *Curr. Drug Abuse Rev.* **2014**, *7*, 67–68. [CrossRef] [PubMed]
56. Papanti, D.; Schifano, F.; Botteon, G.; Bertossi, F.; Mannix, J.; Vidoni, D.; Bonavigo, T. "Spiceophrenia": A systematic overview of "Spice"-related psychopathological issues and a case report. *Hum. Psychopharmacol.* **2013**, *28*, 379–389. [CrossRef] [PubMed]
57. Schifano, F.; Orsolini, L.; Papanti, G.D.; Corkery, J. Novel psychoactive substances of interest for psychiatry. *World Psychiatry* **2015**, *14*, 15–26. [CrossRef] [PubMed]
58. Zimmermann, U.S.; Winklemann, P.R.; Pilhatsch, M.; Nees, J.A.; Spanagel, R.; Schulz, K. Withdrawal phenomena and dependence syndrome after the cousumption of "spice gold". *Dtsch. Arztebl. Int.* **2009**, *106*, 464–467. [PubMed]
59. Herrmann, E.S.; Weerts, E.M.; Vandrey, R. Sex differences in cannabis withdrawal symptoms among treatment-seeking cannabis users. *Exp. Clin. Psychopharmacol.* **2015**, *23*, 415–421. [CrossRef] [PubMed]
60. Wagner, F.A.; Anthony, J.C. From First Drug Use to Drug Dependence–Developmental Periods of Risk for Dependence upon Marijuana, Cocaine, and Alcohol. *Neuropsychopharmacology* **2002**, *26*, 479–488. [CrossRef]
61. Terry, P.; Wright, K.A.; Cochrane, R. Factors contributing to changes in frequency of cannabis consumption by cannabis users in England: A structured interview study. *Addict. Res. Theory* **2007**, *15*, 113–119. [CrossRef]
62. Silins, E.; Horwood, L.J.; Patton, G.C.; Fergusson, D.M.; Olsson, C.A.; Hutchinson, D.M.; Mattick, R.P. Young adult sequelae of adolescent cannabis use: An integrative analysis. *Lancet Psychiatry* **2014**, *1*, 286–293. [CrossRef]
63. Selye, H. *The Stress of Life*; McGraw Hill: New York, NY, USA, 1956.
64. Lovallo, W.R. *Stress and Health: Biological and Psychological Interactions*; Sage: Kern County, CA, USA, 1997.
65. Parrott, A.C. Cortisol and MDMA (3,4-methylenedioxymethamphetamine): Neurohormonal aspects of bioenergetic-stress in Ecstasy users. *Neuropsychobiology* **2009**, *60*, 148–158. [CrossRef] [PubMed]
66. Parrott, A.C. Oxytocin, cortisol and MDMA (3,4-methylenedioxymethamphetamine): Neurohormonal aspects of recreational 'Ecstasy'. *Behav. Pharmacol.* **2016**, *27*, 649–658. [CrossRef] [PubMed]
67. Harris, D.S.; Baggott, M.; Mendelson, J.H.; Mendelson, J.E.; Jones, R.T. Subjective and hormonal effects of 3,4-methylenedioxymethamphetamine (MDMA) in humans. *Psychopharmacology* **2002**, *162*, 396–405. [CrossRef] [PubMed]
68. Parrott, A.C.; Adnum, L.; Evans, A.; Kissling, C.; Thome, J. Heavy Ecstasy/MDMA use at cool house parties: Substantial cortisol release and increased body temperature. *J. Psychopharmacol.* **2007**, *21*, 35.
69. Wetherell, M.A.; Montgomery, C. Basal functioning of the hypothalamic-pituitary-adrenal (HPA) axis and psychological distress in recreational ecstasy polydrug users. *Psychopharmacology* **2013**, *231*, 1365–1375. [CrossRef] [PubMed]

70. Ogeil, R.P.; Rajaratnam, S.M.; Broadbear, J.H. Male and female ecstasy users: Differences in patterns of use, sleep quality and mental health outcomes. *Drug Alcohol Depend.* **2013**, *132*, 223–230. [CrossRef] [PubMed]
71. Freedman, R.R.; Johanson, C.E.; Tancer, M.E. Thermoregulatory effects of 3,4-methylenedioxymethamphetamine (MDMA) in humans. *Psychopharmacology* **2005**, *183*, 248–256. [CrossRef] [PubMed]
72. Parrott, A.C. MDMA and temperature: A review of the thermal effects of 'Ecstasy' in humans. *Drug Alcohol Depend.* **2012**, *121*, 1–9. [CrossRef] [PubMed]
73. Parrott, A.C.; Young, L. Saturday night fever in ecstasy/MDMA dance clubbers: Heightened body temperature and associated psychobiological changes. *Temperature* **2015**, *3*, 1–6. [CrossRef] [PubMed]
74. Canazza, I.; Ossato, A.; Trapella, C.; Fantinati, A.; De Luca, M.A.; Margiani, G.; Vincenzi, F.; Rimondo, C.; Di Rosa, F.; Gregori, A. Effect of the novel synthetic cannabinoids AKB48 and 5F-AKB48 on "tetrad", sensorimotor, neurological and neurochemical responses in mice. In vitro and in vivo pharmacological studies. *Psychopharmacology* **2016**, *233*, 3685–3709. [CrossRef] [PubMed]
75. Alsufyani, H.A. Cardiovascular and Temperature Actions of Cathinones. Ph.D. Thesis, Royal College of Surgeons in Ireland, Dublin, Ireland, 2017.
76. Parrott, A.C.; Sands, H.R.; Jones, L.; Clow, A.; Evans, P.; Downey, L.; Stalder, T. Increased cortisol levels in hair of recent Ecstasy/MDMA users. *Eur. Neuropsychopharmacol.* **2014**, *24*, 369–374. [CrossRef] [PubMed]
77. Ranganathan, M.; Braley, G.; Pittman, B.; Cooper, T.; Perry, E.; Krystal, J.; D'Souza, D.C. The effects of cannabinoids on serum cortisol and prolactin in humans. *Psychopharmacology* **2009**, *203*, 737–744. [CrossRef] [PubMed]
78. King, G.R.; Ernst, T.; Deng, W.; Stenger, A.; Gonzales, R.M.K.; Nakama, H.; Chang, L. Effects of chronic active cannabis use on visuomotor integration, in relation to brain activation and cortisol levels. *J. Neurosci.* **2011**, *31*, 17923–17931. [CrossRef] [PubMed]
79. Parrott, A.C. MDMA in humans: Factors which affect the neuropsychobiological profiles of recreational ecstasy users, the integrative role of bio-energetic stress. *J. Psychopharmacol.* **2006**, *20*, 147–163. [CrossRef] [PubMed]
80. Nung, S. *The Divine Farmer's Materia Medica Classic*; Blue Poppy Press: Boulder, CO, USA, 1998.
81. Ashton, C.H. Pharmacology and effects of cannabis: A brief review. *Br. J. Psychiatry* **2001**, *178*, 101–106. [CrossRef] [PubMed]
82. D'Souza, D.C.; Perry, E.; MacDougall, L.; Ammerman, Y.; Cooper, T.; Yu-Te, W.; Krystal, J.H. The psychotomimetic effects of intravenous delta-9-tetrahydrocannabinol in healthy individuals: Implications for psychosis. *Neuropsychopharmacology* **2004**, *29*, 1558–1572. [CrossRef] [PubMed]
83. Nottage, J.; Stone, J.; Murray, R.; Sumich, A.; Bramon-Bosch, E.; Ffytche, D.; Morrison, P. Delta-9-tetrahydrocannabinol, neural oscillations above 20 Hz and induced acute psychosis. *Psychopharmacology* **2015**, *232*, 519–528. [CrossRef] [PubMed]
84. Paparelli, A.; Di Forti, M.; Morrison, P.D.; Murray, R.M. Drug-induced psychosis: How to avoid star gazing in schizophrenia research by looking at more obvious sources of light. *Front. Behav. Neurosci.* **2011**, *5*. [CrossRef] [PubMed]
85. Andréasson, S.; Engström, A.; Allebeck, P.; Rydberg, U. Cannabis and schizophrenia: A longitudinal study of Swedish conscripts. *Lancet* **1987**, *330*, 1483–1486. [CrossRef]
86. Le Bec, P.Y.; Fatséas, M.; Denis, C.; Lavie, E.; Auriacombe, M. Cannabis and psychosis: Search of a causal link through a critical and systematic review. *L'Encephale* **2009**, *35*, 377–385. (In French) [CrossRef] [PubMed]
87. Henquet, C.; Krabbendam, L.; Spauwen, J.; Kaplan, C.; Lieb, R.; Wittchen, H.-U.; Van Os, J. Prospective cohort study of cannabis use, predisposition for psychosis, and psychotic symptoms in young people. *Br. Med. J.* **2005**, *330*, 11. [CrossRef] [PubMed]
88. Bovasso, G.B. Cannabis abuse as a risk factor for depressive symptoms. *Am. J. Psychiatry* **2014**, *158*, 2033–2037. [CrossRef] [PubMed]
89. Richardson, T. Cannabis use and mental health: A review of recent epidemiological research. *Int. J. Pharmacol.* **2010**, *6*, 796–807. [CrossRef]
90. Feyissa, A.M.; Kelly, J.P. A review of the neuropharmacological properties of khat. *Prog. Neuro Psychopharmacol. Biol. Psychiatry* **2008**, *32*, 1147–1166. [CrossRef] [PubMed]
91. Vearrier, D.; Greenberg, M.I.; Miller, S.N.; Okaneku, J.T.; Haggerty, D.A. Methamphetamine: History, pathophysiology, adverse mental health effects, current trends, and hazards associated with the clandestine manufacture of methamphetamine. *Dis. Mon.* **2012**, *58*, 38–89. [CrossRef] [PubMed]

92. Brière, F.N.; Fallu, J.S.; Janosz, M.; Pagani, L.S. Prospective associations between meth/amphetamine (speed) and MDMA (ecstasy) use and depressive symptoms in secondary school students. *J. Epidemiol. Community Health* **2012**, *66*, 990–994. [CrossRef] [PubMed]
93. MacInnes, N.; Handley, S.L.; Harding, G.F. Former chronic methylenedioxymethamphetamine (MDMA or ecstasy) users report mild depressive symptoms. *J. Psychopharmacol.* **2001**, *15*, 181–186. [CrossRef] [PubMed]
94. Parrott, A.C.; Montgomery, C.A.; Wetherell, M.A.; Downey, L.A.; Stough, C.; Scholey, A.B. MDMA, cortisol, and heightened stress in recreational Ecstasy/MDMA users. *Behav. Pharmacol.* **2014**, *25*, 458–472. [CrossRef] [PubMed]
95. Parrott, A.C.; Milani, R.M.; Parmar, R.; Turner, J.J.D. Recreational Ecstasy/MDMA and other drug users form the UK and Italy: Psychiatric symptoms and psychobiological problems. *Psychopharmacology* **2001**, *159*, 77–82. [CrossRef] [PubMed]
96. Schifano, F.; Di Furia, L.; Forza, G.; Minicuci, N.; Bricolo, R. MDMA ('ecstasy') consumption in the context of polydrug abuse: A report on 150 patients. *Drug Alcohol Depend.* **1998**, *52*, 85–90. [CrossRef]
97. Scholey, A.B.; Owen, L.; Gates, J.; Rodgers, J.; Buchanan, T.; Ling, J.; Heffernan, T.; Swan, P.; Stough, C.; Parrott, A.C. Hair MDMA samples are consistent with reported Ecstasy use: Findings from an internet study investigating effects of Ecstasy on mood and memory. *Neuropsychobiology* **2011**, *63*, 15–21. [CrossRef] [PubMed]
98. Taurah, L.; Chandler, C.; Sanders, G. Depression, impulsiveness, sleep and memory in past and present polydrug users of 3,4-methylenedioxymethamphetamine (MDMA, ecstasy). *Psychopharmacology* **2014**, *231*, 737–751. [CrossRef] [PubMed]
99. Turner, J.J.D.; Singer, L.T.; Moore, D.G.; Min, M.O.; Goodwin, J.; Fulton, S.; Parrott, A.C. Psychiatric profiles of mothers who take Ecstasy/MDMA during pregnancy: Reduced depression one year after giving birth and quitting Ecstasy. *J. Psychopharmacol.* **2014**, *28*, 55–66. [CrossRef] [PubMed]
100. Downey, L.A.; Tysse, B.; Ford, T.C.; Samuels, A.C.; Wilson, R.P.; Parrott, A.C. Psychomotor tremor and proprioceptive control problems in current and former stimulant drug users: An accelerometer study of heavy users of amphetamine, MDMA, and other recreational stimulants. *J. Clin. Pharmacol.* **2017**, *57*, 1330–1337. [CrossRef] [PubMed]
101. Vonmoos, M.; Hulka, L.M.; Preller, K.H.; Jenni, D.; Baumgartner, M.R.; Stohler, R.; Bolla, K.I.; Quednow, B.B. Cognitive dysfunction in recreational and dependent cocaine users: Role of attention-deficit hyperactivity disorder, craving and early age at onset. *Br. J. Psychiatry* **2014**, *203*, 35–43. [CrossRef] [PubMed]
102. Fisk, J.E.; Montgomery, C.; Wareing, M.; Murphy, P.N. Reasoning deficits in ecstasy (MDMA) polydrug users. *Psychopharmacology* **2005**, *181*, 550–559. [CrossRef] [PubMed]
103. Fox, H.; Parrott, A.C.; Turner, J.J.D. Ecstasy/MDMA related cognitive deficits: A function of dosage rather than awareness of problems. *J. Psychopharmacol.* **2001**, *15*, 273–281. [CrossRef] [PubMed]
104. Fox, H.C.; McLean, A.; Turner, J.J.D.; Parrott, A.C.; Rogers, R.; Sahakian, B.J. Neuropsychological evidence of a relatively selective profile of temporal dysfunction in drug-free MDMA ("ecstasy") polydrug users. *Psychopharmacology* **2002**, *162*, 203–214. [CrossRef] [PubMed]
105. Laws, K.R.; Kokkalis, J. Ecstasy (MDMA) and memory function: A meta-analytic update. *Hum. Psychopharmacol.* **2007**, *22*, 381–388. [CrossRef] [PubMed]
106. Montgomery, C.; Hatton, N.P.; Fisk, J.E.; Ogden, R.S.; Jansari, A. Assessing the functional significance of ecstasy-related memory deficits using a virtual reality paradigm. *Hum. Psychopharmacol.* **2010**, *25*, 318–325. [CrossRef] [PubMed]
107. Parrott, A.C.; Lees, A.; Garnham, N.J.; Jones, M.; Wesnes, K. Cognitive performance in recreational users of MDMA or "ecstasy": Evidence for memory deficits. *J. Psychopharmacol.* **1998**, *12*, 79–83. [CrossRef] [PubMed]
108. Parrott, A.C.; Downey, L.A.; Roberts, C.A.; Montgomery, C.; Bruno, R.; Fox, H.C. Recreational 3,4-methylenedioxymethamphetamine or 'ecstasy': Current perspective and future research needs. *J. Psychopharmacol.* **2017**, *31*, 959–966. [CrossRef] [PubMed]
109. Bolla, K.I.; Brown, K.; Eldreth, D.; Tate, K.; Cadet, J.L. Dose-related neurocognitive effects of marijuana use. *Neurology* **2002**, *59*, 1337–1343. [CrossRef] [PubMed]
110. Grant, I.; Gonzalez, R.; Carey, C.L.; Natarajan, L.; Wolfson, T. Non-acute (residual) neurocognitive effects of cannabis use: A meta-analytic study. *J. Int. Neuropsychol. Soc.* **2003**, *9*, 679–689. [CrossRef] [PubMed]

111. Jager, G.; Block, R.I.; Luijten, M.; Ramsey, N.F. Cannabis use and memory brain function in adolescent boys: A cross-sectional multicenter fMRI study. *J. Am. Acad. Child Adolesc. Psychiatry* **2010**, *49*, 561–572. [CrossRef] [PubMed]
112. Meier, M.H.; Caspi, A.; Ambler, A.; Harrington, H.; Houts, R.; Keefe, R.S.E.; Moffitt, T.E. Persistent cannabis users show neuropsychological decline from childhood to midlife. *Proc. Nat. Acad. Sci. USA* **2012**, *109*, E2657–E2664. [CrossRef] [PubMed]
113. Pope, H.G.; Gruber, A.J.; Hudson, J.I.; Huestis, M.A.; Yurgelun-Todd, D. Neuropsychological performance in long-term cannabis users. *Arch. Gen. Psychiatry* **2001**, *58*, 909–915. [CrossRef] [PubMed]
114. Yücel, M.; Solowij, N.; Respondek, C.; Whittle, S.; Fornito, A.; Pantelis, C.; Lubman, D.I. Regional brain abnormalities associated with long-term heavy cannabis use. *Arch. Gen. Psychiatry* **2008**, *65*, 694–701. [CrossRef] [PubMed]
115. Mandelbaum, D.E.; de la Monte, S.M. Adverse structural and functional effects of marijuana on the brain: Evidence reviewed. *Pediatric Neurol.* **2017**, *66*, 12–20. [CrossRef] [PubMed]

# 14

# Abuse of Prescription Drugs in the Context of Novel Psychoactive Substances (NPS)

**Fabrizio Schifano, Stefania Chiappini *, John M. Corkery and Amira Guirguis**

Psychopharmacology, Drug Misuse and Novel Psychoactive Substances Research Unit, School of Life and Medical Sciences, University of Hertfordshire, Hertfordshire AL10 9AB, UK; f.schifano@herts.ac.uk (F.S.); j.corkery@herts.ac.uk (J.M.C.); a.guirguis2@herts.ac.uk (A.G.)

* Correspondence: stefaniachiappini9@gmail.com

**Abstract:** Recently, a range of prescription and over-the-counter drugs have been reportedly used as Novel Psychoactive Substances (NPS), due to their potential for abuse resulting from their high dosage/idiosyncratic methods of self-administration. This paper provides a systematic review of the topic, focusing on a range of medications which have emerged as being used recreationally, either on their own or in combination with NPS. Among gabapentinoids, pregabalin may present with higher addictive liability levels than gabapentin, with pregabalin being mostly identified in the context of opioid, polydrug intake. For antidepressants, their dopaminergic, stimulant-like, bupropion activities may explain their recreational value and diversion from the therapeutic intended use. In some vulnerable clients, a high dosage of venlafaxine ('baby ecstasy') is ingested for recreational purposes, whilst the occurrence of a clinically-relevant withdrawal syndrome may be a significant issue for all venlafaxine-treated patients. Considering second generation antipsychotics, olanzapine appears to be ingested at very large dosages as an 'ideal trip terminator', whilst the immediate-release quetiapine formulation may possess proper abuse liability levels. Within the image- and performance-enhancing drugs (IPEDs) group, the beta-2 agonist clenbuterol ('size zero pill') is reported to be self-administered for aggressive slimming purposes. Finally, high/very high dosage ingestion of the antidiarrhoeal loperamide has shown recent increasing levels of popularity due to its central recreational, anti-withdrawal, opiatergic effects. The emerging abuse of prescription drugs within the context of a rapidly modifying drug scenario represents a challenge for psychiatry, public health and drug-control policies.

**Keywords:** drug abuse; novel psychoactive substances; NPS; pharmacovigilance; prescribing drugs' abuse

---

## 1. Introduction

Novel Psychoactive Substances (NPS; 'legal highs' or 'research chemicals') are molecules designed to mimic the effects of legal traditional recreational drugs with intense psychoactive effects and virtual non-detectability in routine drug screenings. NPS include synthetic cannabinoids, cathinone derivatives, psychedelic phenethylamines, novel stimulants, synthetic opioids, tryptamine derivatives, phencyclidine-like dissociatives, piperazines, psychoactive plants/herbs and a range of prescribed medications [1]. The term NPS was first used by United Nations Office on Drugs and Crime (UNODC) to refer to "substances of abuse, either in a pure form or a preparation, that are not controlled by the 1961 Single Convention on Narcotic Drugs or the 1961 Convention on Psychotropic Substances, but which may pose a public health threat" [2]. At present, the emergence of NPS, typically from outside Western countries [3], represents a considerable public health challenge. Moreover, in order to circumvent the present controls and regulations, NPS are constantly diversifying and being replaced [4]. This is being facilitated by the growing number of anonymous online marketplaces, called 'cryptomarkets', which host many anonymous sellers whilst using untraceable cryptocurrencies [5]. NPS users report a range of reasons behind their preference for NPS as opposed to traditional drugs such as cannabis, cocaine and heroin, including typical lack of detectability, greater affordability, lack of stigma, and relative ease of online acquisition [6]. Recently, however, the phenomenon of using prescription drugs in an idiosyncratic way to resemble, or counteract, the effects of NPS, has increasingly been described. This phenomenon refers not only to high potency opioids (e.g., fentanyl) and 'exotic'/designer benzodiazepines—molecules already having been reported to be addictive [1]—but also: gabapentinoids [7], a range of stimulants [1], antipsychotics [8], antidepressants [9] and image- and performance-enhancing drugs (IPEDS, e.g., anabolic steroids, vitamins, clenbuterol and salbutamol) [10]. Among over-the-counter drugs, the two most common agents reportedly ingested in intentional abuse cases are the antitussive, dextromethorphan [11], and loperamide, a common antidiarrhoeal drug [12].

Any pharmacovigilance approach aims to detect, assess, understand and hopefully prevent adverse effects or any other medicine-related problems. From this point of view, there is a growing attention on prescription drugs and their addictive liability levels/diversion potential [7,8,10,12]. As the intended and the actual use of medicines differ between clinical trials and real-world use, pharmacovigilance activities are well placed to focus on the post-marketing phase. In Europe, those activities are coordinated by the European Medicines Agency (EMA) [13] through EudraVigilance (EV), which is the system for collecting, managing and analyzing information on suspected adverse reactions to medicines which have been authorized in the European Economic Area (EEA) [14].

This paper aims to provide a systematic review of the available literature relating to a preselected range of prescription medicines (pregabalin, gabapentin, quetiapine, olanzapine, venlafaxine, bupropion, loperamide, clenbuterol and salbutamol) previously reported as possibly being misused as NPS. For each molecule, a range of preclinical, epidemiological, and clinical pharmacological data will be provided.

## 2. Materials and Methods

A systematic review was carried out, consistent with the Preferred Reporting Items for Systematic Reviews and Meta-Analysis (PRISMA) guidelines [15]. A literature search was performed on PubMed, Medline/OvidSP (includes Embase), and Web-of-Science; the current search was completed in February 2018 and was not associated with any time restrictions. We focused on pregabalin, gabapentin, quetiapine, olanzapine, venlafaxine, bupropion, clenbuterol, salbutamol and loperamide [Title/Abstract]. For each molecule, a number of search terms [Title/Abstract] were considered as follows: 'misuse', 'abuse', 'dependence', 'withdrawal', 'off-label use' and 'non-medical use'. In addition, the authors performed further secondary searches by using the reference listing of all eligible papers. All titles/abstracts were examined, and full texts of potentially relevant papers obtained. Relevant works were selected in order to obtain a full representation of the available literature data on the selected topic. Eligible studies were identified if they possessed a range of characteristics, including (1) peer-reviewed clinical/human studies; (2) at least an abstract with estimates and/or full availability of results; and (3) focusing on the misuse/abuse/dependence/withdrawal of pregabalin; gabapentin; quetiapine; olanzapine, venlafaxine, bupropion, loperamide, clenbuterol and salbutamol. The entire range of literature papers were included, e.g., experimental and observational studies; case reports; case series; and fatalities' reports. Although letters to the editor, conference proceedings, and book chapters were excluded from the systematic review, they were still considered in the retrieval of further secondary searches. SC independently extracted and collected relevant data; FS contributed to the analysis of the results and discussed possible issues and disagreements during the revision of the paper with SC.

From an initial list of 171 studies, 151 were identified as relevant and appropriate in terms of quality according to PRISMA checklists. Following this, duplicates, papers lacking an English abstract, letters to the editor, animal studies and papers unrelated to the topic were excluded, and 128 papers were finally considered for the current study. A flow diagram (Figure 1) describes the reasons for study inclusion/exclusion at each stage, is here provided.

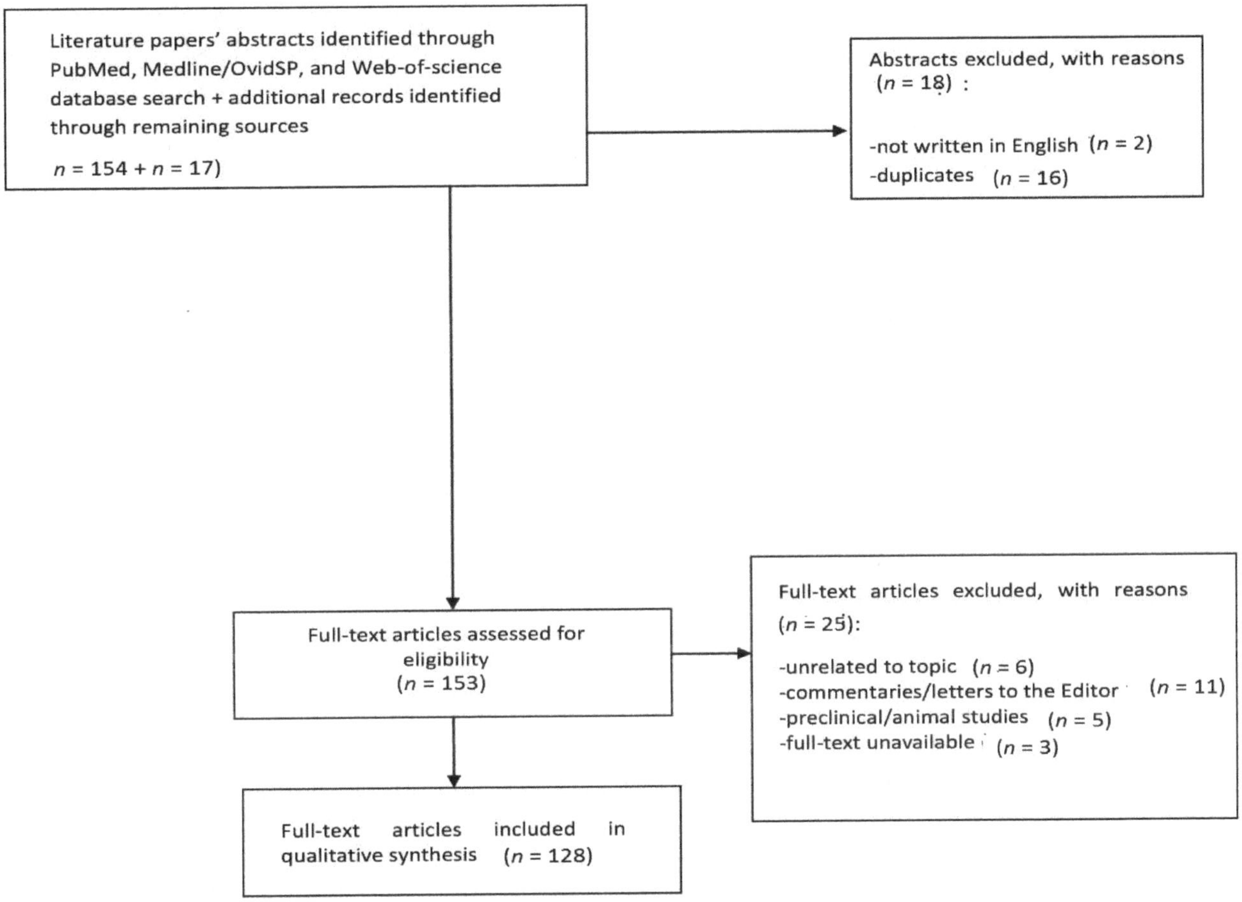


**Figure 1.** Selection of retrieved studies.

## 3. Results

### *3.1. Gabapentinoids*

Recently, the gabapentinoids, pregabalin and gabapentin, have increasingly been reported to be abused at the EU-wide level, in parallel with increasing levels of prescriptions, related fatalities and a growing black market [16–19]. Gabapentinoids are anticonvulsants but are also prescribed for a range of clinical conditions in neurology, psychiatry and rheumatology, whilst being used off-label for the treatment of benzodiazepine and alcohol dependence. Their effects are the result of calcium channel binding, resulting in decreased central excitability levels. Compared to gabapentin, pregabalin's binding affinity and potency are six times higher; pregabalin's more significant misuse potential may also be due to its more rapid absorption, faster onset of action, much faster attainment of maximum plasma concentration and higher bioavailability (>90%, irrespective of the dosage). Furthermore, gabapentinoids are thought to possess GABA-mimetic properties, whilst possibly having direct/indirect effects on the dopaminergic 'reward' system [7]. Gabapentionoid web enthusiasts report the ingestion of this compound alone or in combination with other drugs (e.g., cannabis, alcohol, opioids and other prescribed drugs), at a dosage range of 1000–4800 mg for gabapentin [20], and 750–12,000 mg for pregabalin [7]. Typical psychoactive effects include a sense of well-being/relaxation, euphoria, and even hallucinations [1]. In 2005, the Drug Enforcement Administration (DEA) placed pregabalin into Schedule V of the Controlled Substances Act (CSA) because of its potential for abuse [21] and a similar scheduling approach has recently been approved in the UK. Chiappini and Schifano [7] recently assessed the EMA EV database of pregabalin and gabapentin misuse-related Adverse Drug Reactions (ADRs) over the last decade. According to the Proportional Reporting Ratio (PRR) computation, abuse/dependence issues were more frequently reported for pregabalin compared with gabapentin, hence confirming its higher addictive liability levels [7,22]. Furthermore, Emergency Department presentations involving intentional drug overdoses recorded by the National Self-Harm Registry (Ireland; 2007–2015), showed that gabapentinoids have been increasingly identified over time, with high dosages and polydrug abuse being reported [23]. Indeed, gabapentinoid fatalities are typically observed when these molecules are associated with other psychoactive drugs, especially opioids and other sedatives whose effects are potentiated by gabapentinoids [24,25].

### 3.2. *Antidepressants*

Consistent with a worldwide rise in antidepressant consumption [26,27], bupropion and venlafaxine have anecdotally emerged as increasingly being abused [1,28,29]. In examining a range of online communities and specialized web services, several antidepressant misusers' experiences may be identified [20]. These reports emphasise both bupropion's stimulant effects and venlafaxine's dissociative properties. Indeed, bupropion described as being ingested in very large quantities (up to 4050 mg/day, roughly 14 times higher than the maximal therapeutic dosage) in order to achieve an 'amphetamine-like high' [30]. In most abuse cases, its recreational use is associated with oral or nasal administration, but intravenous use has also been reported [28,30–34]. Bupropion pharmacology relies on its action both as a selective inhibitor of catecholamines (noradrenaline and DA) reuptake [35,36], and as a non-competitive antagonist of nicotinic acetylcholine receptors, hence being prescribed as well as an aid in smoking cessation [36]. Bupropion is known to be a cathinone derivative, that is, a beta-ketone amphetamine analogue with dopaminergic and noradrenergic effects, which may explain its misuse potential [37,38]. This is a reason for concern since bupropion is also used 'off-label' in a range of conditions, including attention-deficit/hyperactivity disorder, chronic fatigue, sexual dysfunction, and obesity. The adverse effects of bupropion misuse range from nasal pain to irritability, agitation, cardiac toxicity, hallucinations and seizures [39,40]. A retrospective review [41] on bupropion cases of intentional abuse reported to the US National Poison Data System highlighted an increase of 75% from 2000 to 2012, with the typical effects reported including tachycardia, seizures, agitation/irritability, hallucinations/delusions, and tremor; similar data were identified by the Toxicology Data Network of the US National Institute of Health (Toxnet) [42]. Typical bupropion abusers may present with a history of drug addiction [38,43,44] and/or are inmates, with bupropion having been removed from some US prison formularies [45–47]. Conversely, venlafaxine is a selective serotonin-norepinephrine reuptake inhibitor (SNRI) antidepressant, indicated [48] for the treatment of major depressive episodes, generalised anxiety disorder and social phobia, with off-label use including obsessive-compulsive disorder and chronic pain syndromes. Its reuptake effects are dose-dependent, with action progressively including serotonin (5-HT), norepinefrine (NE) and dopamine (DA). Venlafaxine's main active metabolite, desvenlafaxine, is highly inhibitive of NE transporter activities, further increasing the rate of DA turnover in the prefrontal cortex [49]. Both venlafaxine and its metabolite are not associated with monoamine oxidase inhibitory activity, which is responsible for the degradation of DA. Hence, venlafaxine abuse may be associated with DA increase in the prefrontal cortex [50], high affinity for D2 receptors adaptive changes in D3 receptors following its chronic administration and, finally, with the desensitisation of both 5-HT1A and beta-adrenergic receptors [51]. Dependence and withdrawal symptoms associated with both SSRIs and SNRIs have already been described, specifically with abrupt discontinuation of venlafaxine (including Extended Release (XR) formulation) after long-term use [9,52–54]. Symptoms range from mild to severe and include nausea, depression, suicidal thoughts, disorientation, stomach cramps, panic attacks, sexual dysfunction, headaches and occasional psychotic symptoms [55–59]; a newborn discontinuation syndrome has been described as well, at times associated with encephalopathy or paroxysmal episodes [60]. The management of venlafaxine withdrawal includes the use of other antidepressants (Ads) or venlafaxine tapering doses [61,62]. Furthermore, venlafaxine/'baby ecstasy' abuse has been reported, typically being the result of the intake of very large doses [63–65]. Consistent with this, studies have assessed drug and pharmaceutical consumption in England through wastewater analysis and comparing it to NHS prescription statistics. Discrepancies have been observed in the case of venlafaxine, suggesting sales of non-prescribed venlafaxine, which are, therefore, not included within NHS data [66]. Furthermore, in a retrospective review of the records of the New Zealand National Poisons Centre over the period 2003-2012, rapidly increasing levels of enquiries were identified for a range of prescription medicines, including venlafaxine [67]. According to the EMA EV database from the last decade [68], the misuse-/abuse-/dependence- and withdrawal-related ADRs reported respectively for bupropion and venlafaxine show that bupropion may possess a higher recreational value due to its dopaminergic and stimulant-like activity, whilst the occurrence of a venlafaxine-withdrawal syndrome may be a significant issue for venlafaxine-treated patients; these data were confirmed by analysis of the UK-based Yellow Card Scheme [68].

### *3.3. Antipsychotics*

Consistent with their increased prescription and availability [69], second-generation antipsychotic (SGA) (e.g., quetiapine and olanzapine) abuse has recently been reported [1,70–72]. Quetiapine appears to be the most documented SGA being abused; it is commonly administered in the 400–800 mg/day range for the treatment of schizophrenia; bipolar disorder; and as an add-on in major depression and anxiety [73–76]. Quetiapine is anecdotally known as 'Susie Q'; 'Quell'; and 'baby heroin' [75–79], with 'Q ball' and 'Maq ball', respectively, being combinations with cocaine, and marijuana. Crushed quetiapine tablets can be self-administered through nasal insufflation [79–81], although both oral [81–84], and intravenous [85–87] routes of administration have been reported. Consistent with these anecdotal clinical observations, post-marketing surveillance reports indicate an increase in quetiapine availability on the black-market [75,79,88–90]. Furthermore, quetiapine, either on its own or in combination with heroin and/or alcohol [91], is consistently associated with high rates of ambulance attendances, indicating greater community-level harm relative to other atypical antipsychotics [92]. Indeed, between 2005 and 2011, quetiapine-related Emergency Department visits increased in the USA by 90%, from 35,581 to 67,497 attendances [93]. A recent US National Poison Data retrospective analysis identified all cases of single-substance SGA exposures coded as 'intentional abuse' [94] during a 10-year period (2003–2013), quetiapine being the most represented molecule, followed by risperidone and olanzapine. Prison inmates and opioid addicts seem to represent the most at-risk populations [24,75,76,95–97]. Quetiapine psychotropic effects [86,87] are associated with both increased levels of DA in the nucleus accumbens (NAc) area [89,98–100] and D2 receptor blockage. As some pharmacodynamic mechanisms are shared by other non-misused SGAs [101–104], other factors [105,106] or pharmacological effects explaining the molecule misuse potential may include norquetiapine-related norepinephrine reuptake blockade [75], 5-HT7 antagonist properties and sigma receptor activation [107,108]. Quetiapine pharmacokinetics, mediated by the cytochrome CYP3A4, may play a part, as well, in facilitating its misuse [109]. Its XR formulation may be less frequently abused, due to the delayed (by approximately 3 h) and blunted (by approximately 67%) serum peak [88]; the tablet coating may also make snorting of the crushed tablets quite problematic [89].

Another SGA, olanzapine, is normally prescribed at a dosage of 5–20 mg oral daily in order to treat schizophrenia, bipolar disorder and resistant depression. Whilst being widely prescribed, it has been anecdotally reported, at dosages up to 50 mg, as the 'ideal trip terminator/modulator' after a psychedelic drug binge [110]. According to discussion forums/specialised websites [111], olanzapine is also being used to treat unwanted 'comedown' symptoms from drug/alcohol intake [112,113]. Consistent with this, clients on methadone maintenance treatment attending the National Drug Treatment Centre (NDTC) in Dublin reported levels of non-medical use of olanzapine, with dosages of up to 100 mg/day, in order to manage anxiety and improve sleep, and in a minority of cases, to 'get stoned' [114]. Olanzapine activity involves GABA-A receptors [115], hence the associated sedation, the rewarding glutamatergic stimulation of the ventral tegmental area DAergic neurons [116], the 5HT2C and histamine/H1 antagonist properties and the potent inhibiting action on the muscarinic M1 receptors [115,116]. In comparing quetiapine with olanzapine through the UK

Prescription Cost Analysis and the Drug Analysis Profiles of the Yellow Card Scheme, quetiapine was shown to be slightly less frequently prescribed but associated with a smaller total number of general reports, and hence, a comparatively higher number of abuse/dependence/withdrawal ADR reports [117,118]. In line with this, the OPPIDUM French addictovigilance network highlighted the emerging misuse of prescription molecules, and this included quetiapine as well [119]. Information from the previous 10 years from the EMA EV database relating to quetiapine and olanzapine misuse/abuse/dependence/withdrawal-related ADR reports [8] shows a higher misuse risk for quetiapine in comparison with olanzapine for the selected ADR reports. Indeed, quetiapine XR formulation was represented in only a smalll proportion of misuse cases, with both nasal and parenteral administration having been identified. Of particular interest was, in comparison with olanzapine, a higher risk of discontinuation/withdrawal syndrome following the abrupt cessation of quetiapine [75,113,120]. Finally, consistent with previous data [75,82–85,90,121–123], the quetiapine- and olanzapine-related fatalities reported on the EMA EV database were typically the result of a polydrug intake, which included opiates/opioids, antidepressants, and over-the-counter drugs [124,125].

### *3.4. Image-And Performance-Enhancing Drugs (IPEDs)*

Over the last few decades, a range of prescribed and non-prescribed enhancement drugs have increasingly been self-administered [72] in order to improve the ageing process, and sexual performances, and to reduce hair loss, fatigue and other physiological conditions which are, at times, considered pathological in a society that strongly emphasises the importance of physical appearance [126]. Prescribed image- and performance-enhancing drugs (IPEDs) include anabolic-androgenic steroids (AAS), human growth hormone (hGH), steroid hormones (e.g., androstenedione), insulin, erythropoietin, diuretics, but also, β-2 agonists (e.g., clenbuterol and salbutamol) [127]. Their misuse is typically carried out within a polypharmacy context [128] with alcohol, cannabis/cannabinoids, cocaine, amphetamines/methamphetamines being ingested as ancillary drugs. Moreover, the recent reporting of IPED injecting practices are a reason for concern [129]; these mostly involve anabolic androgenic steroids, non-steroidal anabolic hormones (e.g., hGH and insulin), tanning peptides, cosmetic injectables such as botox and dermal fillers, etc. [130–132]. Among non-steroidal anabolic hormones, insulin seems to be misused for performance-enhancement purposes through several administration routes (intravenous, intramuscular and subcutaneous); indeed, insulin may help in achieving a decrease in fat deposition, an increase in muscle mass and positive mood changes, although serious hypoglycaemic episodes and other medical sequelae can occur as well [133,134]. Within the IPED group, anti-asthmatic beta-2 agonists have recently emerged as having potential for misuse, e.g., salbutamol for its performance-enhancing effects and clenbuterol for its hypertrophic and lipolytic effects. They are both included in the list of prohibited substances released by the World Anti-Doping Agency (WADA) [135], with salbutamol being allowed only as a component in the treatment regimen for athletes with asthma. Clenbuterol, even if different from anabolic steroids, has been also prohibited as an anabolic agent since 2006. In parallel with this, the Food and Drug Administration (FDA) banned the use of clenbuterol in food animals in 1991 and the European Union (EU) followed suit in 1996 [136]. Beta-2 agonists are synthetic molecules with sympathomimetic activity, prescribed as bronchodilators for the treatment of asthma. Clenbuterol is licensed for human use only in a few countries (Austria, Germany, Italy, Spain and Mexico), but not in the UK or the USA [137]. Clenbuterol, as a 'size zero pill', is popular and widely available on the web, being considered an ergo/thermogenic drug and hence, an anabolic burner [138], similar to caffeine, ephedrine, and thyroid hormones. Clenbuterol-associated lypolisis can occur via both β-2 adrenergic agonism and its specific action on the adipocytes' β-3 adrenergic receptors, which further facilitates lipolysis and weight loss [139–141]. While anti-asthmatic clenbuterol dosage ranges between 20 and 40mcg daily, the typical 'fat burning' dose is in the 120–160 mcg daily range; dosage starts at 40 mcg daily, gradually increases, and then remains at the highest dosage for a duration of 2–4 weeks [142]. In parallel with this, recent years have seen an increase in clenbuterol exposure reported to poison control centres [143], with the molecule being used either as a dietary supplement [144] or as an adulterant in illicit drugs, such as cocaine [145]. Its adverse effects are dose-dependent and may include dysrhythmias and myocardial injury, headache, abdominal pain, nausea, and rhabdomyolysis [136,146–148]. Reports relating to salbutamol misuse have been less frequently mentioned [149–151]. Similar to clenbuterol, salbutamol's adverse effects are dose-related and may include tremor, restlessness, anxiety/agitation, tachycardia, atrial fibrillation, and myocardial ischaemia, especially in cases of overdosage, chronic use, or intravenous injection [152]. With respect to salbutamol, clenbuterol's higher levels of abuse potential could be associated with its pharmacological characteristics [143], such as its prolonged elimination half-life (35 h) and its higher lipophilicity, which can be associated with a fast transition through the blood–brain barrier. Consistent with this, salbutamol has been described as significantly less potent on a reinforcement schedule than clenbuterol [149,152–154]. Clenbuterol abuse-related fatalities have consistently been reported in the literature [136,140,147,155], whilst salbutamol is considered safer [156]. In this regard, Milano et al. [10] studied the 2006–2016 EMA clenbuterol- and salbutamol-related, misuse/abuse/dependence/withdrawal/overdose/off-label spontaneous reports. They found that clenbuterol, in comparison with salbutamol, had higher levels of misuse/abuse. These clenbuterol-related data were most typically from males and were associated with the intake of steroids [10], hence confirming previous reports [157,158].

### 3.5. Over-The-Counter (OTC) Medicines—Loperamide

Currently, over-the-counter (OTC) abuse ('pharming') is an internationally recognised problem, and the recent emergence of new forms, including online, of medicine supply, is alarming clinicians and health authorities nationwide. The EU introduced a strong legal framework for the licensing, manufacturing and distribution of medicines [159], but no measures have been taken so far for the distribution of OTC drugs, and it is hence, difficult to quantify their actual misuse and abuse [159–168]. Over previous years, the OTC antidiarrhoeal medicine loperamide has increasingly been reported as being diverted and used to achieve recreational effects [159–162]. Loperamide acts as a potent mu-opioid receptor agonist, albeit with predominantly peripheral activity on the myenteric plexus, hence primarily increasing the intestinal transit time by decreasing propulsive activity. Secondary peripheral effects are seen at κ-opioid and δ-opioid receptors as well [169,170]. Loperamide was initially placed by the US FDA in Schedule V of the Controlled Substance Act but then, after having assessed its safety profile with the conclusion of low levels of physical dependence risk, in 1988, it was made available for OTC use. In the 2–16 mg daily dosage, loperamide is considered safe and devoid of misuse abuse potential because of its rapid metabolism and poor blood–brain barrier (BBB) penetration. In doses of 50–300 mg, however, loperamide ingestion has been associated with euphoria, central nervous system depression [171–174] and even death [175]. Its diversion potential may be associated with its use as a relief from opioid withdrawal [176]. Anecdotally described as the 'poor's' methadone' [177], detailed loperamide dosage titration regimens are being reported online [20]. Related misuse case series [178] have reported both extremely high daily intakes (up to 1200 mg), and associated cardiotoxicity issues, such as QTc prolongation and torsades de pointes, QRS prolongation, ventricular dysrhythmias [179–182], syncope, and cardiac arrest [12,179,183,184]. The cardiotoxicity mechanism of loperamide is not clearly understood, although it may be due to potent inhibition of cardiac ion channels which is, in turn, associated with delayed repolarisation and QT prolongation [185–187]. Consequently, the FDA [175] has recently warned clinicians and users about the combination of loperamide with other drugs or herbal products that are known to prolong the QT interval, including Class 1A (e.g., quinidine, procainamide) or Class III drugs (e.g., amiodarone, sotalol) antiarrhythmics, antipsychotics (e.g., chlorpromazine, haloperidol, thioridazine, ziprasidone), antibiotics (e.g., moxifloxacin), and methadone. Loperamide ingestion has also been reported in association with P-glycoprotein (P-gp) substrates (e.g., quetiapine, cetirizine, oxycodone) or inhibitors (e.g., fluoxetine, citalopram, sertraline, omeprazole, quinine, quinidine, propranolol, ritonavir). These associations are associated with an increase in the low bioavailability of loperamide, normally being <2%; plasmatic concentration; levels of euphoric effects; the capacity of possible contrasting opioid withdrawal symptoms [186–189]; and toxicity effects [175]. Concurrent use of loperamide with CYP3A4 inhibitors (e.g., itraconazole, grapefruit juice, omeprazole, tonic water and cimetidine) or CYP2C8 inhibitors (e.g., gemfibrozil) can increase its plasma levels as well, with recurrent ventricular tachycardia having been reported in a patient who was taking large recreational doses of both loperamide and the CYP3A4 inhibitor, famotidine [190]. Treatment of loperamide intoxication involves the use of naloxone, which may not be able to directly reverse loperamide cardiotoxic effects [191,192].

## 4. Discussion

The ever-increasing number of NPS emerging worldwide and the parallel changes in drug scenarios represent a challenge for psychiatric, public health and drug-control policies [193]. In line with this, the current systematic review has focused on a different range of prescribed medications which are indeed being used as NPS [1]. Within both online drug forum communities and social networks, there are some educated/informed users (the 'psychonauts') [194] who typically 'test' a range of psychotropics, including prescribed drugs, to achieve specific mindsets and eventually, share this information with peers [193]. However, in parallel with recently increased levels of access to the web, a large number of vulnerable subjects, including both children/adolescents and psychiatric patients, have been exposed to a range of 'pro-drug' information, and this is a reason for concern [193]. Although a number of online 'rogue' pharmacies have been shut down, this typically prompts the sellers to move to servers in overseas countries, leading to a growing black market [195].

It is intriguing that, for the range of prescription molecules discussed, including the fairly recently introduced gabapentinoids, pre-marketing processes were not been able to appropriately identify their abuse/misuse potential. However, similar to what happened with benzodiazepines and z-hypnotics, this potential has finally emerged over time. Present data seem to suggest that abuse liability-focused, pre-marketing laboratory testing may need to consider interaction studies with alcohol and/or other drugs [194,196]. Furthermore, post-marketing surveillance for substance abuse [197] should routinely be carried out to assess the abuse potential of newly released drugs, especially those with activity on the central nervous system (CNS) [198]. Indeed, lack of information on the abuse/misuse potential of a new medicine's interaction with the CNS does not mean that a specific medicine does not actually produce these effects. Furthermore, in order to look at how medicines are actually used in real life, modern pharmacovigilance should identify a range of technical tools and approaches to go beyond spontaneous reporting systems. Physicians should be vigilant when prescribing drugs with an abuse/misuse/diversion potential and carefully evaluate the possibility for some clients (inmates; people with a personal history of misuse or abuse) to be more vulnerable to these misuse activities. Finally, while a continuum of related professional training is needed, it may be important to consider a strategy to increase clients' access to treatment services, possibly through enhanced links between community pharmacists, who are the first professionals to identify a repeat supply issue, and prescribers/clinicians [198].

**Author Contributions:** F.S. devised the paper, the main conceptual ideas and the proof outline. He contributed to the analysis of the results and the revision of the paper. S.C. performed the systematic literature review and drafted the initial version of the manuscript. J.M.C. and A.G. contributed to the interpretation of related data.

**Acknowledgments:** No sources of funding for the study are disclosed.

## References


1. Schifano, F.; Orsolini, L.; Papanti, D.; Corkery, J.M. Novel psychoactive substances of interest for psychiatry. *World Psychiatry* **2015**, *14*, 15–26. [CrossRef] [PubMed]
2. United Nations Office for Drugs and Crime (UNODC). Early Warning Advisory on New Psychoactive Substances. Available online: https://www.unodc.org/LSS/Page/NPS (accessed on 20 January 2018).
3. European Monitoring Centre for Drugs and Drug Abuse (EMCDDA). *European Drug Report. Trends and Developments*; EMCDDA: Lisbon, Portugal, 2017. Available online: http://www.emcdda.europa.eu/system/files/publications/4541/TDAT17001ENN.pdf (accessed on 2 March 2018).
4. Zawilska, J.B.; Andrzejczak, D. Next generation of novel psychoactive substances on the horizon—A complex problem to face. *Drug Alcohol Depend.* **2015**, *157*, 1–17. [CrossRef] [PubMed]
5. Van Hout, M.C.; Hearne, E. New psychoactive substances (NPS) on crypto market fora: An exploratory study of characteristics of forum activity between NPS buyers and vendors. *Int. J. Drug Policy* **2017**, *40*, 102–110. [CrossRef] [PubMed]
6. Soussan, C.; Andersson, M.; Kjellgren, A. The diverse reasons for using Novel Psychoactive Substances—A qualitative study of the users' own perspectives. *Int. J. Drug Policy* **2018**, *52*, 71–78. [CrossRef] [PubMed]
7. Chiappini, S.; Schifano, F. A decade of gabapentinoid misuse: An analysis of the European Medicines Agency's 'suspected adverse drug reactions' database. Assessment of gabapentinoid misuse/dependence as reported to the EMA. *CNS Drugs* **2016**, *30*, 1–8. [CrossRef] [PubMed]
8. Chiappini, S.; Schifano, F. Is there a potential of misuse for quetiapine? Literature review and analysis of the European Medicines Agency/EMA Adverse Drug Reactions' database. *J. Clin. Psychopharmacol.* **2018**, *38*, 72–79. [CrossRef] [PubMed]
9. Carvalho, A.F.; Sharma, M.S.; Brunoni, A.R.; Vieta, E.; Fava, G.A. The safety, tolerability and risks associated with the use of newer generation antidepressant drugs: A critical review of the literature. *Psychother. Psychosom.* **2016**, *85*, 270–288. [CrossRef] [PubMed]
10. Milano, G.; Chiappini, S.; Mattioli, F.; Martelli, A.; Schifano, F. β-2 agonists as misusing Drugs? Assessment of both Clenbuterol- and Salbutamol-related European Medicines Agency (EMA) Pharmacovigilance Database Reports. *Basic Clin. Pharmacol. Toxicol.* **2018**, *2*. [CrossRef]
11. Sheridan, D.C.; Hendrickson, R.G.; Beauchamp, G.; Laurie, A.; Fu, R.; Horowitz, B.Z. Adolescent Intentional Abuse Ingestions: Overall 10-Year Trends and Regional Variation. *Pediatr. Emerg. Care* **2016**. [CrossRef] [PubMed]
12. Lasoff, D.R.; Koh, C.H.; Corbett, B.; Minns, A.B.; Cantrell, F.L. Loperamide Trends in Abuse and Misuse Over 13 Years: 2002–2015. *Pharmacotherapy* **2017**, *37*, 249–253. [CrossRef] [PubMed]
13. European Medicines Agency (EMA). Pharmacovigilance. Available online: http://www.ema.europa.eu/ema/index.jsp?curl=pages/regulation/general/general_content_000258.jsp (accessed on 20 January 2017).
14. European Medicines Agency (EMA). EudraVigilance. Available online: http://www.ema.europa.eu/ema/index.jsp?curl=pages/regulation/general/general_content_000679.jsp (accessed on 3 March 2018).
15. Prisma. Transparent Reporting of Systematic Reviews and Meta-Analyses. Available online: http://www.prisma-statement.org/ (accessed on 21 December 2017).
16. Schifano, F. Misuse and Abuse of Pregabalin and Gabapentin: Cause for Concern? *CNS Drugs* **2014**, *28*, 491. [CrossRef] [PubMed]
17. Evoy, K.E.; Morrison, M.D.; Saklad, S.R. Abuse and Misuse of Pregabalin and Gabapentin. *Drugs* **2017**, *77*, 403–426. [CrossRef] [PubMed]
18. Schjerning, O.; Rosenzweig, M.; Pottegård, A.; Damkier, P.; Nielsen, J. Abuse Potential of Pregabalin: A Systematic Review. *CNS Drugs* **2016**, *30*, 9–25. [CrossRef] [PubMed]
19. Schjerning, O.; Pottegård, A.; Damkier, P.; Rosenzweig, M.; Nielsen, J. Use of Pregabalin—A Nationwide Pharmacoepidemiological Drug Utilization Study with Focus on Abuse Potential. *Pharmacopsychiatry* **2016**, *49*, 155–161. [CrossRef] [PubMed]
20. Erowid. Experiences. Available online: https://erowid.org/experiences/ (accessed on 16 January 2018).
21. Drug Enforcement Administration. Schedules of Controlled Substances: Placement of Pregabalin into Schedule V. Available online: https://www.deadiversion.usdoj.gov/fed_regs/rules/2005/fr0728.htm (accessed on 16 January 2018).

22. Bonnet, U.; Scherbaum, N. How addictive are gabapentin and pregabalin? A systematic review. *Eur. Neuropsychopharmacol.* **2017**, *27*, 1185–1215. [CrossRef] [PubMed]
23. Daly, C.; Griffin, E.; Ashcroft, D.M.; Webb, R.T.; Perry, I.J.; Arensman, E. Intentional Drug Overdose Involving Pregabalin and Gabapentin: Findings from the National Self-Harm Registry Ireland, 2007–2015. *Clin. Drug Investig.* **2017**, *20*. [CrossRef] [PubMed]
24. Reeves, R.R.; Ladner, M.E. Potentiation of the effect of buprenorphine/naloxone with gabapentin or quetiapine. *Am. J. Psychiatry* **2014**, *171*, 691. [CrossRef] [PubMed]
25. Greater use of gabapentinoids in intentional drug overdose. Available online: https://doi.org/10.1007/s40278-018-40617-3 (accessed on 21 April 2018).
26. OECD Indicators. Health at a Glance. 2015. Available online: http://www.keepeek.com/Digital-Asset-Management/oecd/social-issues-migration-health/health-at-a-glance-2015_health_glance-2015-en#page187 (accessed on 20 January 2018).
27. Kantor, E.D.; Rehm, C.D.; Haas, J.S.; Chan, A.T.; Giovannucci, E.L. Trends in prescription drug use among adults in the US from 1999–2012. *JAMA* **2015**, *314*, 1818–1831. [CrossRef] [PubMed]
28. Anderson, L.S.; Bell, H.G.; Gilbert, M.; Davidson, J.E.; Winter, C.; Barratt, M.J.; Win, B.; Painter, J.L.; Menone, C.; Sayegh, J.; et al. Using Social Listening Data to Monitor Misuse and Nonmedical Use of Bupropion: A Content Analysis. *JMIR Public Health Surveill.* **2017**, *3*, e6. [CrossRef] [PubMed]
29. Evans, E.A.; Sullivan, M.A. Abuse and misuse of antidepressants. *Subst. Abuse Rehabil.* **2014**, *5*, 107–120. [CrossRef] [PubMed]
30. McCormick, J. Recreational bupropion abuse in a teenager. *Br. J. Clin. Pharmacol.* **2002**, *53*, 211–214. [CrossRef]
31. Welsh, C.J.; Doyon, S. Seizure-induced by insufflation of bupropion. *N. Engl. J. Med.* **2002**, *347*, 951. [CrossRef] [PubMed]
32. Glaxo Smith and Kline (GSK). 2012 35 Clinical Study Result Summary. PRJ2215: Assessment of Buproprion Misuse/Abuse 2004–2011. Updated August 2016. Available online: https://www.gsk-clinicalstudyregister.com/files2/201235-Clinical-Study-Result-Summary.pdf (accessed on 20 October 2017).
33. Reeves, R.R.; Ladner, M.E. Additional evidence of the abuse potential of bupropion. *J. Clin. Psychopharmacol.* **2013**, *33*, 584–585. [CrossRef] [PubMed]
34. Baribeau, D.; Araki, K.F. Intravenous bupropion: A previously undocumented method of abuse of a commonly prescribed antidepressant agent. *J. Addict. Med.* **2013**, *7*, 216–217. [CrossRef] [PubMed]
35. Stahl, S.M.; Pradko, J.F.; Haight, B.R.; Modell, J.G.; Rockett, C.B.; Learned-Coughlin, S. A Review of the Neuropharmacology of Bupropion, a Dual Norepinephrine and DA Reuptake Inhibitor. *J. Clin. Psychiatry* **2004**, *6*, 159–166. [CrossRef]
36. Guzman, F. The Psychopharmacology of Bupropion: An Illustrated Overview. Available online: http://psychopharmacologyinstitute.com/antidepressants/bupropion-psychopharmacology/ (accessed on 7 October 2017).
37. Prosser, J.M.; Nelson, L.S. The toxicology of bath salts: A review of synthetic cathinones. *J. Med. Toxicol.* **2012**, *8*, 33–42. [CrossRef] [PubMed]
38. Vento, A.E.; Schifano, F.; Gentili, F.; Pompei, F.; Corkery, J.M.; Kotzalidis, G.D.; Girardi, P. Bupropion perceived as a stimulant by two patients with a previous history of cocaine misuse. *Ann. Super Sanita* **2013**, *49*, 402–405. [CrossRef]
39. Rettew, D.C.; Hudziak, J.J. Bupropion. In *Essentials of Clinical Psychopharmacology*, 2nd ed.; Schatzberg, A.F., Nemeroff, C.B., Eds.; American Psychiatric Publishing Inc.: Arlington, VA, USA, 2001; ISBN 1585624195.
40. Stall, N.; Godwin, J.; Juurlink, D. Bupropion abuse and overdose. *CMAJ* **2014**, *186*, 1015. [CrossRef] [PubMed]
41. Stassinos, G.L.; Klein-Schwartz, W. Bupropion "Abuse" Reported to US Poison Centers. *J. Addict. Med.* **2016**, *10*, 357–362. [CrossRef] [PubMed]
42. Toxnet, Toxicology Data Network. Bupropion; National Library of Medicine HSDB Database. 2015. Available online: https://toxnet.nlm.nih.gov/cgi-bin/sis/search/a?dbs+hsdb:@term+@DOCNO+6988 (accessed on 19 October 2017).
43. Hill, S.; Sikand, H.; Lee, J. Letter to the editor. A case report of seizure induced by bupropion nasal insufflation. *J. Clin. Psychiatry* **2007**, *9*, 67–69.
44. Yoon, G.; Westermeyer, J. Intranasal bupropion abuse case report. *Am. J. Addict.* **2013**, *22*, 180. [CrossRef] [PubMed]

45. Hilliard, W.T.; Barloon, L.; Farley, P.; Penn, J.V.; Koranek, A. Bupropion diversion and misuse in the correctional facility. *J. Correct. Health Care* **2013**, *19*, 211–217. [CrossRef] [PubMed]
46. Phillips, D. Wellbutrin: Misuse and abuse by incarcerated individuals. *J. Addict. Nurs.* **2012**, *23*, 65–69. [CrossRef] [PubMed]
47. Laird, G.; Narayan, P. Formulary Controls: Abuse of Psychotropics, and Dispensary Costs in the Incarceration Environment. Available online: http://www.fmhac.net/Assets/Documents/2009/Presentations/Laird%20Formulary%20Controls.pdf (accessed on 6 October 2017).
48. European Medicines Agency (EMA). Venlafaxine. 2007. Available online: http://www.ema.europa.eu/ema/index.jsp?curl=pages/medicines/human/referrals/Efexor/human_referral_000020.jsp (accessed on 20 December 2017).
49. Harvey, A.T.; Rudolph, R.L.; Preskorn, S.H. Evidence of the dual mechanisms of action of venlafaxine. *Arch. Gen. Psychiatry* **2000**, *57*, 503–509. [CrossRef] [PubMed]
50. Weikop, P.; Kehr, J.; Scheel-Krüger, J. The role of alpha1- and alpha2-adrenoreceptors on venlafaxine-induced elevation of extracellular serotonin, noradrenaline and DA levels in the rat prefrontal cortex and hippocampus. *J. Psychopharmacol.* **2004**, *18*, 395–403. [CrossRef] [PubMed]
51. Maj, J.; Rogoz, Z. Pharmacological effects of venlafaxine, a new antidepressant, given repeatedly, on the alpha 1-adrenergic, DA and serotonin systems. *J. Neural Transm.* **1999**, *106*, 197–211. [CrossRef] [PubMed]
52. Sabljić, V.; Ružić, K.; Rakun, R. Venlafaxine withdrawal syndrome. *Psychiatr. Danub.* **2011**, *23*, 117–119. [PubMed]
53. Fava, M.; Mulroy, R.; Alpert, J.; Nierenberg, A.; Rosenbaum, J. Emergence of adverse events following discontinuation of treatment with extended-release venlafaxine. *Am. J. Psychiatry* **1997**, *12*, 1760–1762. [CrossRef] [PubMed]
54. Stahl, S.M.; Grady, M.M.; Moret, C.; Briley, M. SNRIs: Their pharmacology, clinical efficacy, and tolerability in comparison with other classes of antidepressants. *CNS Spectr.* **2005**, *10*, 732–747. [CrossRef] [PubMed]
55. Sir, A.; D'Souza, R.F.; Uguz, S.; George, T.; Vahip, S.; Hopwood, M.; Martin, A.J.; Lam, W.; Burt, T. Randomized Trial of Sertraline Versus Venlafaxine XR in Major Depression: Efficacy and Discontinuation Symptoms. *J. Clin. Psychiatry* **2005**, *66*, 1312–1320. [CrossRef] [PubMed]
56. Taylor, D.; Stewart, S.; Connolly, A. Antidepressant withdrawal symptoms-telephone calls to a national medication helpline. *J. Affect. Disord.* **2006**, *95*, 129–133. [CrossRef] [PubMed]
57. Llorca, P.M.; Fernandez, J.L. Escitalopram in the treatment of major depressive disorder: Clinical efficacy, tolerability and cost-effectiveness vs. venlafaxine extended release formulation. *Int. J. Clin. Pract.* **2007**, *61*, 702–710. [CrossRef] [PubMed]
58. Kotzalidis, G.D.; de Pisa, E.; Patrizi, B.; Savoja, V.; Ruberto, G.; Girardi, P. Similar discontinuation symptoms for withdrawal from medium-dose paroxetine and venlafaxine. *J. Psychopharmacol.* **2008**, *22*, 581–584. [CrossRef] [PubMed]
59. Koga, M.; Kodaka, F.; Miyata, H.; Nakayama, K. Symptoms of delusion: The effects of discontinuation of low-dose venlafaxine. *Acta Psychiatr. Scand.* **2008**, *120*, 329–331. [CrossRef] [PubMed]
60. Holland, J.; Brown, R. Neonatal venlafaxine discontinuation syndrome: A mini-review. *Eur. J. Paediatr. Neurol.* **2017**, *21*, 264–268. [CrossRef] [PubMed]
61. Cutler, N. Severe Venlafaxine Withdrawal Successfully Treated With a Short Course of Duloxetine. *Prim. Care Companion CNS Disord.* **2017**, 19. [CrossRef] [PubMed]
62. Groot, P.C. Consensus group Tapering. [Tapering strips for paroxetine and venlafaxine]. *Tijdschr. Psychiatr.* **2013**, *55*, 789–794. [PubMed]
63. Francesconi, G.; Orsolini, L.; Papanti, D.; Corkery, J.M.; Schifano, F. Venlafaxine as the 'baby ecstasy'? Literature overview and analysis of web-based misusers' experiences. *Hum. Psychopharmacol.* **2015**, *30*, 255–261. [CrossRef] [PubMed]
64. Sattar, S.P.; Grant, K.M.; Bhatia, S.C. A case of venlafaxine abuse. *N. Engl. J. Med.* **2003**, *348*, 764–765. [CrossRef] [PubMed]
65. Venlafaxine overdose. Available online: https://doi.org/10.1007/s40278-018-40604-4 (accessed on 21 April 2018).
66. Baker, D.R.; Barron, L.; Kasprzyk-Hordern, B. Illicit and pharmaceutical drug consumption estimated via wastewater analysis. Part A: Chemical analysis and drug use estimates. *Sci. Total Environ.* **2014**, *487*, 629–641. [CrossRef] [PubMed]

67. Fountain, J.S.; Slaughter, R.J. TOXINZ, the New Zealand Internet poisons information database: The first decade. *Emerg. Med. Australas.* **2016**, *28*, 335–340. [CrossRef] [PubMed]
68. Schifano, F.; Chiappini, S. Is there a potential of misuse for venlafaxine and bupropion? *Front. Neuropharmacol.* **2018**, *9*. [CrossRef] [PubMed]
69. Health and Social Care Information Centre (HSCIC). Prescriptions Dispensed in the Community. England 2004–2014. Available online: http://content.digital.nhs.uk/catalogue/PUB17644/pres-disp-com-eng-2004-14-rep.pdf (accessed on 20 February 2017).
70. Bogart, G.T.; Ott, C.A. Abuse of second-generation antipsychotics: What prescribers need to know. *Curr. Psychiatry* **2011**, *10*, 77–79. [CrossRef]
71. Sarker, A.; O'Connor, K.; Ginn, R.; Scotch, M.; Smith, K.; Malone, D.; Gonzalez, G. Social Media Mining for Toxicovigilance: Automatic Monitoring of Prescription Medication Abuse from Twitter. *Drug Saf.* **2016**, *39*, 231–240. [CrossRef] [PubMed]
72. Advisory Council on the Misuse Drugs (ACMD). ACMD Report on Diversion and Illicit Supply of Medicines. 2016. Available online: https://www.gov.uk/government/uploads/system/uploads/attachment_data/file/580296/Meds_report-_final_report_15_December_LU__2_.pdf (accessed on 26 February 2018).
73. Food and Drug Administration (FDA). Seroquel Prescribing Information. 2010. Available online: http://www.accessdata.fda.gov/drugsatfda_docs/label/2011/020639s049s054lbl.pdf (accessed on 20 February 2017).
74. Terán, A.; Majadas, S.; Galan, J. Quetiapine in the treatment of sleep disturbances associated with addictive conditions: A retrospective study. *Subst. Use Misuse* **2008**, *43*, 2169–2171. [CrossRef]
75. Srivastava, A.; Patil, V.; Da Silva Pereira, Y. A Case Series of Quetiapine Addiction/Dependence. *Ger. J. Psychiatr.* **2013**, *16*, 152–155.
76. Kim, S.; Lee, G.; Kim, E.; Jung, H.; Chang, J. Quetiapine Misuse and Abuse: Is it an Atypical Paradigm of Drug-Seeking Behavior? *J. Res. Pharm. Pract.* **2017**, *6*, 12–15. [CrossRef] [PubMed]
77. Di Chiara, G.; Imperato, A. Drugs abused by humans preferentially increase synaptic DA concentrations in the mesolimbic system of freely moving rats. *Proc. Natl. Acad. Sci. USA* **1988**, *85*, 5274–5278. [CrossRef] [PubMed]
78. Waters, B.M.; Joshi, K.G. Intravenous Quetiapine-Cocaine Use ("Q-Ball"). *Am. J. Psychiatry* **2007**, *164*, 173–174. [CrossRef] [PubMed]
79. Pierre, J.M.; Shnayder, I.; Wirshing, D.A.; Wirshing, W.C. Intranasal quetiapine abuse. *Am. J. Psychiatry* **2004**, *61*, 1718. [CrossRef] [PubMed]
80. George, M.; Haasz, M.; Coronado, A.; Salhanick, S.; Korbel, L.; Kitzmiller, J.P. Acute dyskinesia, myoclonus, and akathisia in an adolescent male abusing quetiapine via nasal insufflation: A case study. *BMC Pediatr.* **2013**, *13*, 187. [CrossRef] [PubMed]
81. Morin, A.K. Possible intranasal quetiapine misuse. *Am. J. Health Syst. Pharm.* **2007**, *64*, 723–725. [CrossRef] [PubMed]
82. Fischer, B.A.; Boggs, D.L. The role of antihistaminic effects in the misuse of quetiapine: A case report and review of the literature. *Neurosci. Biobehav. Rev.* **2010**, *34*, 555–558. [CrossRef] [PubMed]
83. Reeves, R.R.; Brister, J.C. Additional evidence of the abuse potential of quetiapine. *South. Med. J.* **2007**, *100*, 834–836. [CrossRef] [PubMed]
84. Paparrigopoulos, T.; Karaiskos, D.; Liappas, J. Quetiapine: Another drug with potential for misuse? A case report. *J. Clin. Psychiatry* **2008**, *69*, 162–163. [CrossRef] [PubMed]
85. Chen, C.Y.; Shiah, I.S.; Lee, W.K.; Kuo, S.C.; Huang, C.C.; Wang, T.Y. Dependence on quetiapine in combination with zolpidem and clonazepam in bipolar depression. *Psychiatry Clin. Neurosci.* **2009**, *63*, 427–428. [CrossRef] [PubMed]
86. Hussain, M.Z.; Waheed, W.; Hussain, S. Intravenous quetiapine abuse. *Am. J. Psychiatry* **2005**, *162*, 1755–1756. [CrossRef] [PubMed]
87. Sansone, R.A.; Sansone, L.A. Is Seroquel developing an illicit reputation for misuse/abuse? *Psychiatry* **2010**, *7*, 13–16.
88. Murphy, D.; Bailey, K.; Stone, M.; Wirshing, W.C. Addictive potential of quetiapine. *Am. J. Psychiatry* **2008**, *165*, 167. [CrossRef] [PubMed]
89. Peyrière, H.; Diot, C.; Eiden, C.; Petit, P. Réseau de centres de d'Addictovigilance. Abuse Liability of Quetiapine (Xeroquel®): Analysis of the literature. *Fundam. Clin. Pharmacol.* **2015**, *29*, 27–28. [CrossRef]

90. Pilgrim, J.L.; Drummer, O.H. The toxicology and comorbidities of fatal cases involving quetiapine. *Forensic Sci. Med. Pathol.* **2013**, *9*, 170–176. [CrossRef] [PubMed]
91. Haller, E.; Bogunovic, O.; Miller, M. Atypical antipsychotics new drugs of abuse. In Proceedings of the American Academy of Addiction Psychiatry (AAAP) 24th Annual Meeting & Symposium, Scottsdale, AZ, USA, 7 December 2013. Abstract 16.
92. Heilbronn, C.; Lloyd, B.; McElwee, P.; Eade, A.; Lubman, D.E. Trends in quetiapine use and non-fatal quetiapine-related ambulance attendances. *Drug Alcohol Rev.* **2013**, *32*, 405–411. [CrossRef] [PubMed]
93. Mattson, M.E.; Albright, V.; Yoon, J.; Council, C.L. Emergency Department Visits Involving Misuse and Abuse of the Antipsychotic Quetiapine: Results from the Drug Abuse Warning Network (DAWN). *Subst. Abuse* **2015**, *9*, 39–46. [CrossRef] [PubMed]
94. Klein, L.; Bang, S.; Cole, J.B. Intentional Recreational Abuse of Quetiapine Compared to Other Second-generation Antipsychotics. *West. J. Emerg. Med.* **2017**, *18*, 243–250. [CrossRef] [PubMed]
95. Pinta, E.R.; Taylor, R.E. Letter to the editor. Quetiapine Addiction? *Am. J. Psychiatry* **2007**, *164*, 1. [CrossRef] [PubMed]
96. McLarnon, M.E.; Fulton, H.G.; MacIsaac, C.; Barrett, S.P. Characteristics of quetiapine misuse among clients of a community-based methadone maintenance program. *J. Clin. Psychopharmacol.* **2012**, *32*, 721–723. [CrossRef] [PubMed]
97. Malekshahi, T.; Tioleco, N.; Ahmed, N.; Campbell, A.N.; Haller, D. Misuse of atypical antipsychotics in conjunction with alcohol and other drugs of abuse. *J. Subst. Abuse Treat.* **2015**, *48*, 8–12. [CrossRef] [PubMed]
98. Cha, H.J.; Lee, H.A.; Ahn, J.I.; Jeon, S.H.; Kim, E.J.; Jeong, H.S. Dependence potential of quetiapine: Behavioral pharmacology in rodents. *Biomol. Ther.* **2013**, *21*, 307–312. [CrossRef] [PubMed]
99. Tanda, G.; Valentini, V.; De Luca, M.A.; Perra, V.; Serra, G.P.; Di Chiara, G. A systematic microdialysis study of DA transmission in the accumbens shell/core and prefrontal cortex after acute antipsychotics. *Psychopharmacology* **2015**, *232*, 1427–1440. [CrossRef]
100. Brutcher, R.E.; Nader, S.H.; Nader, M.A. Evaluation of the reinforcing effect of Quetiapine, alone and in combination with cocaine, in Rhesus monkeys. *J. Pharmacol. Exp. Ther.* **2016**, *356*, 244–250. [CrossRef] [PubMed]
101. Kapur, S.; Seeman, P. Antipsychotic agents differ in how fast they come off the DA D2 receptors. Implications for atypical antipsychotic action. *J. Psychiatry Neurosci.* **2000**, *25*, 161–166. [PubMed]
102. Tauscher, J.; Hussain, T.; Agid, O.; Verhoeff, N.P.; Wilson, A.A.; Houle, S.; Remington, G.; Zipursky, L.P.; Kapur, S. Equivalent occupancy of DA D1 and D2 receptors with clozapine: Differentiation from other atypical antipsychotics. *Am. J. Psychiatry* **2004**, *161*, 1620–1625. [CrossRef] [PubMed]
103. Kuroki, T.; Nagao, N.; Nakahara, T. Neuropharmacology of second-generation antipsychotic drugs: A validity of the serotonin-DA hypothesis. *Prog. Brain Res.* **2008**, *172*, 199–212. [CrossRef] [PubMed]
104. Kapur, S.; Remington, G. Atypical antipsychotics: New directions and new challenges in the treatment of schizophrenia. *Ann. Rev. Med.* **2001**, *52*, 503–517. [CrossRef] [PubMed]
105. Montebello, M.E.; Brett, J. Misuse and Associated Harms of Quetiapine and Other Atypical Antipsychotics. *Curr. Top. Behav. Neurosci.* **2017**, *34*, 125–139. [CrossRef] [PubMed]
106. Navailles, S.; De Deurwaerdère, P. Presynaptic control of serotonin on striatal DA function. *Psychopharmacology* **2011**, *213*, 213–242. [CrossRef] [PubMed]
107. Kotagale, N.R.; Mendhi, S.M.; Aglawe, M.M.; Umekar, M.J.; Taksande, B.G. Evidences for the involvement of sigma receptors in antidepressant-like effect of quetiapine in mice. *Eur. J. Pharmacol.* **2013**, *702*, 180–186. [CrossRef] [PubMed]
108. Yasui, Y.; Su, T.P. Potential Molecular Mechanisms on the Role of the Sigma-1 Receptor in the Action of Cocaine and Methamphetamine. *J. Drug Alcohol Res.* **2016**, *5*. [CrossRef] [PubMed]
109. Grabowski, K. Quetiapine abuse and dependence: Is pharmacokinetics important? *Acta Clin. Belg.* **2017**, *13*, 1. [CrossRef] [PubMed]
110. Dahr, R.; Sidana, A.; Singh, T. Olanzapine Dependence. *Ger. J. Psychiatry* **2010**, *13*, 51–53.
111. Valeriani, G.; Corazza, O.; Bersani, F.S.; Melcore, C.; Metastasio, A.; Bersani, G.; Schifano, F. Olanzapine as the ideal "trip terminator"? Analysis of online reports relating to antipsychotics' use and misuse following occurrence of novel psychoactive substance-related psychotic symptoms. *Hum. Psychopharmacol.* **2015**, *30*, 249–254. [CrossRef] [PubMed]
112. Reeves, R.R. Abuse of olanzapine by substance abusers. *J. Psychoact. Drugs* **2007**, *39*, 297–299. [CrossRef] [PubMed]

113. Kumsar, N.A.; Erol, A. Olanzapine abuse. *Subst. Abuse* **2013**, *34*, 73–74. [CrossRef] [PubMed]
114. James, P.D.; Fida, A.S.; Konovalov, P.; Smyth, B.P. Non-medical use of olanzapine by people on methadone treatment. *BJPsych Bull.* **2016**, *40*, 314–317. [CrossRef] [PubMed]
115. Skilbeck, K.J.; O'Reilly, J.N.; Johnston, G.A.; Hinton, T. The effects of antipsychotic drugs on GABAA receptor binding depend on period of drug treatment and binding site examined. *Schizophr. Res.* **2007**, *90*, 76–80. [CrossRef] [PubMed]
116. Egerton, A.; Ahmad, R.; Hirani, E.; Grasby, P.M. Modulation of striatal DA release by 5-HT2A and 5-HT2C receptor antagonists: [11C]raclopride PET studies in the rat. *Psychopharmacology* **2008**, *200*, 487–496. [CrossRef] [PubMed]
117. National Health Service (NHS) Prescription Cost Analysis (PCA) Data. 2016. Available online: http://www.nhsbsa.nhs.uk/PrescriptionServices/3494.aspx (accessed on 11 July 2017).
118. Medicines and Health Regulatory Agency (MHRA). Drug Analysis Profiles. The Yellow Card Scheme. 2016. Available online: Https://yellowcard.mhra.gov.uk/the-yellow-card-scheme/ (accessed on 11 July 2017).
119. Frauger, E.; Pochard, L.; Boucherie, Q.; Chevallier, C.; Daveluy, A.; Gibaja, V.; Caous, A.S.; Eiden, C.; Authier, N.; Le Boisselier, R.; et al. Le Réseau français d'addictovigilance. Surveillance system on drug abuse: Interest of the French national OPPIDUM program of French addictovigilance network. *Therapie* **2017**. [CrossRef] [PubMed]
120. Cerovecki, A.; Musil, R.; Klimke, A.; Seemüller, F.; Haen, E.; Schennach, R.; Kühn, K.U.; Volz, H.P.; Riedel, M. Withdrawal symptoms and rebound syndromes associated with switching and discontinuing atypical antipsychotics: Theoretical background and practical recommendations. *CNS Drugs* **2013**, *27*, 545–572. [CrossRef] [PubMed]
121. Parker, D.R.; McIntyre, I.M. Case studies of postmortem quetiapine: Therapeutic or toxic concentrations? *J. Anal. Toxicol.* **2005**, *29*, 407–412. [CrossRef] [PubMed]
122. Skov, L.; Johansen, S.S.; Linnet, K. Postmortem Quetiapine Reference Concentrations in Brain and Blood. *J. Anal. Toxicol.* **2015**, *39*, 557–561. [CrossRef] [PubMed]
123. Vance, C.; McIntyre, I.M. Postmortem Tissue Concentrations of Olanzapine. *J. Anal. Toxicol.* **2009**, *33*, 15–26. [CrossRef] [PubMed]
124. Aspirin/paracetamol/quetiapine overdose. Available online: https://doi.org/10.1007/s40278-018-40658-z (accessed on 21 April 2018).
125. Quetiapine/trazodone overdose. Available online: https://doi.org/10.1007/s40278-018-40528-4 (accessed on 21 April 2018).
126. McVeigh, J.; Evans-Brown, M.; Bellis, M.A. Human enhancement drugs and the pursuit of perfection. *Adicciones* **2012**, *24*, 185–190. [CrossRef] [PubMed]
127. Corazza, O.; Bersani, F.S.; Brunoro, R.; Valeriani, G.; Martinotti, G.; Schifano, F. The diffusion of Performance and Image-Enhancing Drugs (IPEDs) on the Internet: The Abuse of the Cognitive Enhancer Piracetam. *Subst. Use Misuse* **2014**, *49*, 1849–1856. [CrossRef] [PubMed]
128. Sagoe, D.; McVeigh, J.; Bjørnebekk, A.; Essilfie, M.; Schou Andreassen, C.; Pallesen, S. Polypharmacy among anabolic-androgenic steroid users: A descriptive metasynthesis. *Subst. Abuse Treat. Prev. Policy* **2015**, *10*, 12. [CrossRef] [PubMed]
129. Brennan, R.; Wells, J.S.G.; Van Hout, M.C. The injecting use of image and performance-enhancing drugs (IPED) in the general population: A systematic review. *Health Soc. Care Community* **2017**, *25*, 1459–1531. [CrossRef] [PubMed]
130. Van Hout, M.C.; Kean, J. An exploratory study of image and performance enhancement drug use in a male British South Asian community. *Int. J. Drug Policy* **2015**, *26*, 860–867. [CrossRef] [PubMed]
131. Rowe, R.; Berger, I.; Yaseen, B.; Copeland, J. Risk and blood-borne virus testing among men who inject image and performance enhancing drugs, Sydney, Australia. *Drug Alcohol Rev.* **2017**, *36*, 658–666. [CrossRef] [PubMed]
132. Van de Ven, K.; Koenraadt, R. Exploring the relationship between online buyers and sellers of image and performance enhancing drugs (IPEDs): Quality issues, trust and self-regulation. *Int. J. Drug Policy* **2017**, *50*, 48–55. [CrossRef] [PubMed]
133. Albertson, T.E.; Chenoweth, J.A.; Colby, D.K.; Sutter, M.E. The Changing Drug Culture: Use and Misuse of Appearance- and Performance-Enhancing Drugs. *FP Essent.* **2016**, *441*, 30–43. [PubMed]

134. Cassidy, E.M.; O'Halloran, D.J.; Barry, S. Insulin as a substance of misuse in a patient with insulin dependent diabetes mellitus. *BMJ* **1999**, *319*, 1417–1418. [CrossRef] [PubMed]
135. World Anti-Doping Agency (WADA). The Prohibited List 2017. Available online: https://www.wada-ama.org/sites/default/files/resources/files/2016-09-29_-_wada_prohibited_list_2017_eng_final.pdf (accessed on 24 January 2018).
136. Grimmer, N.M.; Gimbar, R.P.; Bursua, A.; Patel, M. Rhabdomyolysis Secondary to Clenbuterol Use and Exercise. *J. Emerg. Med.* **2016**, *50*, e71–e74. [CrossRef] [PubMed]
137. Mottram, D.R.; Chester, N. *Drugs in Sports*, 6th ed.; Routledge: Abington-on-Thames, UK, 2014; ISBN 9780415715287.
138. Quinley, K.E.; Chen, H.Y.; Yang, H.S.; Lynch, K.L.; Olson, K.R. Clenbuterol causing non-ST-segment elevation myocardial infarction in a teenage female desiring to lose weight: Case and brief literature review. *Am. J. Emerg. Med.* **2016**, *34*, 1739. [CrossRef] [PubMed]
139. Al-Majed, A.A.; Khalil, N.Y.; Khbrani, I.; Abdel-Aziz, H.A. Clenbuterol Hydrochloride. *Profiles Drug Subst. Excip. Relat. Methodol.* **2017**, *42*, 91–123. [CrossRef] [PubMed]
140. Spiller, H.A.; James, K.J.; Scholzen, S.; Borys, D.J. A descriptive study of adverse events from clenbuterol misuse and abuse for weight loss and bodybuilding. *Subst. Abuse* **2013**, *34*, 306–312. [CrossRef] [PubMed]
141. Howard, R. The Size Zero Pill. Available online: http://www.dailymail.co.uk/femail/article-409347/The-size-zero-pill.html (accessed on 13 November 2017).
142. Steroidal.com. Clenbuterol Dosage. Available online: Https://www.steroidal.com/fat-loss-agents/clenbuterol/clenbuterol-dosage/ (accessed on 2 November 2017).
143. Brett, J.; Dawson, A.H.; Brown, J.A. Clenbuterol toxicity: A NSW poisons information centre experience. *Med. J. Aust.* **2014**, *200*, 219–221. [CrossRef] [PubMed]
144. Van der Bijl, P.; Tutelyan, V.A. Dietary supplements containing prohibited substances. *Vopr. Pitan* **2013**, *82*, 6–13. [PubMed]
145. Solimini, R.; Rotolo, M.C.; Pellegrini, M.; Minutillo, A.; Pacifici, R.; Busardò, F.P.; Zaami, S. Adulteration Practices of Psychoactive Illicit Drugs: An Updated Review. *Curr. Pharm. Biotechnol.* **2017**, *18*, 524–530. [CrossRef] [PubMed]
146. Barry, A.R.; Graham, M.M. Case report and review of clenbuterol cardiac toxicity. *J. Cardiol. Cases* **2013**, *8*, 131–133. [CrossRef]
147. Huckins, D.S.; Lemons, M.F. Myocardial ischemia associated with clenbuterol abuse: Report of two cases. *J. Emerg. Med.* **2013**, *44*, 444–449. [CrossRef] [PubMed]
148. Daubert, G.P.; Mabasa, V.H.; Leung, V.W.; Aaron, C. Acute clenbuterol overdose resulting in supraventricular tachycardia and atrial fibrillation. *J. Med. Toxicol.* **2007**, *3*, 56–60. [CrossRef] [PubMed]
149. Ferrua, S.; Varbella, F.; Conte, M.R. Acute myocardial infarction due to coronary vasospasm and salbutamol abuse. *Heart* **2009**, *95*, 673. [CrossRef] [PubMed]
150. Patanè, S.; Marte, F.; La Rosa, F.C.; La Rocca, R. Atrial fibrillation associated with chocolate intake abuse and chronic salbutamol inhalation abuse. *Int. J. Cardiol.* **2010**, *145*, e74–e76. [CrossRef] [PubMed]
151. Boucher, A.; Payen, C.; Garayt, C.; Ibanez, H.; Dieny, A.; Doche, C.; Chuniaud, C.; Descotes, J. Salbutamol misuse or abuse with fatal outcome: A case report. *Hum. Exp. Toxicol.* **2011**, *30*, 1869–1871. [CrossRef] [PubMed]
152. O'Donnell, J.M. Effects of clenbuterol and prenalterol on performance during differential reinforcement of low response rate in the rat. *J. Pharmacol. Exp. Ther.* **1987**, *241*, 68–75. [PubMed]
153. Edwards, J.G.; Holgate, S.T. Dependency upon salbutamol inhalers. *Br. J. Psychiatry* **1979**, *134*, 624–626. [CrossRef] [PubMed]
154. Morgan, D.J.; Paull, J.D.; Richmond, B.H.; Wilson-Evered, E.; Ziccone, S.P. Pharmacokinetics of intravenous and oral salbutamol and its sulphate conjugate. *Br. J. Clin. Pharmacol.* **1986**, *22*, 587–593. [CrossRef] [PubMed]
155. Pope, H.G.; Wood, R.I.; Rogol, A.; Nyberg, F.; Bowers, L.; Bhasin, S. Adverse health consequences of performance-enhancing drugs: An Endocrine Society scientific statement. *Endocr. Rev.* **2013**, *35*, 341–375. [CrossRef] [PubMed]
156. Lewis, L.D.; Essex, E.; Volans, G.N.; Cochrane, G.M. A study of self- poisoning with oral salbutamol-laboratory and clinical features. *Hum. Exp. Toxicol.* **1993**, *12*, 397–401. [CrossRef] [PubMed]
157. Nicoli, R.; Petrou, M.; Badoud, F.; Dvorak, J.; Saugy, M.; Baume, N. Quantification of clenbuterol at trace level in human urine by ultra-high pressure liquid chromatography-tandem mass spectrometry. *J. Chromatogr. A* **2013**, *1292*, 142–150. [CrossRef] [PubMed]

158. Vaso, M.; Weber, A.; Tscholl, P.M.; Junge, A.; Dvorak, J. Use and abuse of medication during 2014 FIFA World Cup Brazil: A retrospective survey. *BMJ Open* **2015**, *5*, E007608. [CrossRef] [PubMed]
159. EMA. Buying Medicine Online. Available online: http://www.ema.europa.eu/ema/index.jsp?curl=pages/regulation/general/general_content_000630.jsp&mid=WC0b01ac05808fd210 (accessed on 11 November 2017).
160. Miller, H.; Panahi, L.; Tapia, D.; Tran, A.; Bowman, J.D. Loperamide misuse and abuse. *J. Am. Pharm. Assoc.* **2017**, *57*, S45–S50. [CrossRef] [PubMed]
161. Daniulaityte, R.; Carlson, R.; Falck, R.; Cameron, D.; Perera, S.; Chen, L.; Sheth, A. "I just wanted to tell you that loperamide WILL WORK": A web-based study of the extra-medical use of loperamide. *Drug Alcohol Depend.* **2013**, *130*, 241–244. [CrossRef] [PubMed]
162. Grey Pages: The Merits of High Dose Loperamide for Opiate Withdrawal. Available online: http://derekwmeyer.blogspot.com/2012/03/merits-of-high-dose-loperamide-for.html (accessed on 30 November 2017).
163. Finch, M. How to Use Loperamide for Opiate Withdrawal. 2015. Available online: http://opiateaddictionsupport.com/how-to-use-loperamidefor-opiate-withdrawal/ (accessed on 30 November 2017).
164. Levine, D.A. "Pharming": The abuse of prescription and over-the-counter drugs in teens. *Curr. Opin. Pediatr.* **2007**, *19*, 270–274. [CrossRef] [PubMed]
165. Cooper, R.J. Over the counter medicine abuse—A review of the literature. *J. Subst. Use* **2013**, *18*, 82–107. [CrossRef] [PubMed]
166. Fox, N.; Ward, K.; O'Rourke, A. The birth of the e-clinic. Continuity or transformation in the UK governance of pharmaceutical consumption? *Soc. Sci. Med.* **2005**, *61*, 1474–1484. [CrossRef] [PubMed]
167. Manchikanti, L. Prescription drug abuse: What is being done to address this new drug epidemic? Testimony before the Subcommittee on Criminal Justice, Drug Policy and Human Resources. *Pain Physician* **2006**, *9*, 287–321. [PubMed]
168. National Association of Board of Pharmacy (NABP). Buying Medicine Online. Available online: https://nabp.pharmacy/initiatives/dot-pharmacy/buying-medicine-online/ (accessed on 11 November 2017).
169. Food and Drug Administration (FDA) Imodium Label. Available online: https://www.accessdata.fda.gov/drugsatfda_docs/label/2016/017690s005lbl.pdf (accessed on 28 January 2018).
170. Baker, D.E. Loperamide: A pharmacological review. *Rev. Gastroenterol. Disord.* **2007**, *7* (Suppl. 3), S11-8. [PubMed]
171. Jaffe, J.H.; Kanzler, M.; Green, J. Abuse potential of loperamide. *Clin. Pharmacol. Ther.* **1980**, *28*, 812–819. [CrossRef] [PubMed]
172. Wightman, R.S.; Hoffman, R.S.; Howland, M.A.; Rice, B.; Binary, R.; Lugassy, D. Not your regular high: Cardiac dysrhythmias caused by loperamide. *Clin. Toxicol.* **2016**, *54*, 454–458. [CrossRef] [PubMed]
173. Borron, S.W.; Watts, S.H.; Tull, J.; Baeza, S.; Diebold, S.; Barrow, A. Misuse and Abuse of Loperamide: A New Look at a Drug with "Low Abuse Potential". *J. Emerg. Med.* **2017**, *53*, 73–84. [CrossRef] [PubMed]
174. Marraffa, J.M.; Holland, M.G.; Sullivan, R.W.; Morgan, B.W.; Oakes, J.A.; Wiegand, T.J.; Hodgman, M.J. Cardiac conduction disturbance after loperamide abuse. *Clin. Toxicol.* **2014**, *52*, 952–957. [CrossRef] [PubMed]
175. Food and Drug Administration (FDA) Drug Safety Communications. FDA Warns about Serious Heart Problems with High Doses of the Anti-Diarrheal Medicine Loperamide (Imodium), Including from Abuse and Misuse. Safety Announcement. 6 July 2016. Available online: https://www.fda.gov/Drugs/DrugSafety/ucm504617.htm (accessed on 22 November 2017).
176. New York Times. Addicts Who Can't Find Painkillers Turn to Anti-Diarrhea Drugs. 10 May 2016. Available online: https://www.nytimes.com/2016/05/11/health/imodium-opioid-addiction.html?_r=0. (accessed on 24 November 2017).
177. Stanciu, C.N.; Gnanasegaram, S.A. Loperamide, the "Poor Man's Methadone": Brief Review. *J. Psychoact. Drugs* **2017**, *49*, 18–21. [CrossRef] [PubMed]
178. Eggleston, W.; Marraffa, J.M.; Stork, C.M.; Mercurio-Zappala, M.; Su, M.K.; Wightman, R.S.; Cummings, K.R.; Schier, J.G. Notes from the Field: Cardiac Dysrhythmias after Loperamide Abuse—New York, 2008–2016. *MMWR Morb. Mortal Wkly. Rep.* **2016**, *65*, 1276–1277. [CrossRef] [PubMed]
179. Eggleston, W.; Clark, K.H.; Marraffa, J.M. Loperamide Abuse Associated With Cardiac Dysrhythmia and Death. *Ann. Emerg. Med.* **2017**, *69*, 83–86. [CrossRef] [PubMed]
180. Bhatti, Z.; Norsworthy, J.; Szombathy, T. Loperamide metabolite-induced cardiomyopathy and QTc prolongation. *Clin. Toxicol.* **2017**, *55*, 659–661. [CrossRef] [PubMed]

181. Kozak, P.M.; Harris, A.E.; McPherson, J.A.; Roden, D.M. Torsades de pointes with high-dose loperamide. *J. Electrocardiol.* **2017**, *50*, 355–357. [CrossRef] [PubMed]
182. Wu, P.E.; Juurlink, D.N. Clinical Review: Loperamide Toxicity. *Ann. Emerg. Med.* **2017**, *70*, 245–252. [CrossRef] [PubMed]
183. Bishop-Freeman, S.C.; Feaster, M.S.; Beal, J.; Miller, A.; Hargrove, R.L.; Brower, J.O.; Winecker, R.E. Loperamide-Related Deaths in North Carolina. *J. Anal. Toxicol.* **2016**, *40*, 677–686. [CrossRef] [PubMed]
184. Swank, K.A.; Wu, E.; Kortepeter, C.; McAninch, J.; Levin, R.L. Adverse event detection using the FDA post-marketing drug safety surveillance system: Cardiotoxicity associated with loperamide abuse and misuse. *J. Am. Pharm. Assoc.* **2017**, *57*, S63–S67. [CrossRef] [PubMed]
185. Church, J.; Fletcher, E.J.; Abdel-Hamid, K.; MacDonald, J. Loperamide blocks high-voltage-activated calcium channels and N-methyl-D-aspartate-evoked responses in rat and mouse cultured hippocampal pyramidal neurons. *Mol. Pharmacol.* **1994**, *45*, 747–757. [PubMed]
186. Nozaki-Taguchi, N.; Yaksh, T.L. Characterization of the antihyperalgesic action of a novel peripheral mu-opioid receptor agonist- loperamide. *Anesthesiology* **1999**, *90*, 225–234. [CrossRef] [PubMed]
187. Kang, J.; Compton, D.R.; Vaz, R.J.; Rampe, D. Proarrhythmic mechanisms of the common anti-diarrheal medication loperamide: Revelations from the opioid abuse epidemic. *Naunyn Schmiedebergs Arch. Pharmacol.* **2016**, *389*, 1133–1137. [CrossRef] [PubMed]
188. Zhou, S.; Lim, L.Y.; Chowbay, B. Herbal modulation of P-glycoprotein. *Drug Metab. Rev.* **2004**, *36*, 57–104. [CrossRef] [PubMed]
189. Loperamide + Black Pepper Exctract = Feeling Really Nice. Available online: www.erowid.com (accessed on 3 January 2018).
190. Corazza, O.; Assi, S.; Simonato, P.; Corkery, J.M.; Bersani, F.S.; Demetrovics, Z.; Stair, J.; Fergus, S.; Pezzolesi, C.; Pasinetti, M.; et al. Promoting innovation and excellence to face the rapid diffusion of novel psychoactive substances in the EU: The outcomes of the ReDNet project. *Hum. Psychopharmacol.* **2013**, *28*, 317–323. [CrossRef] [PubMed]
191. Larsen, T.R.; McMunn, J.; Ahmad, H.; AlMahameed, S.T. Ventricular Tachycardia Triggered by Loperamide and Famotidine Abuse. *Drug Saf. Case Rep.* **2018**, *5*, 11. [CrossRef] [PubMed]
192. Sehring, M.; Chambers, J. Letter to the editor. Loperamide abuse and cardiotoxicity. *J. Community Hosp. Intern. Med. Perspect.* **2017**, *7*, 275. [CrossRef]
193. Orsolini, L.; Papanti, G.D.; Francesconi, G.; Schifano, F. Mind navigators of chemicals' experimenters? A web-based description of e-psychonauts. *Cyberpsychol. Behav. Soc. Netw.* **2015**, *18*, 296–300. [CrossRef] [PubMed]
194. Johanson, C.E.; Balster, R.L.; Henningfield, J.E.; Schuster, C.R.; Anthony, J.C.; Barthwell, A.G.; Coleman, J.J.; Dart, R.C.; Gorodetzky, C.W.; O'Keeffe, C.; et al. Risk management post-marketing surveillance for the abuse of medications acting on the central nervous system: Expert panel report. *Drug Alcohol Depend.* **2009**, *105* (Suppl. 1), S65–S71. [CrossRef] [PubMed]
195. Mackey, T.K.; Nayyar, G. Digital danger: A review of the global public health, patient safety and cybersecurity threats posed by illicit online pharmacies. *Br. Med. Bull.* **2016**, *118*, 110–126. [CrossRef] [PubMed]
196. McColl, S.; Sellers, E.M. Research design strategies to evaluate the impact of formulations on abuse liability. *Drug Alcohol Depend.* **2006**, *83* (Suppl. 1), S52–S62. [CrossRef] [PubMed]
197. FDA's Role in Preventing Prescription Drug Abuse. Statement of Robert J. Meyer, M.D. before the House Committee on Government Reform, September 13, 2005. Available online: http://www.fda.gov/NewsEvents/Testimony/ucm112718.htm (accessed on 30 November 2017).
198. Schifano, F.; Papanti, G.D.; Orsolini, L.; Corkery, J.M. The consequences of drug misuse on post-marketing surveillance. *Exp. Rev. Clin. Pharmacol.* **2016**, *9*, 867–871. [CrossRef] [PubMed]

# 15

# Novel Synthetic Opioids: The Pathologist's Point of View

**Paolo Frisoni [1], Erica Bacchio [1], Sabrine Bilel [2], Anna Talarico [3], Rosa Maria Gaudio [1], Mario Barbieri [1], Margherita Neri [4,*] and Matteo Marti [4,5]**

1 Department of Medical Sciences, University of Ferrara, 44121 Ferrara, Italy; paolo.frisoni@unife.it (P.F.); erica.bacchio@unife.it (E.B.); rosamaria.gaudio@unife.it (R.M.G.); mario.barbieri@unife.it (M.B.)

2 Department of Life Sciences and Biotechnology (SVeB), University of Ferrara, 44121 Ferrara, Italy; bllsrn@unife.it

3 Department of Chemical and Pharmaceutical Sciences, University of Ferrara, 44121 Ferrara, Italy; anna.talarico@unife.it

4 Department of Morphology, Surgery and Experimental Medicine, Section of Legal Medicine, University of Ferrara, 44121 Ferrara, Italy; matteo.marti@unife.it

5 Collaborative Center for the Italian National Early Warning System, Department of Anti-Drug Policies, Presidency of the Council of Ministers, 00184 Roma, Italy

* Correspondence: margherita.neri@unife.it

**Abstract:** Background: New Psychoactive Substances (NPS) constitute a broad range of hundreds of natural and synthetic drugs, including synthetic opioids, synthetic cannabinoids, synthetic cathinones, and other NPS classes, which were not controlled from 1961 to 1971 by the United Nations drug control conventions. Among these, synthetic opioids represent a major threat to public health. Methods: A literature search was carried out using public databases (such as PubMed, Google Scholar, and Scopus) to survey fentanyl-, fentanyl analogs-, and other synthetic opioid-related deaths. Keywords including "fentanyl", "fentanyl analogs", "death", "overdose", "intoxication", "synthetic opioids", "Novel Psychoactive Substances", "MT-45", "AH-7921", and "U-47700" were used for the inquiry. Results: From our literature examination, we inferred the frequent implication of fentanyls and synthetic opioids in side effects, which primarily affected the central nervous system and the cardiovascular and pulmonary systems. The data showed a great variety of substances and lethal concentrations. Multidrug-related deaths appeared very common, in most reported cases. Conclusions: The investigation of the contribution of novel synthetic opioid intoxication to death should be based on a multidisciplinary approach aimed at framing each case and directing the investigation towards targeted toxicological analyses.

**Keywords:** fentanyl; NPS; synthetic opioids; MT-45; AH-7921; U-47700; forensic pathology

---

## 1. Introduction

New Psychoactive Substances (NPS) are a heterogeneous class of non-controlled substances available on the global illicit drug market (e.g., smart shops, internet, "darknet"). The use of NPS, often consumed along with other drugs of abuse and alcohol, has resulted in a significantly growing number of emergency admissions due to overdoses and a high number of deaths. By July 2017, 739 different NPS were reported to United Nations Office on Drugs and Crime (UNODC) [1]. According to the The European Monitoring Centre for Drugs and Drug Addiction (EMCDDA)report, with an overall total of 38 substances, synthetic opioids have become the fourth largest group of substances monitored in 2017, after synthetic cannabinoids (179 substances), cathinones (130), and phenethylamines (94) [2].

The class of synthetic opioids include fentanyl, its analogs used in medical therapy (e.g., sufentanil, alfentanil, and remifentanil) [3], and novel non-pharmaceutical fentanyls not approved for human medical use (e.g., acetylfentanyl, acryloylfentanyl, carfentanil, α-methylfentanyl, 3-methylfentanyl, furanylfentanyl, 4-fluorobutyrylfentanyl, 4-methoxybutyrylfentanyl, 4-chloroisobutyrylfentanyl, 4-fluoroisobutyrylfentanyl, tetrahydrofuranylfentanyl, valerylfentanyl, cyclopentylfentanyl, and ocfentanil), and compounds with different chemical structures, such as MT-45 (1-cyclohexyl-4-(1,2-diphenylethyl)piperazine), AH-7921 (3,4-dichloro-*N*-{[1(dimethylamino) cyclohexyl]methyl} benzamide) and U-47700 (3,4-dichloro- *N*-[(1R,2R)-2-(dimethylamino)cyclohexyl]-*N*-methylbenzamide) [4,5]. They are used on their own or more often in combination with heroin or other opioids [6,7]. This paper critically examines the literature on deaths related to fentanyls and synthetic opioid overdose, alone or in combination with other psychoactive drugs (i.e., cocaine, benzodiazepine, alcohol, and other opioids) and investigates the characteristics and complexity of such deaths, analyzing all data useful for the forensic pathologist.

## 2. Materials and Methods

A literature search was carried out using public databases (such as PubMed, Google Scholar, and Scopus) to revise fentanyl-, fentanyl analogs- and others synthetic opioids-related deaths. Keywords including "fentanyl", "fentanyl analogs", "death", "overdose", "intoxication", "synthetic opioids", "Novel Psychoactive Substances", "MT-45", "AH-7921", and "U-47700" were used for the inquiry. The data were collected from 1990 to June 2018. Only deaths were considered. There were no language restrictions. All types of papers were included. We also reviewed the reference lists of the identified publications and PubMed suggestions. The full texts of all the eligible papers were obtained. Finally, 128 articles were included in this review. The examined data included the circumstances of death (e.g., trauma, external injuries) and drug exposure (pharmaceutical versus illicit drug use). With regard to the concentrations of the compounds, blood and, when stated, liver, urine, stomach content, kidney, brain, vitreous humor, and nasal swab concentrations were reported.

## 3. Results

### *3.1. Synthetic Opioid Overview*

Novel synthetic opioids, similar to the classical opioids morphine and heroin, selectively bind to the μ-, δ-, and κ-opioid receptors in the peripheral and central nervous system (CNS), thereby simulating the effects of endogenous opiates. However, they generally show greater selectivity towards the μ-opioid receptor subtype than morphine [8]. Stimulation of the μ-opioid receptor promotes the exchange of GTP (Guanosine Triphosphate) for GDP (Guanosine Diphosphate) in the G-protein complex and subsequently inhibits adenylate cyclase in cells causing a decrease in intracellular cAMP (Cyclic Adenosine Monophosphate). In addition, the activation of the μ-opioid receptors inhibits calcium and potassium ion channel conductance [8]. All these molecular events cause cellular membrane hyperpolarization and inhibit tonic neural activity with a consequent reduction in the release of several neurotransmitters, such as substance P, GABA, dopamine, acetylcholine, and noradrenaline [9].

These neurochemical changes are mainly responsible for the pharmaco-toxicological effects induced by synthetic opioids. Typically, acute intoxication induced by "classical" and novel synthetic opioids is characterized by miosis (but later the pupils may become dilated), a reduced level of consciousness (CNS (central nervous system) depression), respiratory depression, hypoxia, acidosis, hypotension, bradycardia, shock, gastric hypomotility, paralytic ileus, pulmonary edema, lethargy, coma, and even death.

In the last few years, the novel fentanyls have become a serious concern. These substances currently dominate the synthetic opioid group, with a total of 28 reports since they first surfaced in 2012. Fentanyl, which is the prototypical compound of this class, is a synthetic, lipophilic phenylpiperidine opioid agonist. It was developed in the 1960s by Paul Janssen in Belgium, and it is now available therapeutically as an intravenous, transbucal, or transdermal preparation, commonly used for surgical anesthesia and to treat severe chronic pain [10]. Because of its highly potent opioid euphoric effects, fentanyl leads addicts to rapidly abuse this drug through a variety of different methods, including the oral abuse of transdermal fentanyl patches [4]. The clinical effects are dose dependent, ranging from the induction of analgesia alone by serum concentrations of 0.3–0.7 ng/mL to the loss of protective airway reflexes and CNS depression by serum concentrations >3 ng/mL [11]. In addition, fentanyl and its analogs produce drowsiness and euphoria [12]. The most common side effects may include nausea, dizziness, vomiting, fatigue, headache, and constipation. The repeated use of fentanyls leads to the development of tolerance and dependence [13]. Typical withdrawal symptoms involve sweating, anxiety, diarrhea, bone pain, abdominal cramps, and shivers or goose "flesh" [12,14].

From a pharmacological point of view, fentanyl and its analogs are significantly more potent than morphine, with effects' magnitudes ranging from 1.5–7 times (butyrylfentanyl) to 10,000 times (carfentanil) those of morphine [14], and are characterized by high lipid solubility, rapid onset of action, and short duration of action. Like other types of opioid analgesics, such as morphine, methadone, and heroin, fentanyls produce their main effects by stimulating at nanomolar affinity the μ-opioid receptor [15–18]. In particular, they induce acute analgesia, relaxation, euphoria, sedation, bradycardia, hypothermia, depression of the central nervous system and respiratory function [16,19–21]. The last of the listed side effects poses the greatest danger to users and it is responsible for fentanyls-related significant morbidity and mortality [22]. The timely administration of the antidote naloxone [23] can rapidly reverse the severe respiratory depression caused by fentanyls [24], although multiple naloxone doses may be required [25]. The rapid administration of naloxone following fentanyl's overuse is essential, because of the rapid onset of action of the drug that can cause respiratory depression within two minutes [26]. The optimal dose range and methods of administration of naloxone are still not clear. The UK Department of Health recommends the following naloxone dose regimen: an initial dose of 0.4 mg intravenously, followed by up to two doses of 0.8 mg. If the latter two doses are ineffective, a further 2 mg dose should be provided [27]. In fact, despite the fact that fentanyl shows an affinity for μ-opioid receptor (Ki ~ 1.346 nM) similar to that of morphine (Ki ~ 1.168 nM) [28], it displays a greater potency ($EC_{50}$ ~ 0.15 nM) than morphine ($EC_{50}$ ~ 2.4 nM) in functional biological assays [29]. On this basis, higher naloxone doses may be necessary to reverse the adverse effects of fentanyls (i.e., lofentanil) with greater μ-opioid receptor affinity (Ki ~ 0.023 nM) [30] and potency (EC50 ~ 0.03 nM) [29].

Because of the narrow therapeutic index of fentanyl (and, presumably, of its analogs) its recreational use is highly dangerous, especially in opioid-intolerant users. High doses might hasten death due to respiratory arrest and pulmonary edema. Fentanyl analogs are clandestinely developed for recreational use [15,30–34]. These compounds have been synthesized by modification or replacement of the fentanyl's propionyl chain or by replacement of its ethylphenyl moiety. The obtained analogs have been further modified by substitution with fluoro, chloro, or methoxy groups at the *N*-phenyl ring. Among fentanyl analogs, carfentanil [methyl 1-(2-phenylethyl)-4-(*N*-propanoylanilino) piperidine-4-carboxylate] is considered one of the most lethal opioids, showing an extremely high clinical potency. It is used in research and, in some countries, as a veterinary medicine to immobilize large animals. Between November 2016 and April 2017, carfentanil was involved in at least 61 deaths in eight European countries. The vast majority of those deaths are related to heroin consumption [2].

Fentanyls have been found in a range of physical and dosage forms in Europe. The most common form is powder, but they have also been detected in liquids and tablets. E-liquids containing fentanyls that can be vaped using electronic cigarettes have also been reported [2].

These forms are easily absorbed through more convenient administration routes than injection, yet provide the consumers with psychoactive effects similar to those obtained with injectable forms. However, their use may pose a high risk of accidental overdose. In fact, nasal sprays and e-liquids could make fentanyls use more attractive and socially acceptable, promoting their spread and usage.

In addition to fentanyls, other novel synthetic opioids with chemical structures different from fentanyl, i.e., MT-45, AH-7921, and U-47700, have appeared on the recreational drug market and are causing intoxication and potentially fatal outcomes in consumers. MT-45 (1-cyclohexyl-4-(1,2-diphenylethyl) piperazine)), also known as IC-6, CDEP, AC1L8SAC, and NSC 299236, has shown particular effects, such as paresthesia in limbs, hand weakness, balance disturbances, vision impairments, and hearing impairment or loss [35]. In three cases, unusual side effects have been reported, such as loss and depigmentation of hair, folliculitis and dermatitis, painful intertriginous dermatitis, and elevated liver enzymes [36]. MT-45 has been associated with many reports of fatal intoxications in Europe; in particular, Sweden reported 28 analytically confirmed deaths between November 2013 and July 2014 [37,38]. In vitro and in vivo metabolism studies have shown that MT-45 is biotransformed into active hydroxylated compounds [39] that may contribute to the overall pharmaco-toxicological profile of MT-45 in vivo [40]. AH-7921 (3,4-dichloro-*N*-[1(dimethylamino) cyclohexyl] methyl benzamide) belongs to a series of compounds known as cyclohexylamines [41]. The drug exhibited similar potency to morphine in preclinical studies [42]. The compound is taken orally, nasally, by smoking, and, less commonly, by intravenous injection [43]. The main clinical effects included hypertension, tachycardia, and seizures. The first death associated with AH-7921 use was reported by Norway in December 2012 [43]. There has been one confirmed fatality from AH-7921 in the United States, but a number of deaths have been associated with this drug in Europe [44,45].

U-47700 (3,4-dichloro-*N*-[(1R,2R)-2-(dimethylamino)yclohexyl]-*N*-methylbenzamide) is a structural isomer of AH-7921. It is also known as "fake morphine" or "U4" in the recreational drug market and it is sometimes also referred to as "pink", because impurities in its synthesis cause the drug powder to be slightly pink in color. In preclinical studies, U-47700 is about 1/10 as potent as fentanyl, but 7.5 times more potent than morphine [46,47]. During 2016, a significant number of U-47700 acute intoxication cases were reported in the USA. The clinical symptoms are consistent with those of traditional opioids [5]. U-47700 has caused at least 46 deaths from overdose in the United States [48–51].

### 3.2. *Circumstantial Data and External Examination*

It is very important to sample any potential drug-containing material in the area around a dead body, taking into account the numerous opioid administration routes (drug paraphernalia, powders, syringes, vials, pills, patches etc.). It is also important to look for signs of administration on the body, considering, however, that about 20% [52] of subjects take fentanyl or analogs by inhalation, ingestion, or, rarely, transdermal route, therefore puncture marks are not always evident.

Even in the absence of external signs specific for opioid intoxication, it is possible to observe non-specific signs of asphyxia, such as petechiae [53].

### 3.3. *Autopsy-Pathological Findings*

The data from the literature review showed that the new synthetic opioids produce similar clinical effects as the traditional ones [54]; therefore, we sought the typical findings of heroin intoxication trying to capture the differences and identify additional typical findings of fentanyl- and synthetic opioid-related deaths. The autopsy findings collected from the case reports treated in the literature were homogeneous with respect to the detected findings. The routine histological data were not very specific and did not reveal indicative signs of intoxication [13,55].

#### 3.3.1. Central Nervous System

The major autoptic relief found in the CNS was cerebral oedema. This finding was reported for several drugs (fentanyl [56,57], acetylfentanyl [58], butyrylfentany [59], furanylfentanyl [60,61], ocfentanil [62], AH-7921 [63], U-47700 [64], MT-45 [65]). A case of fatal cerebral hemorrhage induced by acetylfentanyl was reported [66], and another case of a 19-month-old girl poisoned by a transdermal administration of fentanyl who developed leukoencephalopathy was described [67]; in this case, the girl survived, however, investigators declared that this is not always the outcome [55].

#### 3.3.2. Cardiovascular System

A reported uncommon intoxication symptom is chest pain mimicking acute coronary syndrome with non-specific T-wave changes on the electrocardiogram [68]. It is necessary to distinguish the alterations induced acutely by the drug from those due to pre-existing pathologies. Most of the observed cardiovascular pathological findings, such as hypertrophy [69], cardiomegaly [56,70,71], cardiac fibrosis [72,73], atherosclerosis [69,74], are not attributable to an acute intoxication but, in some cases, they may be compatible with chronic drug intake. The presence of pericardial petechiae [53] can be interpreted as a generic sign of asphyxia, due to opioid-related respiratory failure.

#### 3.3.3. Pulmonary

The main effect of fentanyl and its analogues on the respiratory system is respiratory depression. Furthermore, fentanyl can cause chest wall rigidity and apnea, particularly with rapid intravenous administration [75], a factor that can contribute to respiratory failure. Rare adverse effects after fentanyl usage include diffuse alveolar hemorrhage immediately after insufflating fentanyl powder [72]. The major pathological findings are pulmonary congestion [53,54,69,70,73,74,76–82] and pulmonary oedema, which are common to all the investigated drugs [57,58,70,73,74,78–81,83]. Signs found occasionally are petechiae on the pleura [57,82] and aspiration of gastric contents inside the trachea and bronchi [57,76,81].

A few cases of fentanyl patch aspiration have been reported, where the patch was found in the airways [71,84]. Microscopically, small amounts of foreign material have been reported in the lungs, consistent with prior intravenous drug abuse [80].

#### 3.3.4. Others

Another common sign is generalized visceral congestion [51,60,65]. Hepatic parenchyma alterations, such as liver cirrhosis [74], chronic active hepatitis [82], fatty degeneration [62,70,84], hepatomegaly [62,70], are common but due to pre-existing conditions or chronic abuse of narcotics.

### *3.4. Sampling*

The samples commonly taken for toxicological analysis consisted of peripheral blood [84], central blood [85], urine, and liver. Less commonly collected samples were vitreous humour [78], brain, kidney, bile, and gastric content.

Among these, the least susceptible site to post-mortem redistribution is the liver (in relation to fentanyl) [86]. However, there is currently no consensus on the ideal sampling site [87].

### *3.5. Lethal Concentrations*

The lethal concentrations found in the literature are reported in Table 1. For each drug, the routes of administration and relative potency compared to morphine are shown, in addition to the dose (and the corresponding tissue). Table 2 shows the concentration data reported in multidrug-associated deaths.

**Table 1.** Lethal concentrations data reported in the literature.

| | Potency Ratio to Morphine [14] | Administration Route Associated with Overdose | Blood Concentration (ng/mL) | Other Concentrations (Site, ng/mL) |
|---|---|---|---|---|
| Acetylfentanyl [53,58,80,88] | 15.7 | Nasal, intravenous | 153–260<br>247.5–285 (heart) | Liver 100–2400 ng/g; urine 2.6–2720 ng/mL; stomach content 880 ng/mL; vitreous humor 131–240 ng/mL. |
| Alpha-Methylfentanyl [89] | 56.9 | Intravenous | 3.1 | liver 78 ng/g; bile 6.4 ng/mL. |
| Butyrylfentanyl [59,71] | 1.5–7.0 | Nasal, rectal, intravenous, sublingual | 66–99 ng/mL;<br>39–220 ng/mL (heart) | liver 41–57 ng/g; kidney 160 ng/g, muscle 100 ng/g; vitreous humor 32 ng/mL; bile 260 ng/mL; urine 64 ng/mL; gastric contents 590 ng/mL; brain 93 ng/g. |
| Carfentanil [90] | 10,000 | | 0.11–0.88 | |
| 4-Fluorobutyrfentanyl [91] | Unknown | By smoking | 91–112 | urine, 200–414 ng/mL; liver, 411–902 ng/g; kidney 136–197 ng/g. |
| Furanylfentanyl [49,60] | Unknown | Nasal, intravenous | 0.43–26 | |
| 3-Methylfentanyl [83,92] | 48.5–7000 | Intravenous | 0.3–1.9 | |
| Ocfentanil [62,93] | 90 | Nasal, by smoking | 9.1–15.3;<br>23.3–27.9 (heart) | vitreous humor 12.5 ng/mL; urine 6.0 ng/mL; bile 13.7 ng/mL; liver 31.2 ng/g; kidney 51.2 ng/g; brain 37.9 ng/g; nasal swabs 2999 ng/swab. |
| AH-7921 [5,44,64,66] | Unknown | Oral, nasal, by smoking, intravenous | 330–6600<br>480–3900 (heart) | urine 760–6000 ng/mL; bile 17,000 ng/mL; liver 530–26,000 ng/g; kidney 7200 ng/g; brain, 7700 ng/g; vitreous humor 190 ng/mL; stomach content, 40 μg/mL. |
| U-47700 [5,49,94,95] | 7.5 | Oral, nasal, intrarectal, smoking, intravenous | 59–525<br>1347 (heart) | Urine 360–1393 ng/mL; liver 430–1700 ng/g; kidney 270 ng/g; lung 320 ng/g; brain 97 ng/g. |
| MT-45 [5,66,96] | Unknown | Oral, nasal, intrarectal, intravenous | 520–660<br>1300 (heart) | Urine 370 ng/mL; vitreous humor 260 ng/mL; gastric content 49 μg/mL; liver 24 μg/g. |
| Fentanyl [70,82,86,87,97,98] | 100 | Oral, transdermal, nasal, intravenous | 0.5–383 | Urine 2.9–895 ng/mL; gastric content 31.6–745 μg/mL; liver 5.8–613 μg/g. |

**Table 2.** Concentrations data reported in multidrug-associated deaths.

| | Associated Drugs | Blood Concentration (ng/mL) | Other Concentrations (Site, ng/mL) |
|---|---|---|---|
| Acetylfentanyl | Butyrylfentanyl [69,81] | Acetylfentanyl: 21–38; 32–95 (heart)<br>Butyrylfentanyl: 3.7–58; 9.2–97 (heart) | Acetylfentanyl: vitreous humor 38–68 ng/mL; bile 330 ng/mL; urine 8–690 ng/mL; gastric contents 170–28,000 ng/mL; brain 200 ng/g; liver 110–160 ng/g.<br>Butyrylfentanyl: vitreous humor 9.8–40 ng/mL; bile 49 ng/mL; urine 2–670 ng/mL; gastric contents 170–4000 ng/mL; brain 63 ng/g; liver 39–320 ng/g. |
| | Fentanyl [85,99] | Acetylfentanyl: 0.13–12<br>Fentanyl: 0.24–21 | |
| | Fentanyl, heroin [100] | Acetylfentanyl: 12<br>Morphine (free): negative<br>Morphine (total): 20<br>Fentanyl: 15 | |
| | Fentanyl, heroin, cocaine [100] | Acetylfentanyl: 9<br>Morphine (free): 30<br>Morphine (total): 60<br>Fentanyl: 20<br>Cocaine: 70<br>Benzoylecgonine: 970 | |
| | Fentanyl, heroin, alprazolam [100] | Acetylfentanyl: 2<br>Morphine (free): 20<br>Morphine (total) <20<br>Alprazolam 30<br>Fentanyl: 19 | |
| | Furanylfentanyl, diphenhydramine [49] | Acetylfentanyl: 0.65<br>Furanylfentanyl: 12.9<br>Diphenhydramine: 140 | |
| | Morphine [100] | Acetylfentanyl: 400<br>Morphine (free): 30<br>Morphine (total): 70 | |
| | Alprazolam [100] | Acetyl Fentanyl 560–600<br>Alprazolam 20–230 | |
| | 4-MethoxyPV8 and others [53] | Acetylfentanyl: 153<br>4-MethoxyPV8: 389<br>7-Aminonitrazepam: 200<br>Phenobarbital: 7700<br>Methylphenidate: 30 | Acetylfentanyl: urine 240 ng/mL; gastric contents 880 ng/mL.<br>4-MethoxyPV8: urine 245 ng/mL; gastric contents 500 ng/mL. |

**Table 2.** *Cont.*

| | Associated Drugs | Blood Concentration (ng/mL) | Other Concentrations (Site, ng/mL) |
|---|---|---|---|
| Butyrylfentanyl | U-47700 [49] | Butyrylfentanyl: 26<br>U-47700: 17 | |
| Furanylfentanyl | U-47700 [49] | Furanylfentanyl: 2.5–26<br>U-47700: 105–490 | |
| | U-47700, Heroin [49] | Furanylfentanyl: 56<br>U-47700: 107<br>Morphine: 48 | |
| | Fentanyl [60] | Furanylfentanyl: 0.4<br>Fentanyl: 1.27 | |
| | Carfentanil [101] | Furanylfentanyl: 0.34<br>Carfentanil: 1.3 | |
| U-47700 | Fentanyl [102] | U-47700: 13.8<br>Fentanyl: 10.9 | U-47700: urine 71 ng/mL |
| | Diphenhydramine [49] | U-47700: 103<br>Diphenhydramine: 694 | |
| | Diphenhydramine, alprazolam, doxylamine [96] | U-4770:190<br>Diphenhydramine: 140<br>Alprazolam: 120<br>Doxylamine: 300 | |
| Fentanyl | Heroin [82,98,100] | Fentanyl: 2.7–16<br>Morphine (free): <20–100<br>Morphine (total): 30–240 | |
| | Heroin, hydromorphone [100] | Fentanyl: 15<br>Morphine (free): 20<br>Morphine (total): 60<br>Hydromorphone (free:) <20<br>Hydromorphone (total): 40 | |
| | Heroin, methamphetamine [100] | Fentanyl: 0.004<br>Morphine (free): 100<br>Morphine (total): 90<br>Methamphetamine: 270 | |
| | Heroin, methadone, alprazolam [100] | Fentanyl 7–38<br>Morphine (free): 20–50<br>Morphine (total): 40–80<br>Methadone: 320–400<br>Alprazolam: 30 | |

**Table 2.** *Cont.*

| | Associated Drugs | Blood Concentration (ng/mL) | Other Concentrations (Site, ng/mL) |
|---|---|---|---|
| Fentanyl | Oxycodone [97] | Fentanyl: 14<br>Oxycodone: 420 | |
| | Oxycodone, citalopram [97] | Fentanyl: 6.7<br>Oxycodone: 500<br>Citalopram: 200 | |
| | Oxycodone, codeine [97] | Fentanyl: 10<br>Oxycodone: 270<br>Codeine: 280 | |
| | Methadone [103] | Fentanyl: 5<br>Methadone: 540<br>Oxycodone: 70<br>Trazodone: 246 | |
| | Hydrocodone [103] | Fentanyl: 90<br>Hydrocodone: 240 | |
| | Morphine [103] | Fentanyl: 10<br>Morphine (total): 3230 | |
| | Cocaine [97,103] | Fentanyl: 12–34<br>Cocaine: 50–780<br>Benzoylecgonine: 31–4100 | |
| | Methanphetamine [71] | Fentanyl: 8.6<br>Methanphetamine: 1456 | |
| | Phenobarbital, nordiazepam, diazepam | Fentanyl: 20<br>Phenobarbital: 7000<br>Nordiazepam: 72<br>Diazepam: 58 | |
| | Bromazepam [55] | Fentanyl: 60.6; 94.1 (heart)<br>Norfentanyl: 19.8; 50.1 (heart)<br>Bromazepam: 874 | Fentanyl: urine 152.2 ng/mL; brain 70.4 ng/g; kidney 161.3 ng/g; stomach content 536.8 ng/mL; liver 203.2 ng/g; bile 274.2 ng/mL<br>Norfentanyl: urine 172.2 ng/mL; brain 5.6 ng/g; kidney 172.9 ng/g; stomach content 54.4 ng/mL; liver 164.6 ng/g; bile 436.4 ng/mL |
| | Alprazolam, tramadol [103] | Fentanyl: 12<br>Alprazolam: 13<br>Tramadol: 1500 | |
| | 7-Aminoclonazepam, Sertraline [82] | Fentanyl: 13.8<br>7-Aminoclonazepam: 57.1<br>Sertraline: 91.9 | |
| Tetrahydrofuranylfentanyl | U-49900, Methoxy-Phencyclidine [104] | Tetrahydrofuranylfentanyl: 339<br>U-49900: 1.5<br>Methoxy-Phencyclidine: 1.0 | Tetrahydrofuranylfentanyl: urine >5000 ng/mL<br>U-49900: urine 2.2 ng/mL<br>Methoxy-Phencyclidine: 31.8 ng/mL |

## 4. Discussion

This review deals with human pathological findings that are directly attributable to the known toxic actions of fentanyls and other synthetic opioids. In the past few years, it has become more and more evident that fentanyls and other synthetic opioids are potentially extremely harmful. Fentanyl-related deaths have increased over the years [47,52], so it is necessary to review the data available on these analog NPS. The results from our literature analysis revealed the lethal potential of fentanyls and other synthetic opioids; a large number of different routes of substance administration have also surfaced, through which all of these compounds are potentially lethal.

In addition, a broad range of side effects associated with fentanyls and other synthetic opioids have emerged, posing serious health issues, which primarily concern the central nervous system, cardiovascular and pulmonary systems, and liver. Macroscopic examinations, autopsy data, and histopathological elements were collected from the literature, leaving evidence that mainly refers to opioid intoxication. The investigation of the cause of death provoked by fentanyl or other synthetic opioid abuse was based on a multidisciplinary approach aimed at framing each case and directing the investigations towards targeted toxicological analyses. This approach should be adopted in all cases of death from uncertain or questionable causes [66,70]. Past medical history and ante-mortem distribution, crime scene investigation, post-mortem toxicology examination, and toxicology findings should be carefully analyzed and considered on a case-by-case basis in light of all other data [11,98,105–107].

The examination of the literature showed that a large number of deaths associated with fentanyl and other synthetic opioids involved the abuse of other psychoactive substances. In a previous review [22] of various case studies of fentanyl-related deaths, it was speculated that the deaths were associated with drugs of abuse such other opiates (up to 64%), cocaine (up to 65%), cannabinoids (up to 50%), amphetamines (up to 40%), but also ethanol (up to 22.9%) and medicines like barbiturates (up to 27%), benzodiazepines (up to 52.2%), antidepressants (up to 48%). These data can lead to a series of considerations. The first is inherent in the contribution to the deaths of the substances detected together with synthetic opioids. Animal studies have shown that some classes of substances, such as benzodiazepines, have a synergistic effect with opioids.

Although the pharmacokinetic and pharmacodynamic interactions between benzodiazepines and opioids are not yet fully understood [108], pre-clinical studies suggest a synergistic effect on opioid-induced respiratory depression (measured as % increase in $pCO_2$) [109]. Forensic data show the risks of this drug combination: the concomitant use of benzodiazepines and "traditional" opioids is associated with the occurrence of opioid overdoses [110,111]. This occurrence is very common, and the co-use of opioid and benzodiazepine could be aimed at amplifying the subjective effects of the opioid [112,113]. However, the current knowledge does not permit to establish the exact contribution of benzodiazepines in opioid-related deaths, considering that many opioid addicts are also chronic benzodiazepine users [114,115].

Regarding the co-administration of ethanol and opioids, it can be dangerous because it enhances the positive subjective effects that contribute to the abuse and affects physical and cognitive functions. It is no coincidence that alcohol and opioid abuses often coexist [116]. Fatal intoxications involving opioids are frequently associated with alcohol use and are likely due to combined CNS- and respiratory-depressant effects [117,118].

Concerning the co-administration of cocaine and synthetic opioids, animal studies have shown that combinations of cocaine and remifentanil can lead to a strong additivity [119], maybe for their synergistic action on the mesolimbic dopaminergic system [120]. Unfortunately, data on humans are not yet reported in the literature. Recently, there has been an increase in cocaine-related overdoses; however, a large part of this increase is due to the simultaneous intake of opioids, especially synthetic ones [121]. Often, the use of a synthetic opioid is accidental, due to an unknown contamination of a cocaine stock [122,123].

The same assumption can be formulated for the deaths from the co-administration of heroin and fentanyl. A recent study showed a strong association between the number of tested samples of seized drugs where fentanyl was detected and unintentional overdose deaths in which fentanyl was also identified [124]. This data are consistent with previous studies that have shown that a significant proportion of drug users unintentionally consume fentanyl, which is present in the substances they are taking [7,122,125]. However, the real diffusion of illicit fentanyl use in the general population is difficult to assess, because routine toxicology screens will not detect synthetic opioids that have little structural homology to morphine and other commonly tested opioids [14].

## 5. Conclusions

In Conclusion, the confirmation or exclusion of opioid overdoses is one of the major challenges for forensic pathologists, considering what has been said and that autopsy findings are not specific. It is therefore necessary that the forensic pathologist have a broader approach and, on the basis of the data collected, request a chemical-analytical analysis to point out NPS [87].

The role of the forensic pathologist in close collaboration with the forensic toxicologist is very important: together, they can identify new cases of fentanyl and synthetic opioid intoxication. The identification of NPS is essential to stop the social problems related to the spread of these new dangerous and highly addictive substances among our population.

**Author Contributions:** Conceptualization, M.M. and M.N.; Methodology, S.B.; Writing—Original Draft Preparation, P.F. and E.B.; Writing—Review & Editing, A.T., M.B., R.M.G.; Supervision, M.M. and M.N.

**Acknowledgments:** We would also like to thank Marina Venturi for her assistance on this project.

## References

1. United Nations Office on Drugs and Crime. 2017 Global Synthetic Drugs Assessment. Available online: https://www.unodc.org/ (accessed on 17 August 2018).
2. European Monitoring Centre for Drugs and Drug Addiction. Fentanils and Synthetic Cannabinoids: Driving Greater Complexity into the Drug Situation—An Update from the EU Early Warning System. Available online: http://www.emcdda.europa.eu/ (accessed on 19 June 2018).
3. Lemmens, H. Pharmacokinetic-pharmacodynamic relationships for opioids in balanced anaesthesia. *Clin. Pharmacokinet.* **1995**, *29*, 231–242. [CrossRef] [PubMed]
4. Armenian, P.; Vo, K.T.; Barr-Walker, J.; Lynch, K.L. Fentanyl, fentanyl analogs and novel synthetic opioids: A comprehensive review. *Neuropharmacology* **2018**, *134*, 121–132. [CrossRef] [PubMed]
5. Zawilska, J.B. An Expanding World of Novel Psychoactive Substances: Opioids. *Front. Psychiatry* **2017**, *8*, 110. [CrossRef] [PubMed]
6. Hempstead, K.; Yildirim, E.O. Supply-side response to declining heroin purity: Fentanyl overdose episode in New Jersey. *Health Econ.* **2014**, *23*, 688–705. [CrossRef] [PubMed]
7. Carroll, J.J.; Marshall, B.D.L.; Rich, J.D.; Green, T.C. Exposure to fentanyl-contaminated heroin and overdose risk among illicit opioid users in Rhode Island: A mixed methods study. *Int. J. Drug Policy* **2017**, *46*, 136–145. [CrossRef] [PubMed]
8. Al-Hasani, R.; Bruchas, M.R. Molecular mechanisms of opioid receptor-dependent signaling and behavior. *Anesthesiology* **2011**, *115*, 1363–1381. [CrossRef] [PubMed]
9. Horsfall, J.T.; Sprague, J.E. The Pharmacology and Toxicology of the 'Holy Trinity'. *Basic Clin. Pharmacol. Toxicol.* **2017**, *120*, 115–119. [CrossRef] [PubMed]
10. Schug, S.A.; Ting, S. Fentanyl Formulations in the Management of Pain: An update. *Drugs* **2017**, *77*, 747–763. [CrossRef] [PubMed]
11. Nelson, L.; Schwaner, R. Transdermal fentanyl: Pharmacology and toxicology. *J. Med. Toxicol.* **2009**, *5*, 230–241. [CrossRef] [PubMed]
12. Stanley, T.H. The fentanyl story. *J. Pain* **2014**, *15*, 1215–1226. [CrossRef] [PubMed]
13. Eiden, C.; Mathieu, O.; Donnadieu-Rigole, H.; Marrot, C.; Peyrière, H. High opioids tolerance due to transmucosal fentanyl abuse. *Eur. J. Clin. Pharmacol.* **2017**, *73*, 1195–1196. [CrossRef] [PubMed]

14. Suzuki, J.; El-Haddad, S. A review: Fentanyl and non-pharmaceutical fentanyls. *Drug Alcohol Depend.* **2017**, *171*, 107–116. [CrossRef] [PubMed]
15. United Nations Office on Drugs and Crime. Fentanyl and Its Analogues—50 Years on. Glob Smart Update. 2017, Volume 17, pp. 3–7. Available online: https://www.unodc.org/documents/scientific/Global_SMART_Update_17_web.pdf (accessed on 19 June 2018).
16. Cox, B.M. Pharmacology of opioid drugs. In *The Opiate Receptors*; Humana Press: New York, NY, USA, 2011; pp. 23–58, ISBN 978-1-60761-993-2.
17. Pasternak, G.W.; Pan, Y.X. Mu opioids and their receptors: Evolution of a concept. *Pharmacol. Rev.* **2013**, *65*, 1257–1317. [CrossRef] [PubMed]
18. Ujváry, I.; Jorge, R.; Christie, R.; Le Ruez, T.; Danielsson, H.V.; Kronstrand, R.; Elliott, S.; Gallegos, A.; Sedefov, R.; Evans-Brown, M. Acryloylfentanyl, a recently emerged new psychoactive substance: A comprehensive review. *Forensic Toxicol.* **2017**, *35*, 232–243. [CrossRef]
19. Dahan, A.; Sarton, E.; Teppema, L.; Olievier, C.; Nieuwenhuijs, D.; Matthes, H.W.; Kieffer, B.L. Anesthetic potency and influence of morphine and sevoflurane on respiration in mu-opioid receptor knockout mice. *Anesthesiology* **2001**, *94*, 824–832. [CrossRef] [PubMed]
20. Kieffer, B.L. Opioids: First lessons from knockout mice. *Trends Pharmacol. Sci.* **1999**, *20*, 19–26. [CrossRef]
21. Pattinson, K.T. Opioids and the control of respiration. *Br. J. Anaesth.* **2008**, *100*, 747–758. [CrossRef] [PubMed]
22. Kuczyńska, K.; Grzonkowski, P.; Kacprzak, L.; Zawilska, J.B. Abuse of fentanyl: An emerging problem to face. *Forensic Sci. Int.* **2018**, *289*, 207–214. [CrossRef] [PubMed]
23. United Nations Office on Drugs and Crime. *Opioid Overdose: Preventing and Reducing Opioid Overdose Mortality*; Discussion Paper UNOCD/WHO 2013; United Nations: New York, NY, USA, 2013. Available online: https://www.unodc.org/docs/treatment/overdose.pdf (accessed on 19 June 2018).
24. Kim, H.K.; Nelson, L.S. Reducing the harm of opioid overdose with the safe use of naloxone: A pharmacologic review. *Expert Opin. Drug Saf.* **2015**, *14*, 1137–1146. [CrossRef] [PubMed]
25. Daniulaityte, R.; Juhascik, M.P.; Strayer, K.E.; Sizemore, I.E.; Harshbarger, K.E.; Antonides, H.M.; Carlson, R.R. Overdose deaths related to fentanyl and its analogs—Ohio, January–February 2017. *MMWR Morb. Mortal Wkly. Rep.* **2017**, *66*, 904–908. [CrossRef] [PubMed]
26. Green, T.C.; Gilbert, M. Counterfeit medications and fentanyl. *JAMA Intern. Med.* **2016**, *176*, 1555–1557. [CrossRef] [PubMed]
27. Abdulahim, D.; Bowden-Jones, O. The Misuse of Synthetic Opioids: Harms and Clinical Management of Fentanyl, Fentanyl Analogues and Other Novel Synthetic Opioids. Available online: https://smmgp.org.uk/media/12031/neptune-fentanyl-clinical-management-mar-18.pdf (accessed on 19 June 2018).
28. Volpe, D.A.; McMahon Tobin, G.A.; Mellon, R.D.; Katki, A.G.; Parker, R.J.; Colatsky, T.; Kropp, T.J.; Verbois, S.L. Uniform assessment and ranking of opioid μ receptor binding constants for selected opioid drugs. *Regul. Toxicol. Pharmacol.* **2011**, *59*, 385–390. [CrossRef] [PubMed]
29. Bot, G.; Blake, A.D.; Li, S.; Reisine, T. Fentanyl and its analogs desensitize the cloned Muopioid receptor. *J. Pharmacol. Exp. Ther.* **1998**, *285*, 1207–1218. [PubMed]
30. Maguire, P.; Tsai, N.; Kamal, J.; Cometta-Morini, C.; Upton, C.; Loew, G. Pharmacological profiles of fentanyl analogs at mu, delta and kappa opiate receptors. *Eur. J. Pharmacol.* **1992**, *213*, 219–225. [CrossRef]
31. Mounteney, J.; Giraudon, I.; Denissov, G.; Griffith, P. Fentanyl: Are we missing the signs? Highly potent and on the rise in Europe. *Int. J. Drug Policy* **2015**, *26*, 626–631. [CrossRef] [PubMed]
32. EMCDDA 2016. Acryloylfentanyl. EMCDDA—Europol Joint Report on a New Psychoactive Substance: *N*-(1-Phenylethylpiperidin-4-yl)-*N*-Phenylacrylamide(Acryloylfentanyl). Available online: http://www.emcdda.europa.eu/publications/joint-reports/acryloylfentanyl (accessed on 19 June 2018).
33. Lucyk, S.N.; Nelson, L.S. Novel synthetic opioids: An opioid epidemic within an opioid epidemic. *Ann. Emerg. Med.* **2017**, *69*, 91–93. [CrossRef] [PubMed]
34. Helander, A.; Bäckberg, M.; Singell, P.; Beck, O. Intoxications involving acrylfentanyl and other novel designer fentanyls–results from the Swedish STRIDA project. *Clin. Toxicol.* **2017**, *55*, 589–599. [CrossRef] [PubMed]
35. Helander, A.; Bäckberg, M.; Beck, O. MT-45, a new psychoactive substance associated with hearing loss and unconsciousness. *Clin. Toxicol.* **2014**, *52*, 901–904. [CrossRef] [PubMed]

36. Helander, A.; Bradley, M.; Hasselblad, A.; Norlén, L.; Vassilaki, I.; Bäckberg, M.; Lapins, J. Acute skin and hair symptoms followed by severe, delayed eye compli-cations in subjects using the synthetic opioid MT-45. *Br. J. Dermatol.* **2017**, *176*, 1021–1027. [CrossRef] [PubMed]
37. EMCDDA. EMCDDA: Europol Joint Report on a New Psychoactive Substance: 1-Cyclohexyl-4-(1,2-diphenylethyl)piperazine ('MT-45') [Risk Assessment Report]. September 2014. Available online: http://www.emcdda.europa.eu/publications/joint-reports/MT-45 (accessed on 19 June 2018).
38. Siddiqi, S.; Verney, C.; Dargan, P.; Wood, D.M. Understanding the availability, prevalence of use, desired effects, acute toxicity and dependence potential of the novel opioid MT-45. *Clin. Toxicol.* **2015**, *53*, 54–59. [CrossRef] [PubMed]
39. Nakamura, H.; Ishii, D.; Yokoyama, Y.; Motoyoshi, S.; Natsuka, K.; Shimizu, M. Analgesic and other pharmacological activities of a new narcotic antagonist analgesic (−)-1-(3-methyl-2-butenyl)-4-[2-(3-hydroxyphenyl)-1-phenylethyl]-piperazine and its enantiomorph in experimental animals. *J. Pharm. Pharmacol.* **1980**, *32*, 635–642. [CrossRef] [PubMed]
40. Montesano, C.; Vannutelli, G.; Fanti, F.; Vincenti, F.; Gregori, A.; Rita Togna, A.; Canazza, I.; Marti, M.; Sergi, M. Identification of MT-45 Metabolites: In silico prediction, in vitro incubation with rat hepatocytes and in vivo confirmation. *J. Anal. Toxicol.* **2017**, *41*, 688–697. [CrossRef] [PubMed]
41. Harper, N.J.; Veitch, G.B.; Wibberley, D.G. 1-(3,4-Dichlorobenzamidomethyl) cyclohexyldimethylamine and related compounds as potential analgesics. *J. Med. Chem.* **1974**, *17*, 1188–1193. [CrossRef] [PubMed]
42. Brittain, R.T.; Kellett, D.N.; Neat, M.L.; Stables, R. Proceedings: Anti-nociceptive effects in N-substituted cyclohexylmethylbenzamides. *Br. J. Pharmacol.* **1973**, *49*, 158–159.
43. EMCDDA. EMCDDA—Europol Joint Report on a New Psychoactive Substance: AH-7921. (2016). Available online: http://www.emcdda.europa.eu/system/files/publications/816/AH-7921_465209.pdf (accessed on 19 June 2018).
44. Karinen, R.; Tuv, S.S.; Rogde, S.; Peres, M.D.; Johansen, U.; Frost, J.; Vindenes, V.; Øiestad, A.M. Lethal poisonings with AH-7921 in combination with other substances. *Forensic Sci. Int.* **2014**, *244*, 21–24. [CrossRef] [PubMed]
45. Kronstrand, R.; Thelander, G.; Lindstedt, D.; Roman, M.; Kugelberg, F.C. Fatal intoxications associated with the designer opioid AH-7921. *J. Anal. Toxicol.* **2014**, *38*, 599–604. [CrossRef] [PubMed]
46. Cheney, B.V.; Szmuszkovicz, J.; Lahti, R.A.; Zichi, D.A. Factors affecting binding of trans-*N*-[2-(methylamino)cyclohexyl]benzamides at the primary morphine receptor. *J. Med. Chem.* **1985**, *28*, 1853–1864. [CrossRef] [PubMed]
47. Narita, M.; Imai, S.; Itou, Y.; Yajima, Y.; Suzuki, T. Possible involvement of mu1-opioid receptors in the fentanyl- or morphine-induced antinociception at supraspinal and spinal sites. *Life Sci.* **2002**, *70*, 2341–2354. [CrossRef]
48. DEA. Schedules of Controlled Substances: Temporary Placement of U-47700 Into Schedule I [Docket No. DEA-440]. Available online: https://www.deadiversion.usdoj.gov (accessed on 19 June 2018).
49. Mohr, A.L.; Friscia, M.; Papsun, D.; Kacinko, S.L.; Buzby, D.; Logan, B.K. Analysis of novel synthetic opioids U-47700, U-50488 and furanyl fentanyl by LC-MS/MS in postmortem casework. *J. Anal. Toxicol.* **2016**, *40*, 709–717. [CrossRef] [PubMed]
50. Ruan, X.; Chiravuri, S.; Kaye, A.D. Comparing fatal cases involving U-47700. *Forensic Sci. Med. Pathol.* **2016**, *12*, 369–371. [CrossRef] [PubMed]
51. Jones, M.J.; Hernandez, B.S.; Janis, G.C.; Stellpflug, S.J. A case of U-47700 overdose with laboratory confirmation and metabolite identification. *Clin. Toxicol.* **2017**, *55*, 55–59. [CrossRef] [PubMed]
52. O'Donnell, J.K.; Halpin, J.; Mattson, C.L.; Goldberger, B.A.; Gladden, R.M. Deaths Involving Fentanyl, Fentanyl Analogs, and U-47700-10 States, July–December 2016. *MMWR Morb. Mortal. Wkly. Rep.* **2017**, *66*, 1197–1202. [CrossRef] [PubMed]
53. Yonemitsu, K.; Sasao, A.; Mishima, S.; Ohtsu, Y.; Nishitani, Y. A fatal poisoning case by intravenous injection of "bath salts" containing acetyl fentanyl and 4-methoxy PV8. *Forensic Sci. Int.* **2016**, *267*, 6–9. [CrossRef] [PubMed]
54. Biedrzycki, O.J.; Bevan, D.; Lucas, S. Fatal overdose due to pre-scription fentanyl patches in a patient with sickle cell/beta-thalassemia and acute chest syndrome: A case report and review of the literature. *Am. J. Forensic Med. Pathol.* **2009**, *30*, 188–190. [CrossRef] [PubMed]

55. Juebner, M.; Fietzke, M.; Beike, J.; Rothschild, M.A.; Bender, K. Assisted suicide by fentanyl intoxication due to excessive transdermal application. *Int. J. Legal. Med.* **2014**, *128*, 949–956. [CrossRef] [PubMed]
56. Denton, J.S.; Donoghue, E.R.; McReynolds, J.; Kalelkar, M.B. An epidemic of illicit fentanyl deaths in Cook County, Illinois: September 2005 through April 2007. *J. Forensic Sci.* **2008**, *53*, 452–454. [CrossRef] [PubMed]
57. Bakovic, M.; Nestic, M.; Mayer, D. Death by band-aid: Fatal misuse of transdermal fentanyl patch. *Int. J. Legal. Med.* **2014**, *129*, 1247–1252. [CrossRef] [PubMed]
58. Cunningham, S.M.; Haikal, N.A.; Kraner, J.C. Fatal intoxication with acetyl fentanyl. *J. Forensic Sci.* **2016**, *61*, 276–280. [CrossRef] [PubMed]
59. Staeheli, S.N.; Baumgartner, M.R.; Gauthier, S.; Gascho, D.; Jarmer, J.; Kraemer, T.; Steuer, A.E. Time-dependent postmortem redistribution of butyrfentanyl and its metabolites in blood and alternative matrices in a case of butyrfentanyl intoxication. *Forensic Sci. Int.* **2016**, *266*, 170–177. [CrossRef] [PubMed]
60. Guerrieri, D.; Rapp, E.; Roman, M.; Druid, H.; Kronstrand, R. Postmortem and toxicological findings in a series of furanylfentanyl-related deaths. *J. Anal. Toxicol.* **2017**, *41*, 242–249. [CrossRef] [PubMed]
61. Martucci, H.F.H.; Ingle, E.A.; Hunter, M.D.; Rodda, L.N. Distribution of furanyl fentanyl and 4-ANPP in an accidental acute death: A case report. *Forensic Sci. Int.* **2018**, *283*, 170–177. [CrossRef]
62. Dussy, F.E.; Hangartner, S.; Hamberg, C.; Berchtold, C.; Scherer, U.; Schlotterbeck, G.; Wyler, D.; Briellmann, T.A. An acute ocfentanil fatality: A case report with post-mortem concentrations. *J. Anal. Toxicol.* **2016**, *40*, 761–766. [CrossRef] [PubMed]
63. Vorce, S.P.; Knittel, J.L.; Holler, J.M.; Magluilo, J., Jr.; Levine, B.; Berran, P.; Bosy, T.Z. A fatality involving AH-7921. *J. Anal. Toxicol.* **2014**, *38*, 226–230. [CrossRef] [PubMed]
64. Fleming, S.W.; Cooley, J.C.; Johnson, L.; Frazee, C.C.; Domanski, K.; Kleinschmidt, K.; Garg, U. Analysis of U-47700, a novel synthetic opioid, in human urine by LC-MS-MS and LC-QToF. *J. Anal. Toxicol.* **2017**, *41*, 173–180. [CrossRef] [PubMed]
65. Fels, H.; Krueger, J.; Sachs, H.; Mussho, F.; Graw, M.; Roider, G.; Stoever, A. Two fatalities associated with synthetic opioids: AH-7921 and MT-45. *Forensic Sci. Int.* **2017**, *77*, 30–35. [CrossRef] [PubMed]
66. Helander, A.; Bäckberg, M.; Beck, O. Intoxications involving the fentanyl analogs acetylfentanyl, 4-methoxybutyrfentanyl and furanylfentanyl: Results from the Swedish STRIDA project. *Clin. Toxicol.* **2016**, *54*, 324–332. [CrossRef] [PubMed]
67. Foy, L.; Seeyave, D.M.; Bradin, S.A. Toxic leukoencephalopathy due to trans-dermal fentanyl overdose. *Pediatr. Emerg. Care* **2011**, *27*, 854–856. [CrossRef] [PubMed]
68. Kucuk, H.O.; Kucuk, U.; Kolcu, Z.; Balta, S.; Demirkol, S. Misuse of fentanyl transdermal patch mixed with acute coronary syndrome. *Hum. Exp. Toxicol.* **2016**, *35*, 51–52. [CrossRef] [PubMed]
69. Poklis, J.; Poklis, A.; Wolf, C.; Hathaway, C.; Arbefeville, E.; Chrostowski, L.; Pearson, J. Two fatal intoxications involving butyryl fentanyl. *J. Anal. Toxicol.* **2016**, *40*, 703–708. [CrossRef] [PubMed]
70. Anderson, D.T.; Muto, J.J. Duragesic transdermal patch: Post- mortem tissue distribution of fentanyl in 25 cases. *J. Anal. Toxicol.* **2000**, *24*, 703–708. [CrossRef]
71. Carson, H.J.; Knight, L.D.; Dudley, M.H.; Garg, U. A fatality involving an unusual route of fentanyl delivery: Chewing and aspirating the transdermal patch. *Leg. Med.* **2010**, *12*, 157–159. [CrossRef] [PubMed]
72. Kronstrand, R.; Druid, H.; Holmgren, P.; Rajs, J. A cluster of fentanyl-related deaths among drug addicts in Sweden. *Forensic Sci. Int.* **1997**, *88*, 185–193. [CrossRef]
73. Takase, I.; Koizumi, T.; Fujimoto, I.; Yanai, A.; Fujimiya, T. An autopsy case of acetyl fentanyl intoxication caused by insufflation of 'designer drugs'. *Leg. Med.* **2016**, *21*, 38–44. [CrossRef] [PubMed]
74. Coopman, V.; Cordonnier, J.; De Leeuw, M.; Cirimele, V. Ocfentanil overdose fatality in the recreational drug scene. *Forensic Sci. Int.* **2016**, *266*, 469–473. [CrossRef] [PubMed]
75. Burns, G.; DeRienz, R.T.; Baker, D.D.; Casavant, M.; Spiller, H.A. Could chest wall rigidity be a factor in rapid death from illicit fentanyl abuse? *Clin. Toxicol.* **2016**, *54*, 420–423. [CrossRef] [PubMed]
76. Chaturvedi, A.K.; Rao, N.G.; Baird, J.R. A death due to self-administered fentanyl. *J. Anal. Toxicol.* **1990**, *14*, 385–387. [CrossRef] [PubMed]
77. Henderson, G.L. Fentanyl-related deaths: Demographics, circumstances, and toxicology of 112 cases. *J. Forensic Sci.* **1991**, *36*, 422–433. [CrossRef] [PubMed]
78. Coopman, V.; Cordonnier, J.; Pien, K.; Van Varenbergh, D. LC-MS/MS analysis of fentanyl and norfentanyl in a fatality due to application of multiple Durogesic transdermal therapeutic systems. *Forensic Sci. Int.* **2007**, *169*, 223–227. [CrossRef] [PubMed]

79. Thomas, S.; Winecker, R.; Pestaner, J.P. Unusual fentanyl patch administration. *Am. J. Forensic Med. Pathol.* **2008**, *29*, 162–163. [CrossRef] [PubMed]
80. McIntyre, I.M.; Trochta, A.; Gary, R.D.; Malamatos, M.; Lucas, J.R. An acute acetyl fentanyl fatality: A case report with postmortem concentrations. *J. Anal. Toxicol.* **2015**, *39*, 490–494. [CrossRef] [PubMed]
81. McIntyre, I.M.; Trochta, A.; Gary, R.D.; Wright, J.; Mena, O. An acute butyr-fentanyl fatality: A case report with postmortem concentrations. *J. Anal. Toxicol.* **2016**, *40*, 162–166. [CrossRef] [PubMed]
82. Lilleng, P.K.; Mehlum, L.I.; Bachs, L.; Morild, I. Deaths after intravenous misuse of transdermal fentanyl. *J. Forensic Sci.* **2004**, *49*, 1364–1366. [CrossRef] [PubMed]
83. Ojanperä, I.; Gergov, M.; Liiv, M.; Riikoja, A.; Vuori, E. An epidemic of fatal 3-methylfentanyl poisoning in Estonia. *Int. J. Legal. Med.* **2008**, *122*, 395–400. [CrossRef] [PubMed]
84. Sinicina, I.; Sachs, H.; Keil, W. Post-mortem review of fentanyl-related overdose deaths among identified drug users in Southern Bavaria, Germany, 2005–2014. *Drug Alcohol Depend.* **2017**, *180*, 286–291. [CrossRef] [PubMed]
85. Dwyer, J.B.; Janssen, J.; Luckasevic, T.M.; Williams, K.E. Report of increasing overdose deaths that include acetyl fentanyl in multiple counties of the southwestern region of the commonwealth of Pennsylvania in 2015–2016. *J. Forensic Sci.* **2018**, *63*, 195–200. [CrossRef] [PubMed]
86. Palamalai, V.; Olson, K.N.; Kloss, J.; Middleton, O.; Mills, K.; Strobl, A.Q.; Thomas, L.C.; Apple, F.S. Superiority of postmortem liver fentanyl concentrations over peripheral blood influenced by postmortem interval for determination of fentanyl toxicity. *Clin. Biochem.* **2013**, *46*, 598–602. [CrossRef] [PubMed]
87. Giorgetti, A.; Centola, C.; Giorgetti, R. Fentanyl novel derivative-related deaths. *Hum. Psychopharmacol.* **2017**, *32*. [CrossRef] [PubMed]
88. Fort, C.; Curtis, B.; Nichols, C.; Niblo, C. Acetyl fentanyl toxicity: Two case reports. *J. Anal. Toxicol.* **2016**, *40*, 754–757. [CrossRef] [PubMed]
89. Gillespie, T.J.; Gandolfi, A.J.; Davis, T.P.; Morano, R.A. Identification and quantification of alpha-methylfentanyl in post mortem specimens. *J. Anal. Toxicol.* **1982**, *6*, 139–142. [CrossRef] [PubMed]
90. Sofalvi, S.; Schueler, H.E.; Lavins, E.S.; Kaspar, C.K.; Brooker, I.T.; Mazzola, C.D.; Dolinak, D.; Gilson, T.P.; Perch, S. An LC-MS-MS Method for the Analysis of Carfentanil, 3-Methylfentanyl, 2-Furanyl Fentanyl, Acetyl Fentanyl, Fentanyl and Norfentanyl in Postmortem and Impaired-Driving Cases. *J. Anal. Toxicol.* **2017**, *41*, 473–483. [CrossRef] [PubMed]
91. Rojkiewicz, M.; Majchrzak, M.; Celiński, R.; Kuś, P.; Sajewicz, M. Identification and physicochemical characterization of 4-fluorobutyrfentanyl (1-((4-fluorophenyl)(1-phenethylpiperidin-4-yl)amino)butan-1-one, 4-FBF) in seized materials and post-mortem biological samples. *Drug Test. Anal.* **2017**, *9*, 405–414. [CrossRef] [PubMed]
92. Ojanperä, I.; Gergov, M.; Rasanen, I.; Lunetta, P.; Toivonen, S.; Tiainen, E.; Vuori, E. Blood levels of 3-methylfentanyl in 3 fatal poisoning cases. *Am. J. Forensic Med. Pathol.* **2006**, *27*, 328–331. [CrossRef] [PubMed]
93. Ruzycki, S.; Yarema, M.; Dunham, M.; Sadrzadeh, H.; Tremblay, A. Intranasal fentanyl intoxication leading to diffuse alveolar hemorrhage. *J. Med. Toxicol.* **2016**, *12*, 185–188. [CrossRef] [PubMed]
94. McIntyre, I.M.; Gary, R.D.; Joseph, S.; Stabley, R. A fatality related to the synthetic opioid U-47700: Postmortem concentration distribution. *J. Anal. Toxicol.* **2016**, *41*, 158–160. [CrossRef] [PubMed]
95. Dziadosz, M.; Klintschar, M.; Teske, J. Postmortem concentration distribution in fatal cases involving the synthetic opioid U-47700. *Int. J. Legal. Med.* **2017**, *131*, 1555–1556. [CrossRef] [PubMed]
96. Papsun, D.; Krywanczyk, A.; Vose, J.C.; Bundock, E.A.; Logan, B.L. Analysis of MT-45, a novel synthetic opioid, in human whole blood by LC-MS-MS and its identification in a drug-related death. *J. Anal. Toxicol.* **2016**, *40*, 313–317. [CrossRef] [PubMed]
97. Martin, T.L.; Woodall, K.L.; McLellan, B.A. Fentanyl-related deaths in Ontario, Canada: Toxicological findings and circumstances of death in 112 cases (2002–2004). *J. Anal. Toxicol.* **2006**, *30*, 603–610. [CrossRef] [PubMed]
98. Wiesbrock, U.O.; Rochholz, G.; Franzelius, C.; Schwark, T.; Grellner, W. Excessive use of fentanyl patches as the only means of suicide. *Arch. Kriminol.* **2008**, *222*, 23–30. [PubMed]
99. Poklis, J.; Poklis, A.; Wolf, C.; Mainland, M.; Hair, L.; Devers, K.; Pearson, J. Postmortem tissue distribution of acetyl fentanyl, fentanyl and their respective nor-metabolites analyzed by ultrahigh performance liquid chromatography with tandem mass spectrometry. *Forensic Sci. Int.* **2015**, *257*, 435–441. [CrossRef] [PubMed]

100. Pearson, J.; Poklis, J.; Poklis, A.; Wolf, C.; Mainland, M.; Hair, L.; Devers, K.; Chrostowski, L.; Arbefeville, E.; Merves, M. Postmortem toxicology findings of acetyl fentanyl, fentanyl, and morphine in heroin fatalities in tampa, florida. *Acad. Forensic Pathol.* **2015**, *5*, 676–689. [CrossRef] [PubMed]
101. Swanson, D.M.; Hair, L.S.; Strauch Rivers, S.R.; Smyth, B.C.; Brogan, S.C.; Ventoso, A.D.; Vaccaro, S.L.; Pearson, J.M. Fatalities involving carfentanil and furanyl fentanyl: Two case reports. *J. Anal. Toxicol.* **2017**, *41*, 498–502. [CrossRef] [PubMed]
102. Coopman, V.; Blanckaert, P.; Van Parys, G.; Van Calenbergh, S.; Cordonnier, J. A case of acute intoxication due to combined use of fentanyl and 3,4-dichloro-*N*-[2-(dimethylamino)cyclohexyl]-*N*-methylben-zamide (U-47700). *Forensic Sci. Int.* **2016**, *266*, 68–72. [CrossRef] [PubMed]
103. Thompson, J.G.; Baker, A.M.; Bracey, A.H.; Seningen, J.; Kloss, J.S.; Strobl, A.Q.; Apple, F.S. Fentanyl concentrations in 23 postmortem cases from the Hennepin County Medical Examiner's Office. *J. Forensic Sci.* **2007**, *52*, 978–981. [CrossRef] [PubMed]
104. Krotulski, A.J.; Papsun, D.M.; Friscia, M.; Swartz, J.L.; Holsey, B.D.; Logan, B.K. Fatality following ingestion of tetrahydrofuranylfentanyl, U-49900 and methoxy-phencyclidine. *J. Anal. Toxicol.* **2018**, *42*, 27–32. [CrossRef] [PubMed]
105. Rudd, R.A.; Seth, P.; David, F.; Scholl, L. Increases in Drug and Opioid-Involved Overdose Deaths–United States, 2010–2015. *MMWR Morb. Mortal Wkly. Rep.* **2016**, *65*, 1445–1452. [CrossRef] [PubMed]
106. Krinsky, C.S.; Lathrop, S.L.; Crossey, M.; Baker, G.; Zumwalt, R. A toxicology-based review of fentanyl-related deaths in New Mexico (1986–2007). *Am. J. Forensic Med. Pathol.* **2011**, *32*, 347–351. [CrossRef] [PubMed]
107. Krinsky, C.S.; Lathrop, S.L.; Zumwalt, R. An examination of the postmortem redistribution of fentanyl and interlaboratory variability. *J. Forensic Sci.* **2014**, *59*, 1275–1279. [CrossRef] [PubMed]
108. Jones, J.D.; Mogali, S.; Comer, S.D. Polydrug abuse: A review of opioid and benzodiazepine combination use. *Drug Alcohol Depend.* **2012**, *125*, 8–18. [CrossRef] [PubMed]
109. Nielsen, S.; Taylor, D.A. The effect of buprenorphine and benzodiazepines on respiration in the rat. *Drug Alcohol Depend.* **2005**, *79*, 95–101. [CrossRef] [PubMed]
110. Darke, S.G.; Ross, J.; Hall, W. Overdose among heroin users in Sydney, Australia: I. Prevalence and correlates of non-fatal overdose. *Addiction* **1996**, *91*, 405–411. [CrossRef] [PubMed]
111. Perret, G.; Déglon, J.J.; Kreek, M.J.; Ho, A.; La Harpe, R. Lethal methadone intoxications in Geneva, Switzerland, from 1994 to 1998. *Addiction* **2000**, *95*, 1647–1653. [CrossRef] [PubMed]
112. Stitzer, M.L.; Griffiths, R.R.; McLellan, A.T.; Grabowski, J.; Hawthorne, J.W. Diazepam use among methadone maintenance patients: Patterns and dosages. *Drug Alcohol Depend.* **1981**, *8*, 189–199. [CrossRef]
113. Spiga, R.; Huang, D.B.; Meisch, R.A.; Grabowski, J. Human methadone self-administration: Effects of diazepam pretreatment. *Exp. Clin. Psychopharmacol.* **2001**, *9*, 40–46. [CrossRef] [PubMed]
114. Darke, S.G.; Ross, J.; Mills, K.; Teesson, M.; Williamson, A.; Havard, A. Benzodiazepine use among heroin users: Baseline use, current use and clinical outcome. *Drug Alcohol Rev.* **2010**, *29*, 250–255. [CrossRef] [PubMed]
115. Ross, J.; Darke, S.; Hall, W. Benzodiazepine use among heroin users in Sydney: Patterns of use, availability and procurement. *Drug Alcohol Rev.* **1996**, *15*, 237–243. [CrossRef] [PubMed]
116. Haukka, J.; Kriikku, P.; Mariottini, C.; Partonen, T.; Ojanperä, I. Non-medical use of psychoactive prescription drugs is associated with fatal poisoning. *Addiction* **2018**, *113*, 464–472. [CrossRef] [PubMed]
117. Hakkinen, M.; Launiainen, T.; Vuori, E.; Ojanpera, I. Comparison of fatal poisonings by prescription opioids. *Forensic Sci. Int.* **2012**, *222*, 327–331. [CrossRef] [PubMed]
118. Webster, L.R.; Cochella, S.; Dasgupta, N.; Fakata, K.L.; Fine, P.G.; Fishman, S.M.; Grey, T.; Johnson, E.M.; Lee, L.K.; Passik, S.D.; et al. An analysis of the root causes for opioid-related overdose deaths in the United States. *Pain Med.* **2011**, *12*, 26–35. [CrossRef] [PubMed]
119. Woolverton, W.L.; Wang, Z.; Vasterling, T.; Tallarida, R. Self-administration of cocaine-remifentanil mixtures by monkeys: An isobolographic analysis. *Psychopharmacology* **2008**, *198*, 387–394. [CrossRef] [PubMed]
120. Leri, F.; Bruneau, J.; Stewart, J. Understanding polydrug use: Review of heroin and cocaine co-use. *Addiction* **2003**, *98*, 7–22. [CrossRef] [PubMed]
121. McCall Jones, C.; Baldwin, G.T.; Compton, W.M. Recent increases in cocaine-related overdose deaths and the role of opioids. *Am. J. Public Health* **2017**, *107*, 430–432. [CrossRef] [PubMed]

122. Klar, S.A.; Brodkin, E.; Gibson, E.; Padhi, S.; Predy, C.; Green, C.; Lee, V. Furanyl-fentanyl overdose events caused by smoking contaminated crack cocaine—British Columbia, Canada, 15–18 July. *Health Promot. Chronic Dis. Prev. Can.* **2016**, *65*, 1015–1016.
123. Marinetti, L.J.; Ehlers, B.J. A series of forensic toxicology and drug seizure cases involving illicit fentanyl alone and in combination with heroin, cocaine or heroin and cocaine. *J. Anal. Toxicol.* **2014**, *38*, 592–598. [CrossRef] [PubMed]
124. Baldwin, N.; Gray, R.; Goel, A.; Wood, E.; Buxton, J.A.; Rieb, L.M. Fentanyl and heroin contained in seized illicit drugs and overdose-related deaths in British Columbia, Canada: An observational analysis. *Drug Alcohol Depend.* **2018**, *185*, 322–327. [CrossRef] [PubMed]
125. Amlani, A.; McKee, G.; Khamis, N.; Raghukumar, G.; Tsang, E.; Buxton, J.A. Why the FUSS (Fentanyl Urine Screen Study)? A cross-sectional survey to characterize an emerging threat to people who use drugs in British Columbia, Canada. *Harm Reduct. J.* **2015**, *12*, 54. [CrossRef] [PubMed]

# Permissions

All chapters in this book were first published by MDPI; hereby published with permission under the Creative Commons Attribution License or equivalent. Every chapter published in this book has been scrutinized by our experts. Their significance has been extensively debated. The topics covered herein carry significant findings which will fuel the growth of the discipline. They may even be implemented as practical applications or may be referred to as a beginning point for another development.

The contributors of this book come from diverse backgrounds, making this book a truly international effort. This book will bring forth new frontiers with its revolutionizing research information and detailed analysis of the nascent developments around the world.

We would like to thank all the contributing authors for lending their expertise to make the book truly unique. They have played a crucial role in the development of this book. Without their invaluable contributions this book wouldn't have been possible. They have made vital efforts to compile up to date information on the varied aspects of this subject to make this book a valuable addition to the collection of many professionals and students.

This book was conceptualized with the vision of imparting up-to-date information and advanced data in this field. To ensure the same, a matchless editorial board was set up. Every individual on the board went through rigorous rounds of assessment to prove their worth. After which they invested a large part of their time researching and compiling the most relevant data for our readers.

The editorial board has been involved in producing this book since its inception. They have spent rigorous hours researching and exploring the diverse topics which have resulted in the successful publishing of this book. They have passed on their knowledge of decades through this book. To expedite this challenging task, the publisher supported the team at every step. A small team of assistant editors was also appointed to further simplify the editing procedure and attain best results for the readers.

Apart from the editorial board, the designing team has also invested a significant amount of their time in understanding the subject and creating the most relevant covers. They scrutinized every image to scout for the most suitable representation of the subject and create an appropriate cover for the book.

The publishing team has been an ardent support to the editorial, designing and production team. Their endless efforts to recruit the best for this project, has resulted in the accomplishment of this book. They are a veteran in the field of academics and their pool of knowledge is as vast as their experience in printing. Their expertise and guidance has proved useful at every step. Their uncompromising quality standards have made this book an exceptional effort. Their encouragement from time to time has been an inspiration for everyone.

The publisher and the editorial board hope that this book will prove to be a valuable piece of knowledge for researchers, students, practitioners and scholars across the globe.

# List of Contributors

**Ana B. Sanchez**
Immunity and Pathogenesis Program, Infectious and Inflammatory Disease Center, Sanford Burnham Prebys Medical Discovery Institute, La Jolla, CA 92037, USA

**Marcus Kaul**
Immunity and Pathogenesis Program, Infectious and Inflammatory Disease Center, Sanford Burnham Prebys Medical Discovery Institute, La Jolla, CA 92037, USA
Department of Psychiatry, University of California San Diego, San Diego, CA 92093, USA

**Stefania Chiappini and John Martin Corkery**
Psychopharmacology, Drug Misuse, and Novel Psychoactive Substances Research Unit, School of Life and Medical Sciences, University of Hertfordshire, Hatfield, Hertfordshire AL10 9AB, UK

**Amira Guirguis**
Psychopharmacology, Drug Misuse and Novel Psychoactive Substances Research Unit, School of Life and Medical Sciences, University of Hertfordshire, Hatfield AL10 9AB, UK
Swansea University Medical School, Institute of Life Sciences 2, Swansea University, Swansea SA2 8PP, UK

**Camille Ramos, Nigel Smeeton and Fabrizio Schifano**
Psychopharmacology, Drug Misuse and Novel Psychoactive Substances Research Unit, School of Life and Medical Sciences, University of Hertfordshire, Hatfield AL10 9AB, UK

**Hadar Zaman**
Bradford School of Pharmacy & Medical Sciences, Faculty of Life Sciences, University of Bradford, Horton Road, Bradford BD7 1DP, UK

**Anna-Marie Felice**
CGL, St Martins House, 14 The Common, Hatfield AL10 0UR, UK

**Stephanie Bancroft**
London North West Local Pharmacy Forum (LNWLPF) of the Royal Pharmaceutical Society, Pinner, Middlesex HA5 3EP, UK

**Rosalind Gittins**
Humankind, Inspiration House, Unit 22 Bowburn North Industrial Estate, Durham DH6 5PF, UK

**Gill Hawksworth**
Royal Pharmaceutical Society, 66-68 E Smithfield, Whitechapel, London E1W 1AW, UK

**Rosalind Gittins**
Addaction, 67-69 Cowcross St., London EC1M 6PU, UK

**Ian Maidment**
Pharmacy Department, School of Life and Health Sciences, Aston University, Birmingham B4 7ET, UK

**Giorgia Miolo and Luca Menilli**
Department of Pharmaceutical and Pharmacological Sciences, University of Padova, 35131 Padova, Italy

**Marianna Tucci, Giulia Stocchero, Susanna Vogliardi, Massimo Montisci and Donata Favretto**
Legal Medicine and Toxicology, University Hospital of Padova, 35121 Padova, Italy

**Salvatore Scrivano**
School of Specialization in Legal Medicine, University Hospital of Padova, 35121 Padova, Italy

**Neil Stewart, Leila Jamal and Naasir-Ud-Dinn Rujully**
Highgate Mental Health Centre, Camden & Islington NHS Foundation Trust, London NW1 0PE, UK

**Stefania Bonaccorso**
Highgate Mental Health Centre, Camden & Islington NHS Foundation Trust, London NW1 0PE, UK
Department of Psychological Medicine, King's College London, London WC2R 2LS, UK

**Angelo Ricciardi**
Highgate Mental Health Centre, Camden & Islington NHS Foundation Trust, London NW1 0PE, UK
Department of Mental Health, ASL Rome 1, 00135 Rome, Italy

**Giuseppe Ducci**
Department of Mental Health, ASL Rome 1, 00135 Rome, Italy

**Christos Theleritis**
Department of Psychosis Studies, King's College London, London WC2R 2LS, UK
National and Kapodistrian University of Athens, Eginition Hospital, 11528 Athens, Greece

**Stefano Ferracuti**
Department of Human Neurosciences, University of Rome 'La Sapienza', 00185 Rome, Italy

**Fabrizio Schifano**
Department of Psychopharmacology, University of Hertfordshire, Hertfordshire AL10 9AB, UK

**Valeria Catalani and Robert Chilcott**
Research Centre for Topical Drug Delivery and Toxicology, University of Hertfordshire, Herts SP9 11FA, UK
Department of Pharmacy, Pharmacology and Clinical Science, University of Hertfordshire, Herts AL10 9AB, UK

**Mire Zloh**
Department of Pharmacy, Pharmacology and Clinical Science, University of Hertfordshire, Herts AL10 9AB, UK

**Ornella Corazza**
Department of Pharmacy, Pharmacology and Clinical Science, University of Hertfordshire, Herts AL10 9AB, UK
Centre for Clinical & Health Research Services, School of Life and Medical Sciences, University of Hertfordshire, Hatfield AL10 9AB, UK

**Mariya Prilutskaya**
Semey State Medical University, Republican Scientific and Practical Center of Mental Health, Pavlodar 140002, Kazakhstan

**Ahmed Al-Imam**
Faculty of Medicine, University of Baghdad, Baghdad 10071, Iraq

**Shanna Marrinan**
Parliamentary Office of Science and Technology, Houses of Parliament, London SW1A 0AA, UK

**Yasmine Elgharably**
Navy General Hospital, Cardiovascular department, Alexandria 21513, Egypt

**Giovanni Martinotti and Rita Santacroce**
Department of Neuroscience, Imaging and Clinical Sciences, University "G. d'Annunzio", 66100 Chieti, Italy
Department of Pharmacy, Pharmacology, Postgraduate Medicine, University of Hertfordshire, Herts AL10 9AB, UK

**Chiara Montemitro, Maria Chiara Spano, Marco Lorusso and Massimo di Giannantonio**
Department of Neuroscience, Imaging and Clinical Sciences, University "G. d'Annunzio", 66100 Chieti, Italy

**Mauro Pettorruso**
Institute of Psychiatry and Psychology, Catholic University of Sacred Heart, 00168 Rome, Italy

**Arturo G. Lerner**
Lev Hasharon Mental Health Medical Center, Pardessya 42100, Israel
Sackler School of Medicine, Tel Aviv University, Ramat Aviv 69121, Israel

**Cristina Miliano, Giulia Margiani and Maria Antonietta De Luca**
Department of Biomedical Sciences, University of Cagliari, Cittadella Universitaria di Monserrato-SP 8, Km 0.700, 09042 Monserrato, Cagliari, Italy

**Liana Fattore**
CNR Institute of Neuroscience-Cagliari, National Research Council, Cittadella Universitaria di Monserrato-SP 8, Km 0.700, 09042 Monserrato, Cagliari, Italy

**Koby Cohen and Aviv Weinstein**
Department of Behavioral Science, Ariel University, Ariel 40700, Israel

**Elle Wadsworth**
School of Public Health and Health Systems, University of Waterloo, Waterloo, ON N2L 3G1, Canada

**Paolo Deluca**
National Addiction Centre, Institute of Psychiatry, Psychology & Neuroscience, King's College London, London SE5 8BB, UK

**Colin Drummond**
National Addiction Centre, Institute of Psychiatry, Psychology & Neuroscience, King's College London, London SE5 8BB, UK
South London and Maudsley NHS Foundation Trust, Maudsley Hospital, London SE5 8AZ, UK

**Antonio Metastasio**
Camden and Islington NHS Foundation Trust, London NW1 0PE, UK
Centre for Clinical & Health Research Services, School of Life and Medical Sciences, University of Hertfordshire, Hatfield AL10 9AB, UK

**Attilio Negri**
Centre for Clinical & Health Research Services, School of Life and Medical Sciences, University of Hertfordshire, Hatfield AL10 9AB, UK

**Sabrine Bilel**
Department of Life Sciences and Biotechnology (SVeB), University of Ferrara, 44121 Ferrara, Italy

**Giovanni Martinotti**
Centre for Clinical & Health Research Services, School of Life and Medical Sciences, University of Hertfordshire, Hatfield AL10 9AB, UK
Department of Neuroscience, Imaging, and Clinical Science, "G. d'Annunzio" University of Chieti-Pescara, 66100 Chieti, Italy

**Andrew C. Parrott**
Department of Psychology, Swansea University, Swansea SA2 8PP, South Wales, UK
Centre for Human Psychopharmacology, Swinburne University, Melbourne, VIC 3122, Australia

**Fabrizio Schifano and John M. Corkery**
Psychopharmacology, Drug Misuse and Novel Psychoactive Substances Research Unit, School of Life and Medical Sciences, University of Hertfordshire, Hertfordshire AL10 9AB, UK

**Paolo Frisoni, Erica Bacchio, Rosa Maria Gaudio and Mario Barbieri**
Department of Medical Sciences, University of Ferrara, 44121 Ferrara, Italy

**Anna Talarico**
Department of Chemical and Pharmaceutical Sciences, University of Ferrara, 44121 Ferrara, Italy

**Margherita Neri**
Department of Morphology, Surgery and Experimental Medicine, Section of Legal Medicine, University of Ferrara, 44121 Ferrara, Italy

**Matteo Marti**
Department of Morphology, Surgery and Experimental Medicine, Section of Legal Medicine, University of Ferrara, 44121 Ferrara, Italy
Collaborative Center for the Italian National Early Warning System, Department of Anti-Drug Policies, Presidency of the Council of Ministers, 00184 Roma, Italy

# Index

www.ingramcontent.com/pod-product-compliance
Lightning Source LLC
LaVergne TN
LVHW082203200926
848484LV00008B/2203